Psychiatry in Learning Disability

Psychiatry in Learning Disability

Edited by

Stephen G. Read MD, FRCPsych
Senior Lecturer – Psychiatry in Learning Disabilities
Learning Disability Services
The Lodge
and University of Leeds
Leeds

W.B. SAUNDERS COMPANY LTD
London   Philadelphia   Toronto   Sydney   Tokyo

W. B. Saunders Company Ltd 24–28 Oval Road
London NW1 7DX

The Curtis Center
Independence Square West
Philadelphia, PA 19106–3399, USA

Harcourt Brace & Company
55 Horner Avenue
Toronto, Ontario M8Z 4X6, Canada

Harcourt Brace & Company, Australia
30–52 Smidmore Street
Marrickville, NSW 2204, Australia

Harcourt Brace & Company, Japan
Ichibancho Central Building, 22–1 Ichibancho
Chiyoda-ku, Tokyo 102, Japan

A catalogue record for this book is available from the British Library

ISBN 0–7020–2119–9

Typeset by Florencetype Ltd, Stoodleigh, Devon.
Printed and bound in Great Britain by WBC Book Manufacturers Ltd,
Bridgend, Mid Glamorgan.

Contents

Contributors

C. Barbara Ballinger BSc, MB ChB, MRCP, FRCPsych
Consultant Psychiatrist, Royal Dundee Liff Hospital, Dundee.

Michael Berger BA(Hons), DipPsych, PhD, FBPsS
Professor of Clinical Psychology, Department of Psychology, Royal Holloway, University of London, Egham, Surrey TW20 0EX.

Thomas P. Berney MB ChB, DPM, FRCPsych
Consultant Psychiatrist, Prudhoe Hospital, Northumberland.

David Clarke MD, MRCPsych
Senior Lecturer in Developmental Psychiatry, University of Birmingham Department of Psychiatry, Queen Elizabeth Psychiatric Hospital, Birmingham B15 2QZ.

Pamela M. Crawford MB ChB, MD, FRCP
Consultant Neurologist and Director, Special Centre for Epilepsy, Department of Neurology, York District Hospital, Wigginton Road, York YO3 7HE.

Kenneth Day FRCPsych
Lately Consultant Psychiatrist and Medical Director, Northgate and Prudhoe NHS Trust, Morpeth, Northumberland; Senior Lecturer, Department of Psychiatry, University of Newcastle-upon-Tyne, Newcastle-upon-Tyne.

Shoumitro Deb MRCPsych MD
Senior Lecturer and Honorary Consultant in Neuropsychiatry, Division of Psychological Medicine, University Hospital of Wales, Heath Park, Cardiff CF4 4XN.

Judith A. Dunstan MB BS, MRCPsych
Senior Registrar in Psychiatry, Newcastle Rotation Scheme, Newcastle-upon-Tyne.

Alexander Esterhuyzen BSc(Hons), MB ChB, MRCPsych
Senior Registrar in Psychotherapy, St George's Hospital Medical School, London.

John Finch BA, BCL
Senior Lecturer in Law, University of Leicester, Leicester.

Sheila Hollins FRCPsych
Professor, Department of Psychiatry of Disability, St George's Hospital Medical School, London.

Kelvin Mackrell BTech, MSc, PhD, CPsychol, AFBPsS
Consultant Clinical Psychologist, Psychology Department, Pontefract General Infirmary, Friarwood Lane, Pontefract WF8 1PL.

Jane M. McCarthy MBChB, MRCGP, MRCPsych
Consultant Psychiatrist in Learning Disabilities, Community Unit, Hinchingbrooke Health Care NHS Trust, Primrose Lane, Huntingdon, Cambridgeshire PE18 6SE.

Stephen G. Read MD, FRCPsych
Senior Lecturer – Psychiatry in Learning Disabilities, Division of Psychiatry and Behavioural Sciences in Relation to Medicine, Clinical Sciences Building, Level 5, St James' University Hospital, Beckett Street, Leeds LS9 7TF.

Andrew H. Reid MD, FRCP, FRCPsych, DPM
Consultant Psychiatrist, Royal Dundee Liff Hospital, Dundee; Honorary Senior Lecturer in Psychiatry, Ninewells Hospital and Medical School, Dundee.

Douglas A. Spencer MB ChB, FRCPsych, DPM, FRSH
Formerly Consultant Psychiatrist, Learning Disability Services, Leeds; The Lodge, Crooked Acres, 1 Spen Lane, Leeds LS5 3EJ.

Stephen Tyrer MA, MB BChir, LMCC, DPM, FRCPsych
Consultant Psychiatrist, Prudhoe Hospital, Prudhoe, Northumberland and Royal Victoria Infirmary, Newcastle-upon-Tyne.

Margaret Walker MBE, MSc, FRCSLT
Chief Research Speech and Language Therapist and Honorary Senior Lecturer, Department of Psychiatry of Disability, St George's Hospital Medical School, London University, Cranmer Terrace, Tooting, London SW1 0RE. Designer of the Makaton Language Programme.

Foreword

All those in mental health professions, especially postgraduate students, frequently complain of the lack of balance in the available literature in different areas of the subject, and particularly the shortage of academically sophisticated and evidence-based work on learning disability. They know where to turn for authoritative, didactic articles and books on other specialties of psychiatry and related disciplines, but there has been a dearth of informative, concise, well-referenced summaries of the psychiatric aspects of learning disability. This fortunately is now no longer true. Dr Read has edited contributions from a number of distinguished authors that will answer the searching questions and fulfil the academic needs both of those working in other areas of mental health and of those specifically providing care for people with learning disability.

There have been pressures over recent years to decrease the link between psychiatry and learning disability, as areas of specialization. A large part of the delivery of care has now appropriately been placed within the responsibility of social services, but there are still considerable psychiatric needs to be met within the field of learning disability; specialists in this subject need to be informed by psychiatry, and those dealing with more general aspects of mental illness need expert opinion, advice and information from experts in learning disability. *Psychiatry in Learning Disability* covers both these fields of knowledge: psychiatry for professionals working with learning disabled people and expertise on learning disability for those more generally concerned with mental illness. It is recommended to the reader not only for finding information on specific subjects but also for re-ordering one's mental set concerning the two areas of specialization. This book will be found to fill an important gap within this important area of professional knowledge.

Professor Andrew Sims MA, MD, FRCPsych, FRCP

Division of Psychiatry and Behavioural Sciences in Relation to Medicine, St James's University Hospital, Leeds.

June 1997

Preface

From time immemorial it would appear that there have been problems associated with people who have what is now called learning disability and what might more precisely be called cerebral impairment. There have been many approaches to these problems, including medical, surgical, genetic, psychological and sociological, and perhaps some others too. The whole variety of primary aetiologies which give rise to a plethora of behavioural symptoms outside the norm do not produce utter chaos in the presentation of such symptoms, but give rise to a spectrum of disorders in which individual hues can usually be detected. It is not chaos that we see but a considerable array of recognizable diagnoses, syndromes and symptom clusters which, taken together, form the basis of psychiatry in learning disability.

What this book aims to do is to describe and even define the limits of the field which is psychiatry in learning disability. The major act of editorship was the conception of the structure of the volume and in the selection of the authors best suited to describe each subspecialty in the most authoritative manner.

The intention is that those who read this book will experience the same fascination with the immensity and variation of the subject as is experienced by the editor and the authors. For those who think this, a lifelong career awaits.

Acknowledgement must go to Helen Osborne, Medical Secretary.

1

IQ, Intelligence and Assessment

Michael Berger

Introduction

One of the main defining characteristics of individuals with learning disabilities is a level of intelligence well below the norm. In many instances, a decisive diagnostic finding is a low IQ (Intelligence Quotient) on an IQ or Intelligence Test.

Such statements seem straightforward enough, yet intelligence as a concept has a variety of definitions and associated theories, a long and often contentious history, and an extensive and diverse empirical research and philosophical literature. There are also many procedures for measuring intelligence with the idea of 'measuring' intelligence itself controversial. Against this background, how are clinicians to understand 'intelligence' and the IQ, and use such knowledge in clinical practice?

This chapter will present some of the main ideas and findings about human intelligence and the measurement of abilities as a background both to this book and to the understanding and uses of 'intelligence' and intelligence tests in working with people with learning disabilities.

Initial Concepts

Intelligence, like so many attributes, is not observable: it is an inference about the nature of people or their characteristics from observations of individual differences. In this instance the conjecture relates to certain classes of behaviour: problem solving skills, knowledge, or in our cultures, variations in school performance and academic attainment. There is no doubt that there are such individual differences. The key question is whether or not these behaviours are a consequence of something real in people – 'intelligence' – that gives rise to the performance differences or whether 'intelligence' is simply an abstraction with pseudo-explanatory powers. For many, it is something real, something that varies quantitatively on a dimension from low to high or little to much, although what it is will also vary within a group of theorists. For others, it is something qualitative. 'Intelligence' and its varied definitions will be discussed later.

An intelligence/IQ test is a standardized procedure aimed at measuring intelligence. It consists of a set of tasks or questions (items) presumed to require the operation of intelligence to be solved. Items are sometimes grouped into subtests, with each subtest sampling a particular domain of function, such as short-term memory or spatial perception. Subtests, made up of homogeneous items, can, in turn, be grouped in sets that are called subscales. The subscales, in turn, are organized so as to measure a more broadly based but still homogeneous set of abilities, such as verbal ability. A test could be made up of a uniform set of items (such as Raven's Matrices),[1] or subscales (exemplified by the Wechsler Adult Intelligence Scale).[2]

The IQ is a transformation of the raw scores, the actual number of problems solved correctly or the time taken to answer a question. In current usage, the IQ is a measure of the distance of an individual's total score from the average scores of comparable individuals. Commonly, the average is set to 100 (unfortunately leading to confusion with percentages), or to 50. The important point about the IQ is that it is a comparison between the score obtained by the testee and the average score of comparable testees or some other criterion group.

The best analogy is with a clinical thermometer. The average body temperature is 37.0° C. An individual can have a temperature at above or below this average value, with the distance measured in degree units. Similarly, but without implying the same precision, the individual IQ can be above or below 100 (or 50, or some other average value). The units of distance will be described in a later section.

Learning disability and its synonyms such as mental retardation, will not be defined here other than in a general, orienting sense, as a clinical term that refers to a heterogeneous physical, psychological and other phenomenology within which there are some identifiable patterns, such as Down's syndrome and the Fragile X syndromes, as well as a common feature – low IQ or a preponderance of poor skills and abilities. Operational and other definitions and diagnosis are covered in greater detail elsewhere in this volume.

The Importance of IQ in Western Cultures

'... one observation that remains that leaves little room for debate: students who score low on tests of intelligence tend to score comparatively low on tests of achievement. ... the correlation is significantly high and difficult to deny.' E.G. Stetson (p. 106)[3]

Although the IQ derives from the measurement of human intelligence, as a measure or index, it could for many purposes survive in isolation from its origins. The reason for this is the body of empirical evidence of its utility. In some ways, the IQ is like a drug whose use is based not on a theoretical rationale but on its efficacy in dealing with disease. The fact that it works can be, and usually is in the first instance, taken as justification for its use. Why it works may then be the subject of subsequent theory and research. In a similar manner, we can discuss the IQ and its usefulness apart from any theoretical justification, although ultimately, the meaning of the IQ will depend on the theoretical framework that informed the construction of the test on which the IQ is based.

A purely empirical approach will be adopted initially as a way of highlighting some of the reasons why the IQ, irrespective of whether or not it is a measure of intelligence, has become such an important and value-laden index in our society.

While there are clear limitations, there is no doubt that the IQ has powerful concurrent and predictive powers. At its best, it has a predictive relationship (correlation) of about 0.6 with other measures. This value should be seen in the context of a potential range of 0.0–1.0 (or 0.0 to –1.0: for predictive purposes, the sign is not important). While 0.6 is not very high, it is among the highest predictive values in psychology.

Individuals with very low scores on IQ tests tend to do poorly on other tests, they show other developmental problems, including poor progress in many areas of functioning and make more limited educational progress than their peers. A low IQ is one of the best indicators of poor concurrent general competence and of limited future competence.

Prediction from developmental tests such as the Bayley Developmental Scales[4] in infancy to childhood IQ and later IQ values is not reliable although severe handicap identified at an early age is predictive of later IQ.[5,6] Among the reasons offered to account for the poor prediction from early developmental testing is the limited overlap between the material in these tests and the reasoning and related tasks found in tests for older age groups. Developmental tests for instance tend to assess basic sensory–motor skills as it is not possible to test more complex skills such as logical reasoning so early in development.

While developmental tests such as the Bayley,[4] Griffiths[7] and Cattell[8] Scales may not be good predictors in the normal range of IQs, it is possible to get fairly strong indicators of later IQ from some experimental tasks administered in infancy. For instance, when shown novel stimuli, together with familiar material, infants who preferred the novel proved later to have higher IQs. Novelty preference was significantly lower in babies for whom there was a significant risk of having learning difficulties.[6,9–11]

The pattern of prediction appears to be that the experimental indices, regarded as indicators of information processing efficiency, correlate better with verbal and general ability measures rather than nonverbal IQs. The methods used in these studies are not routinely used in developmental assessments but, given the strength of the relationship, may come to be so.

The IQ has some other important clinical uses, particularly as an aid to formulation. Some individuals reported to be behaviourally or otherwise difficult, or who have poor reading or other abilities, are occasionally found to have high IQs, suggesting that their environments had not perceived their competence and this leads or contributes to their difficulties. It is also the case that individuals in mainstream schools who present with behaviour difficulties or poor progress may be found to have abilities that are more limited than anticipated by teachers or parents. Again, this may account for their behaviour difficulties.

Although a high IQ does not guarantee educational success, completion of higher education and entry to and progress within undergraduate settings and subsequently are commonly associated with higher than average IQ scores.

It has also been documented that people with differing levels of IQ end up in different occupations. A good predictor of the job status of an adult male is childhood IQ; it is at least as good as how many years he went to school.[12] Further, IQ becomes more important the more intellectually rigorous the job, and that within jobs, the higher the IQ the more productive the individuals usually are in nonmanual and in manual occupations.[12] However, the relationship between job status and IQ, while not denied, is also not seen as that powerful. Sternberg *et al.*[13] point out that IQ tests are less predictive of success out of school and that practical intelligence otherwise known as common sense can supplement the predictive contribution of the conventional IQ.

In summary, the IQ is a very useful index for a variety of purposes, complementing other information in various forms of assessment, decision-making and diagnosis, pointing the way to explanations that might not otherwise have been considered, or if thought about, not tested in a standardized way that allows systematic comparison with an appropriate normal group.

While the utility of the IQ would in itself probably be sufficient justification for its valued status, there is also little doubt that it has become more exceptional because of the assumption that the IQ measures intelligence, a human attribute highly valued in our culture. These attributions have also made it amenable to being used carelessly, or for malicious purposes, among the consequences of which are the prevailing contrasting attitudes to the IQ and intelligence testing,[14] as well as the occasional acrimonious debates and far-reaching legal rulings, the latter particularly in the USA (see [3] for example), associated with intelligence testing.

The use of the IQ in the assessment of learning difficulties has been questioned on a variety of grounds, particularly in relation to individuals from ethnic backgrounds that differ from those of the dominant, usually white culture. It is also recognized that IQ tests sample a limited range of behaviours and do not necessarily indicate the extent of individual adaptation to the environment. This has led to the development of complementary approaches, in particular, adaptive behaviour scales[14] such as the Vineland Adaptive Behavior Scales.[15] Such scales play an important role in a comprehensive clinical assessment and are seen as complementing rather than supplementing conventional IQ tests.[16] This chapter will not consider adaptive behaviour scales further.

Historical Perspectives

The foundations of our interest in intelligence and its measurement, and also the controversies, have important historical roots. A detailed history of the scientific study of intelligence is available from many sources.[17–19]

Among the early landmarks are Galton's research on individual differences and statistical techniques in England in the mid-nineteenth century, the work of Binet and Simon in France, whose research, key papers and tests were published in the period spanning the turn of the century, and the statistical and conceptual work of Spearman on general intelligence. Most of the developments (and controversies) since that time arise from these beginnings.[12,17]

Galton was interested, among other things, in the nature and inheritance of human abilities. He devised various statistical procedures to help develop his views and believed that intelligence was essentially a generic trait: good at one, good at many or most. Galton was also a proponent of eugenics, a topic that has consistently been associated with IQ and is a source of concern because of the ease with which it lends itself to racist and other demeaning ideologies.

Binet and Simon, because of their pre-existing interest in children's intelligence, were asked to provide a solution to an important educational problem – that of identifying children who were not making academic progress and who would benefit from a different education. Whereas Galton tended to use tests or measurements of basic functions such as sensory discrimination and simple reaction times as indices of human intelligence, Binet and Simon devised tests of higher mental functions, such as reasoning, memory and pattern identification. (Similar tasks were being used at the same time, but for a different purpose, by Ebbinghaus in Germany.) By the turn of the century, it was obvious that Galton had lost out in so far as test content was concerned[17] and that the procedures devised by Binet and Simon to test the higher processes became, and remain, established, as basic to the measurement of mental abilities, although other approaches to intelligence continue the Galton tradition.

Binet and Simon also combined all the tasks into a single scale and expressed the outcome using a single number, subsequently known as the IQ, following a procedure devised some time earlier by their compatriots, Blin and Damaye, for the diagnosis of subnormality.[19]

The development of the first scale of intelligence was not a 'fortuitous event'.[19] For over two decades, Binet had been searching for a procedure that would enable a reliable discrimination among the then three accepted grades of mental deficiency. It is important to note that the tasks devised and used by Binet and Simon were introduced because they satisfied several requirements: sampling complex or higher level thought processes, consistent with the theoretical preconceptions of the authors about the nature of intelligence; that the tasks should not compromise the individual simply because of social circumstances or education;[20] and finally that administration of these tasks should be objective. This last requirement derived from the observation that the judgements of doctors and teachers had proved a poor basis for identifying children with low abilities.

The only other landmark that needs to be noted here is the publication by Spearman in 1904[21] of what Herrnstein and Murray[12] describe as 'a conceptual and statistical breakthrough that has shaped both the development and much of the controversy about mental tests ever since'. Spearman documented an observation that has withstood the test of time, namely, that individuals who do well in one set of mental tests tend to do well in others and vice versa.

Evidence for these patterns of association was found through the use of the correlation coefficient. This statistical procedure, devised by Galton, provides a quantitative index of the strength of association between two measures – for instance the number of correct items on a test of word definitions and a test of abstract reasoning. A positive correlation indicates that when one variable increases so does the comparison variable, with a correlation coefficient of +1.0 indicating a strength of relationship such that increase in one invariably leads to an increase in the other. A correlation of 0.0 means that there is no association whatever between them and a correlation of –1.0 means that when one variable increases the other decreases. Intermediate values indicate less than perfect strengths of the association.

Spearman noticed that if a number of mental tests is given and the correlations between each test with the others is computed, the coefficients in the resulting matrix are all positive but of varying magnitudes. Spearman proposed that the correlations were all positive because they were tapping the same underlying ability but were of differing magnitudes because their relationship with this underlying ability varied.

Using a procedure that later came to be called factor analysis, which he applied to the matrix of correlations, Spearman was able to identify what he called 'g', a unitary factor common to all mental tests, which came to be regarded as evidence of 'general intelligence'. He used the statistical pattern of positive intercorrelations to support his view that human intelligence comprises two structural elements: general ability and an ability specific to a particular test. For example, high scores on a task that requires verbal reasoning (in what way are motor car and aeroplane similar?) are, according to Spearman's model, due to the operation of general intelligence and particular skills in carrying out verbal reasoning tasks of the type illustrated by the test. Spearman further contended that individuals differed in the amount of 'g' they possessed: in essence, individual differences in performance were a reflection of individual differences in 'g'.

As will be seen, Spearman's view of the structure of human intelligence, the two-component model, 'g' and task-specific abilities, was subsequently challenged by a range of other structural models that covered a spectrum of alternatives, such as 'no 'g' but many (or a few) abilities', to a model of two forms of 'g', or a hierarchical structure with 'g' at the peak and several layers of increasingly specific abilities beneath.

In summary, it is worth noting the key developments that had come about before the end of the first decade of this century. It was clear that tasks to provoke the operation of 'intelligence' needed to tap higher mental processes involving reasoning, problem solving and other complex thinking and knowledge, that such tasks needed to be administered in a systematic manner to ensure objectivity, and finally, that when such tasks were intercorrelated, the resulting matrix contained positive coefficients, presumed to come about through the operation of a unitary factor known as 'g' which, in turn, came to be identified with general intelligence, subsequently presumed to be measured by the IQ.

The Case For and Against 'g'

The 'g' factor found through correlating mental tests has been dismissed on a number of grounds, two of the most important being that it is essentially a tautology and that it is an artefact of the statistical procedures used to analyse the correlations.

Anderson (pp. 18–19)[20] has presented detailed arguments to refute these two notions. He states that the tautology arises because the 'construct of 'intelligence' is only meaningful ... if it shows some stability across heterogeneous tasks that we would consider to require intelligence.' Tasks on tests of intelligence are chosen initially because they are assumed to sample intelligence. Subsequent tasks are then chosen to correlate with the originals. If they do not correlate, they are not sampling intelligence.

The argument is compounded because of assertions that the selection of the tasks is also either arbitrary or politically motivated.[20] Without going into the details here, Anderson[20] is able to show quite convincingly that none of these assertions hold and that there 'has been a conspicuous failure to discover tests of cognitive ability that do not correlate with already established tests of intelligence.'

What of the argument that 'g' is a statistical artefact? Some of the alternative conceptualizations of the structure of abilities are presented in the section on Theories of Intelligence below. The main finding is that the structural model that emerges when the correlation matrix is analysed depends very much on the theoretical orientation of the person analysing the matrix – 'g' can be retained if the theoretical view favours a unitary general ability or it can be broken down in various ways into two or more factors if the person undertaking the analysis has a multifactor view.

Anderson,[20] in defence of 'g' as general intelligence gives three reasons 'for believing that general intelligence is real'. First, 'g' can only be made to disappear by using an incomplete analysis of the matrix. Jensen and Weng[22] have experimented with different models and methods of analysis on both real and simulated data and found that 'g' is 'remarkably robust'. Second, attempts to construct a test with independent dimensions have all failed. Anderson's[20] third point is somewhat more complex. He draws the important distinction between a statistical pattern which is what 'g' is to begin with, and a psychological or other mechanism that exists and is responsible for the statistical pattern. Positive correlations on their own cannot constitute the evidence. However, to say that a factor does not necessarily correspond to a psychological attribute does not mean, correspondingly, that it cannot.[20] What is needed is independent evidence. This has begun to emerge from recent research and appears to provide independent confirmation of the reality of general intelligence, although, as Anderson recognizes, the outcome is not as yet clear-cut.[20]

By way of summary of the current understanding of 'g', Herrnstein and Murray[12] list six statements about 'g' that they describe as 'beyond technical dispute', of which the first three are as follows (the others will be considered shortly):

(1) There is such a thing as a general factor of cognitive ability on which human beings differ.
(2) All standardized tests of academic aptitude or achievement measure this general factor to some degree, but IQ tests expressly designed for that purpose measure it most accurately.
(3) IQ scores match, to a first degree, whatever it is that people mean when they use the word intelligent or smart in ordinary language.

Definitions of 'Intelligence'

At least from the time of Binet onwards, definitions of intelligence have tended to focus on the higher level processes – 'the superior faculties' – (Binet, quoted in[20]) in one form or another as the central characteristic. Binet and Simon, writing in 1905 stated that 'To judge well, to comprehend well, to reason well, these are the essential activities of intelligence'(quoted in[23]).

For Spearman, intelligence concerned the identification of correlates and the grasping of relationships.[21]

After the publication of the Binet–Simon test and its translation into the American version, the Stanford–Binet, testing and the development of tests grew rapidly, as did definitions of intelligence. At a symposium in 1921, a group of psychologists each proposed definitions that overlapped but which also stressed different aspects, such as abstract thinking, planning capacity or educability, among other views.[23] Somewhat later, Wechsler[24] operationally defined intelligence as the 'aggregate or global capacity of the individual to act purposefully, to think rationally and to deal effectively with his or her environment'.

Vernon's[23] view is that intelligence 'refers to the more generalized skills, strategies of thinking, and overall conceptual level, which apply in a wide range of cognitive abilities or in new learning'.

Kaufman and Kaufman[25] define intelligence as measured by the Kaufman Ability Battery for Children in terms of an individual's style of solving problems and processing information.

Gardner,[26] who proposes a model of 'multiple intelligences' (to be considered in more detail later), views intelligence as the 'ability to solve problems, or to fashion products'. Gardner's views are among a set of influential contemporary approaches to intelligence that focus on higher level concepts, influenced by the writings of Piaget (see also [15]). These approaches attempt to account for intelligence in terms of cognitive mechanisms underlying mental processes. As Anderson[20] states, high-level theorists view intelligence as 'a culturally determined, experientially driven attribute of *cognitive* functions.'

In contrast are the approaches that seek theories based on physiological and other low-level processes, with 'speed' of functioning as an attribute of the nervous system being the key process (e.g. Eysenck).[28,29] The research paradigm is the simple or choice reaction time or related procedure (see section on Reaction and Inspection Times on p. 14).

In general, more recent views recognize that it is difficult to arrive at a definition that captures the essence of intelligence. One approach proposes, as a consequence, the need to specify what it is that the intelligent person does.[16] Butterworth[30] suggests a set of criteria that definitions of intelligence must incorporate, such as the need to refer in part to the way in which knowledge is represented internally – 'the psychological processes which give rise to knowledge'. As a second criterion he suggests that definitions also need to refer to the social and physical context, in that what is perceived as intelligent in one context may not be so in another, or at another time.

Contemporary definitions and theories have also been strongly influenced by information processing theory and concepts. Murphy and Davidshofer[16] for instance, state that ' "general mental ability" – a term to be preferred to the ... value laden concept of "intelligence" – refers to the existence of systematic individual differences in the performance of tasks that involve the manipulation, retrieval, evaluation, or processing of information'.

While it is not going to be possible to come up with a single definition of intelligence, the views presented in this section give some flavour of the ways in which psychologists and others approach the definition of intelligence.

All definitions derive from overt or covert theories of intelligence. A number of these are described briefly in the next section.

Theories of Intelligence

Over the decades since the emergence of the scientific study of intelligence, various theories have been proposed. Among this diversity several sub-types can be discerned. For instance, Kail and Pellegrino[31] identify the 'Psychometric Approach', the 'Information Processing Approach', the developmental perspective of Piaget and what they called then, the 'Emerging Perspectives', referring to the writings of Sternberg[27] and Gardner.[26]

The classification proposed by Herrnstein and Murray[12] describes three major approaches, namely, 'The Classicists: Intelligence as Structure', 'The Revisionists: Intelligence as Information Processing' and 'The Radicals, The Theory of Multiple Intelligences'. These broad systems are not adequate in that they ignore the idea of level of analysis and in doing so, miss out the important work of those (e.g. Eysenck[28] and Jensen[32]) who have sought to introduce a neurophysiological dimension to theory and research. Also, none of the classifications affords a home for the relatively recent and interesting theory of Anderson[20] which, as will be seen, spans levels and attempts to accommodate some of the stable findings and core ideas of a number of the other approaches.

Approaches via the Structure of Abilities

Structural models are attempts to account for the patterns in the matrices of test intercorrelations. They generally begin by accepting 'g' but differ in their views of the remaining underlying structure of abilities. Use is made of the techniques of factor analysis to decompose the matrix into components, the factor 'structures of the mind'. This approach dominated the psychology of intelligence for many years.

Hierarchical Structure

Spearman's initial model of 'g', a general factor plus a test-specific ability (the two-factor model) constituted one of the earliest structural views of intelligence. This model was not generally accepted. Spearman later changed his view, to be consistent with the hierarchical system of Burt and Vernon.

The hierarchical model proposes that while 'g' is the most general factor, it can be decomposed into two broad constellations of other abilities. Hence, at the next level down, the 'Major Group' level, are two factors, verbal:educational (v:ed) and the spatial:mechanical (k:m). These factors, in effect, state that abilities in the verbal/educational domain tend to cluster together (individuals tend to get similar score levels on such tasks), and tend to differ from the second cluster at this level, the spatial/mechanical group. This structure reflects the fact that individuals doing well on v:ed will not always do as well, or may do much better on k:m tests. Below this are the 'Minor Group' abilities, which are subcomponents of the abilities at the Major level. Minor Group factors are composed of separable clusters concerned with verbal and educational abilities. At the base of the hierarchy are the test-specific factors – those abilities tapped by particular tests.

In the organization of test content and structure, the Wechsler Intelligence Scales resemble this hierarchical model. The Full Scale IQ derived from the scores across all subtests corresponds to 'g'. The Verbal Scale IQ, which taps both Verbal and some educational content (e.g. the word knowledge Vocabulary subtest and the Arithmetic subtest, respectively), corresponds to the verbal:educational component. Recent scoring systems for the Wechsler Scales enable purer measures to be obtained. The Verbal Comprehension Factor in the Wechsler Intelligence Scale for Children–III[33] more closely resembles the Verbal component of the Burt–Vernon hierarchy. The Performance Scale IQ corresponds to the spatial:mechanical component and there is a procedure for obtaining a purer spatial measure, the Perceptual Organization Factor, separate from the Motor Speed Factor. Finally, the individual subtests can be seen to correspond to the Burt–Vernon specific component level.

Primary Mental Abilities

In the USA, alternative structural models emerged. In the 1930s Thurstone, while accepting 'g', argued that correlations among tests 'could not be completely explained by their relationship to "g" '.[16] He went on to develop a structural model that became known as the 'Primary Mental Abilities', comprising seven group factors: Verbal Comprehension, Word Fluency, Number, Space, Associative (rote) Memory, Perceptual Speed, and Reasoning, Inductive and Deductive. Interestingly, some of these primary abilities are generated by the Wechsler Tests, as illustrated above.

The Thurstone approach tended to play down the 'g' factor although it was shown by Eysenck[34] that the seemingly independent Primary Mental Abilities were all fairly highly correlated with 'g'. As Anderson[20] states, 'no one has been able to construct a test battery to measure a collection of independent abilities where no general factor can be extracted'. He goes on to note that even the British Ability Scales, constructed to measure heterogeneous mental abilities still yield a large general factor.

Structure of Intellect

Another variation of a fractionated structural model was proposed by Guilford,[35] partly as a rejection of 'g'. In his view, intelligence is organized in three dimensions according to what a person does (Operations), the material on which the operations are performed (Contents) and the form for processing and storing information (Products). Each of these dimensions has a number of components that, when taken together, lead to 180 elements. Although exemplar tests have been devised, as Murphy and Davidshofer[16] note, the theory has not survived critical analysis and finds little, if any, utility in 'the practice of intelligence testing'.

Fluid and Crystallized Abilities

The work of Cattell[36] is regarded as important for a number of reasons: because of the attempt to link the work of Spearman and Thurstone and the attempt at integration of hereditary and environmental influences.[23] In essence, Cattell proposes that 'g' comprises of two components, the Gf or 'fluid' and Gc, 'crystallized' intelligences. Gf is biological in origin and enables us to solve novel problems and grasp novel relationships. It is this aspect of intelligence that is thought to decline with age. Gc consists of an accumulation of skills, strategies and information gained through the learning experiences provided in the culture. It tends to remain stable in the processes of ageing.

Cattell has developed his theory by elaborating several levels of factors in order to account for the patterns in the matrix of test intercorrelations. However, some of his proposals for factors are not especially different from some of the established factors in other models.[23]

Cognitive Psychology and Information Processing Approaches

Cognitive psychology is concerned with the structures and processes of the human mind such as attention, perception, memory, understanding, thinking and intelligence. The study of intelligence was strongly influenced by cognitive psychology and involved attempts to identify the operation and types of mental events needed to produce intelligent actions. This approach, combined with an interest in computers and how they operate, with a particular emphasis on internal mechanisms between input and the output, exercised a strong influence on theory and research that came to the fore in the 1960s. The study of intelligence influenced by the computational analogy became known as information processing approach[37] 'typified by the analysis of problem solving' as described by Kail and Pellegrino.[31]

Triarchic Theory

The most influential of the more recent approaches is that developed by Sternberg.[27] Called the Triarchic or three process theory, its main feature is the combination of three subtheories that together attempt to encompass the complex nature of human intelligence as it is applied in adapting to individual environments.

The first of the subtheories is concerned with the internal architecture of the system of intellectual functioning: the componential subtheory that identifies the internal mental or cognitive mechanisms which underlie intelligent behaviour. This involves the processes of incorporating information from sensory inputs, retrieval and use of the information, including the allocation of resources and inferring conclusions.

A second subtheory is concerned with the routinization of performance: how resources are deployed for dealing with novel tasks and how these processes eventually lead to automatic behaviour. This part of the theory is primarily concerned with the utilization of past experience to deal with current adaptations.

The third subtheory is an attempt to link intelligence to the adaptive real-world actions of people: how people go about identifying contexts for living and their reasons for doing so. This part of the theory, in effect, gives intelligence its purpose within the context of the culture. Sternberg,[27] identifies three mechanisms for doing so, adapting as best they can, shaping the environment to meet their needs or selecting a new environment.

Sternberg[27] also proposes a number of components of mental functioning with their associated processes. Acquisition components are concerned with incorporating new information; retention components that are involved in remembering or retrieving of information from memory; transfer components make the information available across situations; performance components are used in executing a problem solving strategy; and, finally, metacomponents are higher-order processes involved in planning and monitoring the implementation of a strategy.

Sternberg's ideas about intelligence continue to be influential and challenging[13] yet they have been strongly criticised. For example, Anderson[20] suggests that his 'componential theory of intelligence seems simply to be a re-description of the data. That is, it is not a theory of the intellect, but a framework for describing problem-solving tasks . . . Sternberg's framework may come to be regarded as a notorious example of confusing an information processing flow diagram with an information-processing theory'.

Multiple Intelligences

Gardner,[26] the creator of the 'Theory of Multiple Intelligences', believes that there is widespread dissatisfaction with 'the concept of the IQ and with unitary views of intelligence'.[26] To counter the domination of this orientation, he proposes what he considers to be a radical view of intelligence, a pluralistic view which recognizes 'many different and discrete facets of cognition . . . that people have different cognitive strengths and contrasting cognitive styles'.[26] To develop his theory, he proposes that we look at naturalistic expressions of skill in different cultures and in manifestations of unusual ability, evidence of brain localization, developmental profile and cultural significance, among a number of criteria. By examining these varied expressions of human knowledge and skill, Gardner and his associates have arrived at seven intelligences:

- Linguistic Intelligence – expressed in its purest form by poets.
- Logical–mathematical Intelligence – covers the skills in logical, mathematical and scientific ability.
- Spatial Intelligence reflects skills in forming mental models of the world and the ability to manipulate such models. Such skills would be expressed in the work of surgeons and sculptors, among others.
- Musical Intelligence is shown in the talents of famous composers or performers.
- Bodily–kinaesthetic Intelligence is the ability for expression through use of the whole body, seen in gymnasts or dancers.
- Interpersonal Intelligence is the ability to understand people.
- Intrapersonal Intelligence is the ability to understand oneself and to use that information to operate effectively in life.

In developing the theory, Gardner notes that the purer forms of these intelligences are seen only in very exceptional people who represent the extremes. In most others, these intelligences are in more or less developed form and they work together to help people solve problems. Gardner believes that individuals are born with particular intelligence profiles – varied abilities – and these are developed differentially over their lives. Multiple intelligences are also used as the foundation for educational programmes, what schools should be able to foster and accomplish – a philosophy that he and his colleagues have elaborated.[26] Gardner's[26] approach will undoubtedly have a strong appeal to those critical of conventional theories and measurement of intelligence, particularly because it also attempts to formulate an approach to education that is potentially attractive.

Anderson's[20] critique of Gardner's approach is too elaborate to detail here. His conclusions are, however, telling in that he believes that within the approach, 'an intelligence has no theoretical status. It is sometimes a behaviour, sometimes a cognitive process and sometimes a structure in the brain',[20] and later: 'Gardner's evidence for multiple intelligences is illusory'.[20] Such comments are unlikely to deter the development of the theory, mainly because of Gardner's negative views of the alternatives. Given the pervasiveness of 'g', it is just possible that Multiple Intelligences will go the way of Primary Mental Abilities. One reason that it may not is that Gardner and his colleagues appear to have developed a marketing and propagation package affirmed in the appendices to his recent book,[26] which may ensure continuation.

Reaction and Inspection Times, Evoked Potentials and Intelligence

Some of the earliest views of intelligence within experimental psychology were founded on basic processes, rather than higher-level cognitive functions. Speed of reaction was seen as a prime index.[29] The acceptance of the complex task proposed by Binet was seen as a retrogressive step by Spearman[21] and others. However, simple reaction times failed to show adequate correlations with other measures of intelligence and it was not until choice reaction times were introduced that the pursuit of a basic speed measure developed further. (In simple reaction times, the interval between a single stimulus and response provided the measures of speed; in choice reaction times, the stimulus can be one of several responses to several stimuli, requiring a differential response.) Choice reaction times are converted into information measures and various indices can be developed relating speed of reaction to information processing speed. The core hypothesis is that individual differences in intelligence result from differences in speed of processing at the neurophysiological level. This approach elaborated by Eysenck, has been developed in greater detail more recently by Jensen.[32]

A major reason for using reaction time was the belief that it was a fundamental process, incapable of being broken down further. Research has not supported this hypothesis so that the search for the basic unit was refocused on a part of the reaction time task, inspection time. In a reaction time task, the speed measure is the time from the onset of the stimulus to the pressing of a response button. In inspection time studies, the participant must make a mental decision of some sort. The decision time forms the basic index of speed. The assumption is that inspection times are dependent on the speed of sensory processing and it is this that is important in individual differences in intelligence. In one form of the experiment the task is to decide whether a stimulus of two unequal length lines has the longer line on the left or right, based on exposures of varying speeds.

Other approaches aimed at identifying low-level neurophysiological explanations include indices based on auditory evoked potentials, with individual differences in these being linked to individual differences in intelligence.

A more detailed exposition of the approaches involving these ideas and an assessment of their empirical and theoretical status can be found in Anderson.[20] The main criticism is that the underlying assumption that the tasks are 'knowledge free' basic measures does not always hold up in practice. Motivation, cognitively based strategies and other explanations contradict the assumptions and such arguments are sometimes difficult to refute. However, the data from various studies do indicate that there is a nontrivial statistically significant relationship between such relatively knowledge-free measures and 'high level differences in cognition measured by psychometric tests of intelligence'.[20]

These observations are used by Anderson[20] as the basis for one of the central components of his model which will be described under A Cognitive Model of Intelligence (p. 16).

Piaget and Intelligence

According to McShane,[37] Piaget has had a greater influence on our thinking about cognitive development than any other theorist. Other than to note some key features of his approach, no attempt will be made to cover Piaget's contributions: the scope and depth of his work are too extensive.[20,31,37]

Piaget began his career with Binet, developing conventional tests. He soon departed from this approach and began studying children's thinking with a primary focus on process. Also, rather than being concerned with individual differences, Piaget became interested in universals in development – what is common across all individuals – and elaborated a stage theory which proposed qualitative shifts in thought as the individual progressed through each of four main stages. Each stage was regarded as having general properties that typified it and had a pervasive impact in all areas of cognitive functioning during its 'reign'. Further, each stage was qualitatively different from its predecessor, with its own cognitive structure, and each was a prerequisite for the next in the sequence.

Some of the key concepts in Piagetian theory are the schemata, 'a complex, organized sequence of activities'[31] that are the core structures of knowledge. These structures are elaborated through the process of assimilation of new knowledge and accommodation as existing structures change because of mismatches between the structure and incoming information. The process is guided through equilibration which balances the relationship between the cognitive schemata and the real world.

The different nature of Piagetian theory is also demonstrated by his concerns, not with what individuals know at a particular point in their development, but rather with how children come to understand notions such as space, time, number, etc. Although many of his central ideas have come to be questioned,[30,38] Piaget played a critical role in changing thinking about development and, as Anderson (p. 116)[20] states, he 'set the agenda' for what cognitive theories of development need to be able to explain.

Piagetian theory has influenced the content and construction of some intelligence tests such as the British Ability Scales[39] and tests have been based on Piagetian stages and ideas. These have not generally been shown to be independent of 'g' and the latter are not in wide clinical use.

Neuropsychologically Based Views and Models of Intelligence

Lezak asserts on the basis of her interpretation of neuropsychological research and clinical findings, that there is 'no general cognitive or intellectual function, but rather many discrete ones that work together so smoothly when the brain is intact that cognition is experienced as a single, seamless attribute'.[40] She believes further that the notion of intelligence has limited application in neuropsychology and rejects the IQ because its composite nature confounds many different kinds of functions. It is 'inherently meaningless and not infrequently misleading ... and should be discarded'.[40] From the perspective of neuropsychological practice, such sentiments are understandable, mainly because of the importance of being able to differentiate functions and abilities in clinical assessment. Other practitioners however, hold different and, as we have seen, more positive views.

The neuropsychology of Luria, in combination with other ideas, has led to several batteries of tests. One is the Kaufman Ability Battery for Children[25] which attempts to amalgamate neuropsychological findings with those of cognitive psychology. In this test, the two major scales, Simultaneous Processing and Sequential Processing, are said to represent two types of mental functioning identified by several independent groups of researchers: sequential processing requires dealing with serial order in the test items, whereas with simultaneous processing, the individual needs to appreciate the spatial wholeness of the task that frequently requires rapid responses.[25]

Another approach, also based in the work of Luria, is called the PASS model – Planning, Attention, Simultaneous, Successive processing.[41,42] Part of the motivation for introducing this test is the view that the Wechsler Test, its underlying theory and its approach are inadequate for educational assessment, particularly in the investigation of learning disabilities.[42] The PASS processes are described as forming a complex, interdependent system that can be used both to assess functioning and to offer remedial techniques based on the theory.

A Cognitive Model of Intelligence

Anderson's model of intelligence,[20] although within the cognitive psychology and information processing family of theories, is presented separately here and in somewhat greater detail as an example of an important recent approach that attempts to build on the basic empirical findings of research on human intelligence, including the acceptance of 'g' and formulated as an information processing theory. The model is more fully articulated in his book, *Intelligence and Development*[20] which, in addition to providing a detailed rationale, also critically examines other theories.

The findings from research on reaction and inspection times and evoked potentials are used to argue that there is a basic processing mechanism operating at a low level, which is essentially 'knowledge-free' but varies in its speed among individuals. This is the first component of the model and is regarded as being primarily responsible for individual differences in 'g'. This 'basic processing mechanism is responsible for implementing thinking',[20] which in turn generates knowledge.

The second set of components are 'modules'. These are described as 'complex computational functions'. Their 'existence' and nature are derived in part from the observation that in all individuals without major brain disorders the ability to perceive three-dimensional space, encode phonological information, parse the language and have a theory of mind are intact. That is, within a very wide range of intelligence, these capacities remain functional at full capacity. Anderson believes that 'these modules have been shaped by evolutionary pressures to provide us with information that would be impossible to obtain using general-purpose problem-solvers'.[20]

The third component of the model consists of two specific processors whose 'existence' is argued for on the basis of a range of studies at different levels of analysis that consistently show that verbal/propositional and visuo-spatial functions are distinguishable, present at each of the main levels, from neuropsychological functions to higher-level cognition, and show the full spectrum of individual differences. These specific processors, called SP1 and SP2 respectively, function as knowledge-acquisition devices within their specific domains, building up verbal and spatial competence. The functioning of these mechanisms is bound up with the speed of the basic processing mechanism and also their own potentialities.

From the structure of the model, Anderson[20] goes on to show that knowledge is acquired by two routes. The first type of knowledge is acquired through development, and is substantially influenced by an individual's experience interacting with specific processors and the basic processing mechanism.

The second system is that of the modules whose contribution is given directly in the sense that we do not have to think in order to acquire such knowledge. Put crudely, babies do not have to learn how to see three-dimensional space.

Anderson[20] also distinguishes two uses of the term 'intelligence'. The first, that measured by intelligence tests, concerns individual differences in knowledge. The second usage, conforming to what he means by intelligence, is the speed of the basic processing mechanism and the power of the basic processors.[20]

The purpose of introducing this rudimentary description of Anderson's[20] model is to illustrate another new type of approach to intelligence, one which not only attempts to encompass and reframe existing knowledge, but one which exploits new ways of thinking (the computational analogy) and also has the power to begin to provide coherent explanations of other phenomena. Anderson's[20] analysis of 'idiot savant' skills would be of particular interest to clinicians in the field of learning difficulties. His recent study involving individuals with learning disabilities lends support to his theory and is useful in showing some of the ways in which individuals with learning disabilities do not differ from those without such disabilities.[43] Finally, it is also useful in showing how a definition of intelligence is very much theory specific.

Controversies

When dealing with the complex phenomena of human behaviour a number of theoretical positions compete for primacy; the study of intelligence is no exception and is also the subject of several controversies. The first is the view that it is not possible to measure something as complex as human intelligence. Second, assuming that the tests are sampling intelligence and identifying individual differences, are such differences predominantly a result of inherited tendencies or are they determined by experience? Related to this issue is the origin of the documented differences in average test scores of different ethnic and social groups. The contentiousness arises from suggestions that the source of differences is primarily genetic and linked to ethnicity; this argument is countered by the view that the tests are biased against minorities.

As a consequence of selective education (for instance, the 11+ examination in the UK), there has been a socio-political dimension to the controversies, with the view that tests were used to reinforce social and ethnic inequalities and consequently should not be used. Finally, it is argued that what tests were measuring was trivial or incomplete.

These controversies are expressed in an enormous literature such as Jensen's monograph[44] and surface from time to time in the public media, a recent example being the withdrawal of Brand's book[45] by its publishers because of alleged perpetuation of racist ideas.

The controversies will not be dealt with in detail here. Instead, the main conclusions as these currently appear will be given, with source references.

Can Intelligence be Measured?

As noted at the beginning of this chapter, IQ tests sample knowledge and skills. The measurement processes, through the use of standardized tests, produce reproducible results with stable scores and have other predictive powers. Are they measuring intelligence? One answer contends that this depends on what is meant by intelligence, a question for which there are, in turn, many answers given the variety of views about the nature of intelligence. Until there is a very strong theory there will be no strong answer. In the interim, one continues to use IQ tests, not necessarily because they measure intelligence but because they are fairly robust indicators of some important real-life functions and have both concurrent and predictive power. Through the educated use of such tests,[46] it becomes possible to reduce much of the abuse and use tests constructively.

There are others who object not to measurement as such but rather to the implication there may be only one type of intelligence. They therefore see the IQ as unacceptable as an index of the diversity of human capacities.[47] Again, what is required is a supported theory and strong evidence.

The Genetic Basis of IQ

It is now more generally accepted that a nontrivial part of human population variation in IQ is a consequence of genetic variation.[16,48] As Herrnstein and Murray[12] state in the last of their six points: '6. Cognitive ability is substantially heritable, apparently no less than 40 per cent and no more than 80 per cent.' The correct interpretation of this conclusion is critical. The ratios are population estimates and say nothing about an individual's IQ. These heritability estimates 'indicate the degree to which, under present circumstances, genetic factors and environmental factors contribute to individual differences in intelligence'.[16]

Genetic data have no immediate translation to individual IQs. It cannot be said, for instance, that an individual's IQ is made up of 40% genetic and 60% environmental influences. The data are population averages and their exact values will vary as a function of the genetic and environmental heterogeneity. While it is now more widely accepted that the IQ has a genetic basis, argued from the evidence of twin studies and other research, 'g' is not necessarily seen as the major or only component that is so influenced. Ceci *et al.*[49] propose that there is 'not one genetically determined force ('g')' that underlies all intelligent performances. Instead, they argue for 'multiple genetically determined cognitive potentialities that are fairly independent of one another'. These conclusions parallel the debate between proponents of one, a few or many IQs. Another view[50] identifies genetic influences on 'g' as well as finding independent genetic influences in performance on a set of tests.

Time and research will move us towards a resolution of the implicit and explicit differences in these views. Whatever the resolution, genetic influences are seen as having a nontrivial role in test performance. How and why such influences are expressed also remain important research questions.

Consistency and Predictability

The genetic basis to the IQ does not mean that it is unchangeable. There is no doubt that in absolute terms, the types of skills that are sampled by IQ tests increase with age: the older a child gets, the more words he or she can define correctly. The IQ is, however, a relative measure. It is a way of contrasting the individual's score on a test with the scores of other individuals of the same age or some other criterion group. The IQ – the position of the individual relative to comparable individuals – tend to remain stable across much of the individual's life span (see the Discussion in [16]). IQs at one age tend to be strongly predictive of IQs at later ages, with the strength of the relationship being greatest for individuals of low IQ.[6] However, none of the predictions are perfect. If 1.0 is taken as an index of perfect predictability, then, over the school-age years, the year-to-year index is 0.9 while over the whole period of schooling it is about 0.7,[51] indicating that changes do occur. The general conclusion, as expressed by Herrnstein and Murray[12] is: '4. IQ scores are stable, although not perfectly so, over much of a person's life'.

Modifiability

Can IQs be modified? Tests to produce an IQ require knowledge and problem-solving skills. Each of the abilities to perform a task can probably be increased by training and practice. There is clear evidence that simply retesting samples of children from the general population on the Wechsler children's scale over a short interval (a few weeks) leads to substantial practice gains, more on nonverbal than on verbal skills.[52] Individual changes in IQ can and do happen, most commonly in the region of 15 points or less.[16] Does this amount to modifying intelligence? The answer again will ultimately depend on the underlying theory about the nature of intelligence and its relationship with the IQ.

There is strong evidence of secular drift to the extent that the major tests need to be 'renormed' (or calibrated), usually in the direction of making them more difficult, one reason for this being the possibility that the population is becoming more 'able'. For instance, on the Wechsler individual intelligence tests, the evidence indicates that the average IQ in the population increases by three points per decade.[52] However, another explanation could be that the population has become more test sophisticated through the influence of children's television programmes such as Sesame Street, preschool education practices and toys, all of which have been strongly influenced by the content of IQ tests.

In contrast to this trend, people with learning difficulties do not show the same changes – if anything, they tend to score even lower.[52]

At the same time, it is recognized that very major changes in individual IQs will not come about because of environmental variations. As Murphy and Davidshofer[16] state, 'it is unlikely that everyone could be a genius, no matter how favourable the environment'.

There have been attempts to modify over the long term, the average IQ of groups, exemplified by the Head Start programme in the USA. There is some evidence of modifiability from such studies, although the basis for the changes is not clear. The focus of such programmes has also changed to the extent that the outcome criteria are now more concerned with school success rather than with IQ.[16]

Bias and Unfairness

Not unsurprisingly, the finding of race, gender and social class differences has led to the assertion that IQ tests are biased and unfair. Some of the debates around these views have arisen because of a failure to clarify the distinction between the two key terms.[16] Bias refers to tests systematically producing either higher or lower scores – in measuring or in predicting from scores. Unfairness refers to the decisions that are taken based on the test scores.

There is no strong evidence that tests are biased in measurement or in prediction. Rather, the differences found between groups appear to be real differences.[16,52] As Herrnstein and Murray[12] state, as their fifth 'beyond technical dispute' point: '5. Properly administered IQ tests are not demonstrably biased against social, economic, ethnic or racial groups'. What remains to be discovered is why such differences occur. It is highly unlikely that there will be a single or even one major reason.

The issue of unfairness is not limited to the use of tests with individuals from minority groups. Rather, it arises from the improper use of tests for any purpose. It is now widely recognized that one test score is an inadequate basis for decision making; rather, decisions need to be based on the confluence of evidence from a number of sources.[16]

Intelligence, IQ and Learning Difficulties

The term learning difficulties, for purposes of this section, refers to the broad range of individuals whose abilities are well below the average but who do not have demonstrable organic pathology.

Theories of intelligence, as documented earlier, have differing orientations and vary in important ways. Associated with each is a view of intelligence that is an inherent part of the theory. Each of these theories will, in turn, have differing implications for how we are to view, assess and understand learning difficulties.

The relationship between learning difficulties and intelligence is made more complex because the clinical term itself encompasses a heterogeneous range of conditions and phenomena. There are substantial individual differences in abilities, even within many of the diagnostic groupings. It does not help to try to operationalize the diagnosis simply by linking it to IQ. The IQ can be derived from any of a number of different tests each requiring different skills, and each test, in turn, has a somewhat different theory of intelligence underlying it. The IQ and what it means cannot ultimately be divorced from the conceptions of intelligence that informed the processes of test design and construction.

Further, the IQ is a compound measure and any given value of the IQ can be reached by a variety of pathways. A similar IQ does not mean that similar abilities have been deployed to achieve it – a point made by Eysenck in 1967.[28]

Although psychometrically an inadequate concept, Mental Age (MA) is sometimes used as an index of ability. MA is the average (or most common) score obtained on a test battery by individuals of a given Chronological Age (CA). The 'Mental' part of the term derives from the use of tests presumed to tap intelligence. Hence, if the average score of individuals aged 10 years is 35, any individual who gets a score of 35 is said to have a MA of 10. If the individual taking the test is 8 years old, they are mentally 'advanced'; if aged 12, they would be identified as being mentally 'retarded'. The MA, like the IQ, is compound, and so testees can achieve the same total scores even though they have deployed quite different abilities.

There are a number of issues relating to the nature of the 'difficulties' or 'retardation' in individuals of low ability, sometimes known as the 'delay versus deviance debate'. That is, are those without and those with learning difficulties following the same developmental trajectory, but with the 'retarded' individual doing so at a slower rate; also, will 'retarded' individuals reach a lower ceiling, or are there qualitative differences in the paths they are following?

A second question is whether an individual who has an MA well below CA is as competent as 'normal' individuals at that chronological age. Does an individual with a mental age of 10 but chronologically 13 have all the competencies found in chronological 10 year olds? These issues are not restricted to mental ability: a similar debate has taken place with regard to autism[53] and language difficulties.[54]

Questions on quantitative versus qualitative differences have generated substantial debate in the academic literature.[54-56] Evidence that children with and without mental retardation achieve similar MAs by differing routes has been provided by Spitz.[57] After studying patterns of performance on a number of standard tests, Spitz[57] concluded that individuals with mental retardation tend to perform more poorly than their MA controls. Their performance was found to be poorer on tasks that involve more 'g'. They are thought to accumulate successes on tasks which are more susceptible to practice because the individuals with mental retardation are older and have had more opportunities or time to exploit their experience.

Studies such as Spitz's[57] highlight several important points. First, they suggest that the differences between those with and without learning difficulties are not simply quantitative differences but reflect real differences in the nature as well as the level of skills. To assume individuals so afflicted will 'catch up' could be quite misleading. This phenomenon also has manifestations at the population level. While the common pattern is for there to be population IQ gains over the decades, the disparity diminishes towards the extremes of the distribution and in the retardation range the pattern becomes reversed, suggesting differences in the nature of abilities in the groups who are not retarded and those who are.[58] Second, it is clear from the foregoing that even a measure with comparatively substantial powers for differentiating among individuals and for prediction nevertheless masks important information. In other words, the same IQ, even on the same test, can refer to individuals with widely differing patterns of skill and deficit. Further, because intelligence tests all yield IQs, the same IQ level on different tests could conceal substantial differences in the patterns of skill and deficit (because of variations in test content). Given that the IQs could stem from different theoretical models, they might mean quite different things. Even when the theoretical model is similar, disparities can be found among individuals with learning disabilities of similar IQ.[59]

Hence, a fundamental issue for clinical practice is not just the level of score, but score patterning and, critically, what the patterns mean. In the next section, we turn to intelligence testing in clinical practice.

Why Test?

Clinicians dealing with the complexity of psychological and psychiatric disorders rely on experience and judgement to gather and organize the information necessary for diagnosis and treatment.

The core clinical processes of information gathering and organization, developing an understanding of the individual and decision making can be enhanced using psychological tests. While adequate for many purposes, clinical judgement may not cover a sufficiently comprehensive or focused range of behaviour and skills, leading to inaccurate or incomplete conclusions. Clinical judgements are also most vulnerable to error in borderline circumstances. Psychological tests are not limited to the same extent and can objectively and systematically provide information to complement, support or even extend clinical opinion.

The grounds on which clinicians make judgements about psychological characteristics may vary between clinicians and the same clinician can vary over time. Lack of consistency creates problems: for example, it makes communication difficult. One of the advantages of psychological tests is that they make clear the basis for statements or characterizations. Tests also provide opportunities for observation and score patterns can lead to alternative hypotheses and explanations, adding to the creative dimension of clinical practice.

Some tests are designed to differentiate among abilities and processes (auditory contrasted with visual memory), and this is also important in practice, for instance in characterizing neuropsychological dysfunctions or making more refined discriminations. Test scores can provide a baseline for assessing deterioration or monitoring treatment. Finally, it is worth highlighting the importance of test data in clinical research, for matching purposes or for providing the main indices in a project. There are thus many good reasons for using tests.[5]

In addition to these advantages, the research associated with particular tests also enables firmer grounds for diagnosis and prognosis, as is well illustrated by the studies of the developmental and educational correlates of the IQ.

Testing in Clinical Practice

Psychological tests are generally simple to administer and score. Manuals provide clear instructions and administration and scoring are technical skills readily acquired. The main challenge is score interpretation. This requires an understanding of the theories, principles and techniques of measurement and knowledge of the related research literature. A good grounding in developmental psychology and psychopathology are required, together with a knowledge of the issues and techniques that are central to individual test score interpretation. All the above must then be synthesized to produce interpretations about individual functioning that are relevant to the reasons for undertaking testing. It is the application of this knowledge, skill base and clinical experience that characterizes the skilled tester and the proper use of tests.

Characteristics of Psychological Tests

A 'psychological test' can be defined as 'any systematic procedure for observing a person's behaviour and describing it with the aid of a numerical scale or category system'.[60]

Intelligence and other tests share the following goals and characteristics.

Test Content

Tests are devised to provoke specific forms of behaviour because it is assumed on various grounds that these will be outward manifestations of the higher level (mental) psychological characteristic. The behaviours are also selected because they can be quantified (defining a word correctly scores 1).

Achieving Uniformity of Procedures

Standardization refers to the rules for administering and scoring and is critical in psychological (and other) measurement. By carefully specifying, and therefore controlling content and procedures, errors are greatly reduced, leading to coherent and consistent interpretation and communication.

Achieving Measurement

Tests quantify psychological variables. The approach is similar to that in medicine, biology and the natural sciences, the main difference being the degree of inference: key psychological concepts are not always directly linked to observable phenomena.

Several forms of quantification such as points for correct answers and time to solve a problem are used. Summation of such scores produces the raw score, for instance, total words correctly defined.

Raw scores become meaningful when compared with a standard, as in all forms of measurement. For intelligence or other tests this is the performance of a criterion group on the same tasks administered in a standard manner. The criterion against which individual test performance is compared is called the test norms and the procedure a norm-referenced test.

Norms are obtained by giving the test to samples from the population of interest. The nature of this population is determined by the intended range of use of the test. One criterion of test quality is the adequacy of sampling to achieve the norms.

Test scores should correspond in magnitude with the characteristic being measured: the higher the score, the more of the characteristic. The process used to assign numbers to levels of performance is called scaling. The purposes of scaling are to ensure that different scores on tests are closely linked with performance differences and that the magnitude of the test score accurately reflects the magnitude of the characteristic. Reckase[61] provides a good introduction to the scaling.

There are several ways of transforming and expressing raw scores. The IQ and MA were described earlier.

The comparison of an individual's score with that of the normative group can be refined by introducing units which then place the score so many units above or below the average. The common practice is to use intervals or steps of standard deviation units to produce these deviation (from the mean or average) scores. Because the average score and variability (standard deviation) at different ages can differ, several conventions have been adopted. These set the averages and standard deviations to common arbitrary but useful values. Such transformations change the numbers but not the numerical relationships or properties and are therefore justifiable. The transformations are particularly convenient for statistical and interpretative purposes, the most common being to set the mean or average at 100 and the standard deviation at 15. Hence, an IQ of 115 indicates that the individual obtained a raw score one standard deviation above the mean for his or her comparison group. Another common measure, the T-score, is set with a mean of 50 and a standard deviation of 10. Scores transformed in this way are called standard scores.

Test Age (MA is an example) may be converted to a ratio score. The ratio of test age to chronological age (TA/CA × 100) is called a ratio quotient but is not commonly used because of poor statistical properties.[62]

Another transformation, useful for communicating and comparing results, is the percentile. These range from 0 to 100 and indicate the percentage of comparable individuals obtaining the same score or less on the test.

Differentiating Individual Characteristics

Measurement or testing is concerned with the objective identification of individual differences in a characteristic behaviour pattern or process. The underlying assumption is the belief that differential levels of the attribute, reflected in different levels of test score, might be associated with other important individual differences.

Diagnostic Testing

The potential of tests as diagnostic instruments (as devices to high-light individual characteristics, pathological or otherwise), has been recognized for many years.[63] Applications include the identification of broad syndromes, particular assets or deficits in cognitive abilities or other specific processes.

Diagnostic testing is based on a variety of techniques:

(1) An extreme score (very much above or below the middle value) can be indicative of either a deficit or an outstanding ability.
(2) A difference between scores on two tests or subtests may indicate a dysfunction or special ability.
(3) The pattern or profile of test scores may match that of an already 'diagnosed' or criterion group.
(4) A change in score (increase or decrease), or the absence of change on repeated testing may also have diagnostic implications, for instance in detecting deterioration of functioning.
(5) Wide variability in a set of scores may also be indicative of dysfunction.

Although appearing as dissimilar these patterns have the common feature that the 'diagnosis' is based on some form of difference between scores.

The interpretation of score patterns or differences poses difficulties and requires special procedures to ensure that it does not simply reflect the operation of chance.[64-67] Further, even when differences are found to be reliable (nonchance), they can exist in the normal population with substantial frequency, as has been found in studies of the Wechsler test Verbal and Performance Scale differences. Commonly occurring differences may be unlikely to be of diagnostic import on their own.

Further, tests have to be able to select individuals more efficiently than would happen by chance (the base rates or normal frequency of occurrence in the population) and do so in ways that minimize wrong decisions.[68]

Criteria against which difference scores or profiles are to be validated can be particularly problematic if, for instance, they consist of clinical judgements which can be unreliable, particularly in the borderline range where the diagnostic utility of tests is likely to be most valuable.

Practical Implications

The foregoing issues make it appear that diagnostic testing is of limited value. This is not the case. The decision to undertake formal testing should be made in the context of a comprehensive and systematic clinical history. Testing is not a routine procedure. The need to test stems directly from uncertainties and unanswered questions in the history.

A cardinal principle in the use of test information is that it should never on its own be taken as some absolute truth. Rather, test information is part of the totality of clinical information and needs to make sense in that context. Inconsistencies should be checked through various other investigations. In such a framework, diagnostic approaches can make an important contribution to assessment.

Influences on Test Performance

Psychological testing is intrusive and engenders reactions: rather than observing natural behaviour, the tester commonly requires the testee to do things. In the process the individual learns about and experiences the demands of the test and situation. Testing also produces 'side-effects' – anxiety about being tested, elation at success or unhappiness and reduced motivation following failure. These are behavioural effects that can distort the test score and undermine the purpose of testing. Some specific influences on test score and performance are considered next.

Effects of Standardization

Standardized procedures have advantages, noted earlier, but also have disadvantages in that many aspects of functioning that influence test performance cannot be followed up because of the constraints of standardized procedures. The tester has to adhere closely to specified forms of further questioning if the answer is not clear enough to be scored, even though posing the question differently might elicit the correct answer.

Constraints of Test Format

Tests designed to measure the same characteristic or skill may have the same label but vary in form and content and may therefore be measuring different things.

Test Difficulty

Tests experienced as difficult can lead to early and continued failures with an adverse effect on motivation or other aspects of performance. This is a particular problem in the assessment of learning difficulties. Tests that are too easy can also have motivational repercussions, making the individual bored or overconfident.

Scores can also incorrectly represent the characteristic being measured through 'floor' and 'ceiling' effects. Most tests are designed to cover a specific ability range. Floor effects occur when the actual ability of the individual is below the lowest score obtainable on the test whereas ceiling effects arise when the actual ability is well above the maximum score possible on the test.

Test Length

Test length is usually a compromise between the need to have as many items as possible to ensure reliability and comprehensiveness of coverage, and as few items as possible to maintain motivation and avoid fatigue. Even then, young or handicapped individuals may have difficulty completing a test.

Tester Effects

In the one-to-one test situation, the characteristics and style of the tester can hamper or facilitate performance through passivity or encouragement, or other aspects of tester style. Testers can also make errors in administration and scoring, despite standardized procedures.

Individual and Setting Effects

The physical setting, for example extraneous noises, and also transient individual characteristics such as ill health can have an impact on test scores through their effects on performance. Intra-individual characteristics also have the potential to influence test behaviour. These may be temperamental, such as the individual who is 'slow to warm up', very active and impulsive people, or individuals who react strongly to failure.[69]

Incomplete Testing

Individuals with handicaps may complete only parts of a test. Hence, in addition to problems of reliability, interpretations have to be constrained and scores should not be given their usual labels (MA or IQ for example) unless it is made quite explicit that the 'IQ' is based on an incomplete or nonstandard administration. Also, some scores have a variety of implications that may not hold if based on nonstandard procedures or if used to generalize about atypical individuals.

Some individuals refuse to be tested (deliberate non-compliance) while there are others whose behaviour and handicaps make them difficult to test. For a given set of circumstances and attempts, the statement that the person is 'untestable' may hold. However, people are not tested with the purpose of getting a test score but as part of the processes of assessment: with the problem clearly articulated, an answer can be arrived at through different means such as direct observation and structured interviews.

Individuals from Different Cultural Groups

Individuals from different ethnic groups require careful consideration particularly because developmental and functional characteristics may mean different things. Expectations may differ, as may the life experiences, even though brought up in a common broader society. Parental or carer interpretations of behaviour can differ and there are likely to be differences in language.

The Role of Observation

With standardized tests, situations and tasks tend to be constant. Hence, individual differences in performance become more apparent to an experienced tester, and these observations are valuable sources of clinical hypotheses. Careful observation of the style and content of answers, and *ad hoc* investigations when testing is completed, can produce information relevant to understanding the findings. For example, errors may arise from impulsive answering, or they may be rule-governed. Clark and Rutter[70] were able to demonstrate that some autistic children made systematic errors in their responses. While the answers were wrong, there was clear evidence of a consistent strategy. Most crucially, observation provides a basis for an evaluation of the findings and the decision about whether or not they should be used.

Test Adequacy and Data Adequacy

Reviews of new tests and relevant research evaluations of existing procedures provide a general guide to the psychometric adequacy of the test. However, a good test may not produce accurate or interpretable test results for an individual whose scores may be adversely influenced by factors such as anxiety, administration and scoring errors.

While it is always important to give the testee the benefit of the doubt, low scores should not be dismissed because of anxiety during testing. An alternative hypothesis is that poor abilities lead to anxiety.

In the final analysis, test scores should always be checked against other data. Test scores must be disregarded if there are reasons to believe the data are of poor quality because of anxiety or other influences. Occasionally, test results may need to be disregarded in favour of information from other sources.

Observing the individual in their natural environment can be advantageous, especially the ways in which they deal with everyday events. Observations could be guided by a schedule such as the Vineland Adaptive Behaviours Scales.[15] It is important to not base judgements solely on what may be well-practised skills, although these can give an idea of a minimal level. Observing the individual facing new challenges or introducing these in order to observe how they are responded to can be useful. Qualitative indicators, such as the exploratory behaviour or curiosity can, at certain ages, give a guide to the way the individual is functioning.

Social interactions and play in younger individuals can be important sources of information. The ability to follow complex conversations or respond to complex instructions and produce long interactive sentences can be markers for estimating abilities, depending on age. Complexity of play and the creation of novel and detailed objects or in drawings, can also indicate competencies, provided that they are not routinized. Evidence should be cumulative, not based on a single instance of a skill, and should be as extensive as possible.

Integration

The ideals of testing are rarely satisfied in clinical practice. Test scores should not be seen as having substantial numerical precision and the numbers are best seen as a guide to a range rather than as a precise level. Findings must be qualified to enable limitations to be taken into account and ensure that the results are seen in context. Detailed and systematic observations of behaviour should be recorded in the test report so that sources of unreliability are identified. Nonstandard procedures should be reported. Finally, an effort should be made to obtain independent confirmation of test results. This can be achieved partly by relating what was seen in the test situation to information given by parents, carers and others, and partly by comparing test scores with developmental and other data. An attempt should be made at the same time to confirm that the behaviour seen during testing was 'typical' of other situations. Major discrepancies should be investigated and the assessment should not be regarded as complete while unresolved discrepancies remain.

Concluding Comments

The primary characteristic of clinical practice is its focus on the individual client. The task in psychological testing is to integrate what is known about tests, score interpretation, and the effects of being tested with the characteristics and demands of clinical practice. This chapter has provided an overview of IQ testing and intelligence as a background for testing in clinical practice in learning disabilities. Such knowledge is the cornerstone of test interpretation.

Despite the use of statistical procedures, test interpretation always entails a varying degree of uncertainty: key words have different meanings, the research on which interpretations are based, like all psychological research, has methodological and other limitations, individual clients may differ from individuals in research samples, test norms may be out of date, etc. In addition, the level of any score does not necessarily reflect the precise level of the characteristic being measured, as tests usually sample the effects of other psychological processes and performance can easily be influenced by individual and situational factors.

Hence, test user and also the user of test results, require an understanding of the theoretical basis of the tests, a knowledge of development and its disorders, an awareness of the multiplicity of factors that can influence test performance and also an awareness of the problems of score interpretation. This information may then be combined with other clinical information to produce an assessment that is relevant to the needs of the individual. It is only in this broader framework that psychological test data and the theories that underlie them make a relevant and constructive contribution to clinical assessment and management.

References

1. Raven J (1965) *Guide to the Standard Progressive Matrices*. London: Lewis.
2. Wechsler D (1981) *Manual for the Wechsler Adult Intelligence Scale – Revised* New York: Psychological Corporation.
3. Stetson EG (1992) Clinical child psychology and child assessment. In Walker CE & Roberts MC (eds) *Handbook of Clinical Child Psychology*, pp. 101–32. New York: Wiley.
4. Bayley N (1993) *Bayley Scales of Infant Development*, 2nd edn. San Antonio: Psychological Corporation.
5. Berger M & Yule W (1985) IQ tests and assessment. In Clarke AM, Clarke ADB & Berg J (eds) *Mental Deficiency: The Changing Outlook*, 4th edn, pp. 53–96. London: Methuen.
6. Slater A (1995) Individual differences in infancy and later IQ. *Journal of Child Psychology and Psychiatry* **36**, 69–112.
7. Griffiths R (1954) *The Abilities of Babies*. London: University of London Press.
8. Cattell P (1960) *Cattell Infant Intelligence Scale*. Cleveland: Psychological Corporation.
9. Fagan JF (1984) The intelligent infant: theoretical implications. *Intelligence* **8**, 1–9.
10. O'Connor N & Hermelin B (1984) Idiot savant calendrical calculators: maths or memory? *Psychological Medicine* **14**, 801–6.
11. Rose DH, Slater AS & Perry H (1986) Prediction of childhood intelligence from habituation in early infancy. *Intelligence* **10**, 251–63.
12. Herrnstein RJ & Murray C (1994) *The Bell Curve: Intelligence and Class Structure in American Life*. New York: The Free Press.
13. Sternberg RJ, Wagner RK, Williams WM & Horvath JA (1995) Testing common sense. *American Psychologist* **50**, 912–27.
14. Sattler JM (1992) Assessment of children's intelligence. In Walker CE & Roberts MC (eds) *Handbook of Clinical Child Psychology*, pp. 85–100. New York: Wiley.
15. Sparrow S, Balla D & Cicchetti D (1984) *Vineland Adaptive Behavior Scale*. Circle Pines: American Guidance Service.
16. Murphy KR & Davidshofer CO (1994) *Psychological Testing: Principles and Applications*, 3rd edn. New Jersey: Prentice Hall.
17. Boring EG (1957) *A History of Experimental Psychology*. New York: Appleton-Century-Crofts.
18. Freeman FN (1939) *Mental Tests: Their History, Principles and Applications*. New York: Harrap.
19. Wolf TH (1973) *Alfred Binet*. Chicago: University of Chicago Press.
20. Anderson M (1992) *Intelligence and Development: A Cognitive Theory*. Oxford: Blackwell.
21. Spearman CE (1904) 'General Intelligence' objectively determined and measured. *American Journal of Psychology* **15**, 201–93.
22. Jensen AR & Weng L (1994) What is a good g? *Intelligence* **18**, 231–58.
23. Vernon PE (1979) *Intelligence: Heredity and Environment*. San Francisco: WH Freeman.
24. Wechsler D (1958) *The Measurement and Appraisal of Adult Intelligence*, 4th edn. London: Baillère, Tindall & Cox.
25. Kaufman AS & Kaufman NL (1983) *Kaufman Assessment Battery for Children: Interpretative Manual*. Circle Pines: American Guidance Service.
26. Gardner H (1993) *Multiple Intelligences: The Theory in Practice*. New York: Basic Books.
27. Sternberg RJ (1984) *Beyond IQ: A Triarchic Theory of Human Intelligence*. Cambridge: Cambridge University Press.

28. Eysenck HJ (1982) Introduction. In Eysenck HJ (ed) *A Model for Intelligence*, pp. 1–12. Berlin: Springer.
29. Berger M (1982) The 'Scientific Approach' to intelligence: an overview of its history with special reference to mental speed. In Eysenck HJ (ed) *A Model for Intelligence*, pp. 13–43. Berlin: Springer.
30. Butterworth G (1994) Infant intelligence. In Khalfa J (ed) *What is Intelligence?* pp. 49–71. Cambridge: Cambridge University Press.
31. Kail R & Pellegrino JW (1985) *Human Intelligence: Perspectives and Prospects*. New York: WH Freeman.
32. Jensen AR (1982) Reaction time and psychometric g. In Eysenck HJ (ed) *A Model for Intelligence*, pp. 93–132. Berlin: Springer.
33. Wechsler D (1992) *Manual for the Wechsler Intelligence Scale for Children – Third UK Edition WISC-III UK*. Kent: Psychological Corporation.
34. Eysenck HJ (1939) Primary mental abilities. *British Journal of Educational Psychology* **9**, 270–5.
35. Guilford JP (1967) *The Nature of Human Intelligence*. New York: McGraw Hill.
36. Cattell RB (1971) The structure of intelligence in relation to the nature–nurture controversy. In Cancrow R (ed) *Intelligence: Genetic and Environmental Influences*. pp. 3–30. New York: Grune and Stratton.
37. McShane J (1991) *Cognitive Development: An Information Processing Approach*. Oxford: Blackwell.
38. Hobson RP (1985) Piaget: On ways of knowing in childhood. In Rutter M & Hersov L (eds) *Child and Adolescent Psychiatry: Modern Approaches*, 2nd edn, pp. 191–203. Oxford: Blackwell.
39. Elliott CD (1986) The factorial structure and specificity of the British Ability Scales. *British Journal of Psychology* **77**, 175–85.
40. Lezak MD (1995) *Neuropsychological Assessment*, 3rd edn. New York: Oxford University Press.
41. Das JP, Naglieri J & Kirby J (1994) *Assessment of Cognitive Processes: the PASS Theory of Intelligence*. Boston: Allyn & Bacon.
42. Naglieri J & Reardon SM (1993) Traditional IQ is irrelevant to learning disabilities – intelligence is not. *Journal of Learning Disabilities* **26**, 127–33.
43. Moore DG, Hobson RP & Anderson M (1995) Person perception: Does it involve IQ-independent perceptual processing? *Intelligence* **20**, 65–86.
44. Jensen AR (1969) *Bias in Mental Testing*. London: Methuen.
45. Brand C (1996) *The g Factor*. Chichester: John Wiley.
46. Berger M (1986) Toward an educated use of IQ Tests: A reappraisal of intelligence testing. In Lahey BB & Kazdin AE (eds) *Advances in Clinical Child Psychology Vol.9*, pp. 1–34. New York: Plenum Press.
47. Gregory R (1994) Seeing intelligence. In Khalfa J (ed) *What is Intelligence?* pp. 13–26. Cambridge: Cambridge University Press.
48. Plomin R & Neiderheiser J (1991) Quantitative genetics, molecular genetics and intelligence. *Intelligence* **15**, 369–87.
49. Ceci SJ, Nightingale NN & Baker JG (1992) The ecologies of intelligence: Challenges to traditional views. In Detterman D (ed) *Is Mind Modular or Unitary? Current Topics in Human Intelligence, Vol. 2*, pp. 61–82. Norwood: Ablex Publishing Corp.
50. Pederson NL, Plomin R & McClearn GE (1994) Is there G beyond g? Is there genetic influence on specific cognitive abilities independent of genetic influence on general cognitive ability? *Intelligence* **18**, 133–43.
51. Hindley CB & Owen CF (1978) The extent of individual changes in IQ for ages between 6 months and 17 years, in a British longitudinal sample. *Journal of Child Psychology and Psychiatry* **19**, 329–50.
52. Kaufman AS (1994) *Intelligent Testing With the WISC-III*. New York: Wiley.
53. Burack J (1992) Debate and argument: clarifying developmental issues in the study of autism. *Journal of Child Psychology and Psychiatry* **33**, 617–21.
54. Rondal JA (1988) Language development in Down's syndrome: A life-span perspective. *International Journal of Behavioural Development* **11**, 212–36.
55. Zigler E & Balla D (1977) *Mental Retardation: The Developmental-Difference Controversy*. New Jersey: Lawrence Erlbaum Associates.
56. Thal DJ (1991) Language and cognition in normal and late-talking toddlers. *Topics in Language Disorders* **11**, 33–42.

57. Spitz HH (1982) Intellectual extremes, mental age, and the nature of human intelligence. *Merrill-Palmer Quarterly* **28**, 167–92.
58. Spitz HH (1982) Variations in Wechsler interscale IQ disparities at different levels of IQ. *Intelligence* **13**, 157–67.
59. Spitz HH (1986) Disparities in mentally retarded persons' IQs derived from different intelligence tests. *American Journal of Mental Deficiency* **90**, 588–91.
60. Cronbach LJ (1970) *Essentials of Psychological Testing*, 3rd edn. New York: Harper and Row.
61. Reckase MD (1990) Scaling techniques. In Goldstein G & Hersen M (eds) *Handbook of Psychological Assessment* 2nd edn, pp. 41–56. New York: Pergamon Press.
62. Anastasi A (1982) *Psychological Testing*, 5th edn. New York: Macmillan.
63. Garfield SL (1974) *Clinical Psychology*. Chicago: Aldine.
64. Payne RW & Jones HG (1957) Statistics for the investigation of individual cases. *Journal of Clinical Psychology* **13**, 115–21.
65. Rosen A (1966) Stability of the new MMPI scales and statistical procedures for evaluating changes and differences in psychiatric patients. *Journal of Consulting Psychology* **30**, 142–5.
66. Silverstein AB (1981) Reliability and abnormality of test score differences. *Journal of Clinical Psychology* **37**, 392–4.
67. Silverstein AB (1989) Reliability and abnormality of scaled-score ranges. *Journal of Clinical Psychology* **45**, 926–9.
68. Ireton H (1990) Developmental screening measures. In Johnson JH & Goldman J (eds) *Developmental Assessment in Clinical Child Psychology*, pp. 78–99. New York: Pergamon Press.
69. Thomas A, Chess S & Birch HG (1968) *Temperament and Behaviour Disorders in Children*. London: University of London Press.
70. Clarke P & Rutter M (1979) Task difficulty and task performance in autistic children. *Journal of Child Psychology Psychiatry* **20**, 271–85.

2

Concept of Learning Disability

Douglas A. Spencer

Historical Background

The Changing Terminology – Professional, Political and Public Aspects

The dictionary definitions of 'concept' include: a general notion, an idea of a class of objects, the product of the faculty of conception, and – 'concepts are merely the results, rendered permanent by language of a previous process of comparison', Sir W. Harrison.[1]

The simple conception of what is currently called Learning Disability in the United Kingdom (UK) depends on comparing an individual's abilities with what is normal, average or expected for comparable people of similar age and culture. This comparison can involve implied or actual measurements and ratings to quantify how disabled a person is compared with the standard used.

Learning Disability, called Mental Retardation by the World Health Organisation (WHO), has been known by various names for as long as human civilization has existed. While this fundamental, basic and universal disability has always affected mankind, the concept of it at different times and in different parts of the world has shown continuing change. The concept of learning disability is not static, but an evolving process. In this process concept and terminology are closely inter-related. Changes in concept influence changes in terminology. Changes in terminology can influence changes in concept.

The many changes in terminology during the twentieth century reflect the importance attached to a name and its impact and implications. There has been a continuing search for expressions that are less stigmatizing and that may inspire new hope. That people vary enormously in their abilities and talents can hardly be disputed; this is a biological fact of human life. The liberal and humanitarian view that has grown in strength over the latter half of the century has been that people should not be devalued or under-valued as people because they have learning and/or physical disabilities.

At least thirty or more names have been used for learning disability. Old or archaic terms, oligophrenia, hypophrenia, amentia, simple primary amentia, mental defect, mental defective, idiot, imbecile, feeble-minded, moron, moral defective, high-grade, low-grade, subnormal, are historical markers and contrast with arguably more euphemistic recent titles. 'Mental

Handicap' was adopted generally in the 1970s, although it had been used by the National Society for Mentally Handicapped Children from 1955. Its superficial similarity to mental illness led to a confusion between handicap and illness. In the press and media mental illness and mental handicap have been used as interchangeable. In its classifications the WHO has continued to use 'mental retardation', a less emotive North American usage. This sense of retardation has to be distinguished from the psychomotor retardation of depressive illness.

Affected children have been called special, exceptional, extraordinary, unusual, different and under-achievers. Names never widely accepted have been developmental handicap, disability or impairment, under-intellectualization, intellectual disability, intellectual insufficiency and cognitive impairment. For the professional study of the subject defectology, retardology, and developmental psychiatry have been proposed. People with learning disability on whom the acronym PLD has become conferred, have been described as 'one in a 100' and 'strangers in their own country'. The 'no-name' school of thought has contended that any name is a label and, once labelled, the person is treated as conforming to that label, so that it is perpetuated. 'Patients' have become 'residents', 'clients', 'consumers', 'service-users' and 'tenants'.

Some parents and relatives of people with 'learning disability' have not favoured this term. They feared that it was a diminishing of the problem, and hence that special services might be merged and lost within the mainstream. An anecdotal solution to mental handicap has been pretending that it does not exist. In the 1990s the Royal Association for Disability and Rehabilitation (RADAR) advised about disability terms and etiquette. People with learning disability should not be described as 'suffering' from their condition, 'the mentally handicapped' should not be used; 'person with restricted growth' should replace 'dwarf'.

Professionals and their organizations have eventually conceded to changing terminology to stay abreast of the fashion. The Royal College of Psychiatrists has chosen 'Psychiatry of Learning Disability'. The International Association has moved from 'mental deficiency' to 'intellectual disability'. The education services use 'learning difficulty', and their term 'mild learning difficulty' equates to clinical 'specific learning disability', and their 'moderate learning difficulty' approximates to clinical 'mild learning disability'. The rest of Europe and North America have retained 'mental retardation' and keep 'learning disability' for 'specific learning disability'.[2]

The Changing Specialism

In the years of the original standard medical textbooks on mental defect and deficiency, such as Tredgold and Soddy,[3] Hilliard and Kirman[4] and Penrose,[5] the subject comprised a distinct and coherent constellation of knowledge that was broadly within the grasp of one medical specialist. This embraced the history, the legal and administrative processes, and the clinical conditions associated with mental retardation and their features,

causes, diagnosis, pathology, genetics, metabolism, treatment and prevention. The biography of the handicapped person through the milestones of
development, infancy, childhood and adolescence had practical relevance.
Incidence (the occurrence of new cases of a particular condition within a
defined population during a particular period, often a year) and prevalence (a function of incidence and chronicity, for instance, frequency
per 1000) were studied. Conditions present in people with mental retardation, epilepsy, physical disability, sensory impairment, mental illness,
psychopathic disorder, offending and criminality were covered. Treatment,
education, employment, rehabilitation and different forms of care in
hospital and community received increasing attention.

Re-specialization

Over the years subjects which seemed simple have become complex, and
the prerogative of specialists developing their own techniques, skills,
professionalism and services. Genetics has become the province of the
clinical geneticist, metabolic disorders the concern of the chemical patholo-
gist. Paediatricians with interests in child development have taken up the
assessment of handicapped children. The role of the medical specialist has
become concentrated on the psychiatric disorders in children and adults
with learning disabilities. Within this subspeciality secondary specialization has focused on neurobiology, emotion and behaviour. The neuropsychiatry of mental handicap/learning disability is a special interest in its own
right, studying, for instance, sensory impairments, cerebral palsy, overactivity, minimal brain damage, reaction time, arousal and inhibition, inter-
hemisphere relationships, learning, language, psychosis, and abnormal
behaviour.[6] Psychotherapy in learning disability has evolved its own body
of expertise, to pursue such topics as the birth of a child with learning disability, coping with loss, psychotherapy with siblings, coming to terms
with learning difficulties, psychotherapy for people with learning disabilities, deviancy, group therapy, sexuality, counselling and secondary mental
handicap – the emotional sequelae of the primary handicap.[7] Forensic
case work, special needs services, secure units, 'difficult to place'
patients, and seriously challenging behaviour have become a third area of
re-specialization.

Early History – An Overview

In ancient times probably only the severest cases of mental defect were
recognized:[8] 'idiot' (from Greek, a private person), was applied to all cases,
'imbecile' (from Latin, bacillus), a stick,[5] 'weakness' and feebleminded
not coming into use until 1847–91. Hippocrates described anencephaly
and some other cranial anomalies. The Spartans allowed weak infants to
perish. The Romans killed malformed children, but used defectives for
amusement. In the Middle Ages superstition, witchcraft and belief in

changelings could result in cruel treatment of idiots. Their murmurings were interpreted as communication with Satan or divine inspiration. The word 'cretin' was a corruption of chrétien (Christian). Idiots may have been sheltered in monasteries.

In England, in the reign of Edward I, 1272–1307, a distinction was made for the first time between the born fool (*fatuus naturalis*) and the lunatic.[8] In the Statute of Prerogatives, 1325, in the reign of Edward II, a similar division was drawn between the born fool and the person of unsound mind who had lucid intervals (non compos mentis, sicut quidem sunt per lucida intervalla). The Crown could take possession of the belongings of the lunatic only during the period of his illness. The property of an idiot could be taken by the Crown subject to an obligation to provide for his person and estate.[9]

Theories of education began with an attempt by a Spanish teacher, J. Rodriguez Périere 1780, to educate the deaf. Itard tried to teach a wild boy, Victor, in the woods of Averyon, 1798.[10] The Poor Law Amendment Act, 1834, resulted in unions of parishes creating workhouses, many of which would later house mental defectives. The first 'Asylum for idiots' was opened at Park House, Highgate, due to the efforts of Andrew Reed in 1847. Essex Hall, Colchester, started as an annex in 1849, and the Park House residents moved to a model asylum at Earlswood in 1855. More asylums followed: Starcross, (Devon, 1864), Caterham and Leavesden (Metropolitan Asylums Act, 1867), Northern Counties Asylum (Lancaster, 1868), Darenth for children (1878), Stoke Park (Bristol, 1901), The Mary Dendy Homes (Cheshire, 1902), and Whittington Hall (Chesterfield, 1908). In 1881 there were 29 000 idiots in public institutions. An Idiots Act was passed in 1886 to care for idiots and imbeciles.

In 1899 the Elementary Education (Defective and Epileptic Children) Act empowered education authorities to ascertain which children were defective and to provide special schools for defectives, and transport, up to age 16. Goddard's studies in America (1912) showed a high birth rate in the section of the population described as the submerged tenth, which, it was thought, threatened to overwhelm future generations. A fear of national degeneracy led A.F. Tredgold to support segregation and a eugenic movement. After the Mental Deficiency Act 1913 the UK put considerable investment into making colonies for mental defectives. To take affected children and adults from overcrowded urban slums to colony parkland, clean beds, baths, regular meals, occupation and routine was seen to be humane and protective action in those days.

History from 1948 – the Hospital (Nosocomial) Period

The National Health Service

Until 1948 local authorities were responsible for all aspects of care of mentally handicapped people. They had a duty to provide supervision and training or occupation for those not living in institutions, and institutions for those who could not be cared for at home. On 5 July, 1948, the National

Health Service (NHS), was introduced. Residential colonies and institutions for mental deficiency became NHS mental deficiency hospitals. The local authorities continued to provide day occupation and training facilities for mentally defective children and adults in the community.

The NHS became responsible for a wide range of accommodation for over 50 000 mentally defective people; there were institutions dating from the previous century, purpose-built colonies, and former mansions, workhouses, fever hospitals and other premises housing people with varying degrees of mental deficiency and associated disabilities. The largest hospitals had over 2000 inpatients, many had between 300 and 1000, and numerous smaller units had 20 to 300 residents. Only the big hospitals had medical superintendents. Some hospitals had nonmedical secretary- or matron-superintendents. Often, a local general practitioner took a special interest in a hospital. Doctors performed intelligence testing with such tests as the Revized Stanford–Binet Form L Vocabulary Test, the Schonell Graded Word Reading Test and the Koh's Blocks Test. The 'inmates' were looked after by 'attendants', and later 'nurses'. The inmates contributed to the economy of the establishment in cleaning, laundry, kitchen-work, farming, gardening and helping care for the most disabled residents.

The 1950s

On 21 January 1952 a circular 5/52[11] regularized the hospital admission of patients for short-stay care without formality for up to 2 months. Other patients were formally detained. To meet the demand for unskilled labour after the war many able men and women went out to jobs 'on licence'. Being the main providers of residential care the hospitals, often already overcrowded, had long waiting lists. Extra accommodation was opened in new or converted buildings. Some waiting lists were operated on a regional or subregional basis. Priority for admission was given to people who were highly dependent or had behavioural problems. Many patients with greater needs put increasing pressure on the existing staff.

The 1960s

Informal Admission
On 6 October 1959 informal admission was introduced by the repeal of Section 315 of the Lunacy Act 1890, over a year before the Mental Health 1959 Act became law on 1 November 1960. The majority of patients became converted to 'informal' status. Most families wanted their handicapped members to remain in hospital, so few were discharged. 'Mental deficiency' became 'mental subnormality'. In the mid-1960s the beds in subnormality hospitals reached their peak of about 64 000. The norm of the time was 1.3 beds per 1000 of the population. The prevalence of severe subnormality was 3–4 per 1000. State enrolment for nurses in mental subnormality was introduced in 1964.

Improving Services

On 2 December, 1965, a Ministry of Health Circular was issued;[12] in paragraph 4 this stated that the general aim of hospital care is, wherever possible, to enable the patient to return to life in the community, either independently or with help from the local authority or from other sources. The circular reflected good practice which many psychiatrists were striving to develop, but few extra resources were forthcoming.

In the typical large comprehensive subnormality hospitals one quarter or more of the beds were occupied by children under 16. More children with multiple handicaps were surviving from birth and in infancy and paediatricians referred them to subnormality hospitals for long-stay care. Ambulant children admitted had behaviour problems, overactivity, epilepsy and autism. Adults admitted had behaviour disorders, mental illness, intractable epilepsy and high dependency requiring nursing care. Referrals came through medical officers of health, general practitioners and mental welfare officers.

After the 1959 Act people with subnormality going into prison or before the courts, were often admitted to hospital under Section 60 or Section 65 (with restriction) of the Act. Other offenders came for treatment as a condition of probation. Special regional units were set up for these patients, then called 'subnormal psychopaths'. About one-third of the patients in the hospitals had epilepsy. Phenobarbitone, phenytoin and primidone were prescribed for tonic–clonic epilepsy, ethosuximide for absences, paraldehyde for status epilepticus. Chlorpromazine and haloperidol were used to target aggression, violence, self-injury and psychotic symptoms. Electroplexy or neurosurgery were sometimes applied as a last resort in unmanageable cases.

Positive actions to improve services set benchmarks of quality for the future, outreach services, clinics, visits to homes and community centres developed to assess patients before admission, to prevent admission by treatment in the community and to follow-up discharged patients. Patients no longer needing hospital care were discharged home or to hostels and flatlets. Overcrowding was gradually reduced, food and clothing improved. Hospital shops, hairdressing facilities, tea-rooms and clothing stores were introduced, accommodation was refurbished and new buildings constructed. Occupational activities were extended and industrial therapy, the 'work ethic', favoured. For less able patients 'play therapy' and 'adult activities' were devised. Social, recreational, leisure and educational activities were broadened. More holidays, excursions and entertainments were arranged. Hospital evening and further education classes were organized by local education authorities.

In 1960, the cost per patient in a large subnormality hospital could be £6.00 per week. This rose to £12.00 in 1964 and to £25.00 in 1972 as hospitals reduced bed numbers and employed more staff. Specialist staff were gradually recruited: psychiatric, medical, nursing, psychology, social work, occupational therapy, physiotherapy, speech therapy, dietetic and dental. Staff training expanded with courses, libraries, and nurse training for the register and roll. Clinical services took more interest in diagnosis, classification, reports, case conferences, medication, teaching and research. Voluntary con-tribution[13] added an 'extra dimension' with 'leagues' of friends, parents and relatives groups, volunteers and organizers of voluntary services. In 1966 the National Society for Mentally Handicapped Children initiated the for-mation of the National Federation of Gateway Clubs to serve the leisure needs of people with mental handicap in community and hospital. Its 200 clubs in 1970 had grown to 600 by 1986. A positive characteristic of the hospitals was the ethos of loyalty and goodwill among long-serving staff, for whom the hospital was a part of their lives. They had a unique knowledge of the histories, talents and foibles of the patients. Ironically, as hospitals were making improvements critical reports were published.

'Put Away'
A study, 'Put Away', financed by the National Society for Mentally Handicapped Children, was published in 1969.[14] It was a national survey of 35 hospitals by a team using questionnaires. The report suggested selling hospital land and unsuitable units and using the proceeds to buy houses in local communities.

The Ely Hospital Inquiry
In March 1969, the report of the Committee of Inquiry into allegations of ill-treatment of patients and other irregularities at the Ely Hospital Cardiff (the Howe Report, the Ely Inquiry)[15] immediately generated widespread media attention and public and political outrage about conditions in subnormality hospitals. The Committee had commented that the hospital had no 'champions' – no one was 'batting for' Ely.

Interim Measures
R.H.S. Crossman, Secretary of State for Social Services, set up a working party which met for 2 years. In 1969 'interim measures' were given to Regional Hospital Boards. Standards for food (a top priority), clothing, space, staffing and accommodation were set. Each patient was to have a minimum of 50 square feet of bed space. Wards of over 50 adults were to be reduced to 30. Prefabricated wards, 'Crossman Units', were erected to relieve serious overcrowding. The plans were to be achieved over 5 years. The Hospital Advisory Service, later to be the Health Advisory Service (HAS), created under A.A. Baker, sent teams to visit hospitals to advise and report. At the time there were 100 consultants and 14 000 nurses in subnormality hospitals. The report of a committee on the functions of the District General Hospital, 1969, the Bonham Carter Report, suggested mentally subnormal patients should be on district hospital sites.

The 1970s

The White Paper – 'Better Services'
A government white paper on better services for the mentally handi-capped was published in June 1971.[16] In the foreword, Sir Keith Joseph, Secretary of State for Social Services, stated that the paper reflected very

substantial increases in expenditure on services for the mentally handicapped. The report stated that a person who is mentally handicapped does
not develop in childhood as quickly as other children nor attain the full
mental capacities of a normal adult. In the report, estimates of the prevalence of mental handicap used information from surveys in Wessex and
Newcastle hospital regions and in the former metropolitan Borough of
Camberwell. The principles of current thinking on mental handicap were
listed. The history of the services was traced, existing services described,
and shortcomings acknowledged. The services required were discussed.
Action to improve services was proposed, including 'sectorization' – the
designation of particular wards or units for patients from one sector of a
hospital's total service area. Voluntary service, research, prevention and
early detection were also covered.

'The Mental Health Service after Unification'

This was a paper published in June 1972 by a tripartite committee with
authorization of the Royal College of Psychiatrists, the Society of Medical
Officers of Health and the British Medical Association.[17] In October 1972,
Sir Keith Joseph, delivering the Hargreaves Memorial Lecture of the Leeds
Regional Psychiatric Association, reported that government funds for
mental handicap had risen from £7.5 million in 1970 to £9.3 million in
1972–73. He pledged that until services had been built up hospitals could
not be closed.[18] The Farleigh Hospital (Flax Bourton, Avon) Inquiry
reported in April 1971[19] and an inquiry on patients at South Ockenden
Hospital (Greater London) was published in 1974.[20] In the 1970s many
patients were discharged to live in adult residential centres, 'hostels', with
usually 20–30 places, and attended adult training centres, ATCs, with often
about 100 places, which were being opened in the community.

NHS Reorganization

On 1 April, 1974, the NHS was reorganized. Regional Health Authorities
replaced the Regional Hospital Boards, Area Health Authorities and
Districts replaced Hospital Management Committees. In the exigences of
the changes much of the recent impetus to advances in mental handicap
was undermined.

New Initiatives

In February 1975 Barbara Castle, Secretary of State for Social Services,
announced four new initiatives. First was the setting up of a National
Development Group for the Mentally Handicapped, Chairman Professor
Peter Mittler. Second was the establishment of the Development Team for
the Mentally Handicapped. Third was an inquiry into mental handicap
nursing and care, Chairman Peggy Jay. Fourth was a reorientation of the
medical role in mental handicap.

The National Development Group

This group began work in March 1975. It produced bulletins and pamphlets
on planning, mentally handicapped children and school leavers, short-term

care and day services. It presented a report to the Secretary of State in 1978,[21] from which chapters 5 and 6 were reproduced in 1979.[22]

The Development Team

This team, under the directorship of Dr G.B. Simon, was set up in 1976 and took over all the functions previously performed by the Hospital Advisory Service in respect of mentally handicapped children in England. The Team visited hospitals and compiled reports. The Community Team and Community Unit were envisaged as essentials of a local service to a sector of population with 80 000 to 100 000 people. Community Mental Handicap Teams, later called Community Learning Disability Teams, with a core membership of nurse and social worker, were gradually introduced.

'Right from the Start'

This was a report produced by the National Society for Mentally Handicapped Children in 1975.[23] This advised early intervention and comprehensive programmes for every young mentally handicapped child. An average health district of 200 000 would have 50 children each year born with congenital malformations recognizable at birth, and a further 32 a year having an abnormality detectable in the first 7 years of life.

The Jay Recommendations

The Report of the Committee of Inquiry into Mental Handicap Nursing and Care was published in March 1979.[24] It recommended a doubling of care staff in mental health and that they should be part of the residential care service, not the nursing service. It was recommended that training should be supervised, not by Nursing Councils, but by the Central Council for Education and Training of Social Workers. Care should be in small group homes.

The 1980s

Care in the Community

The Department of Health and Social Security published a Green Paper in July 1981.[25] The policy became operational in 1982. Hospital Managements began to move patients into accommodation in the community. Some reprovided NHS facilities were created but most people discharged went to the independent sector. Small group homes for four or five residents were a favoured style of care.

The Restructuring of the NHS

In April 1982, the NHS was restructured, establishing District Health Authorities as Area Health Authorities disappeared. Districts became responsible for their own NHS mental handicap provision. The use of the term 'educationally subnormal' (ESN), which had included mild and severe handicaps, was discontinued in 1981.

Enfranchisement
In 1983, Circular HC(83)14 clarified the law on the enfranchisement of patients living in psychiatric hospitals. Patients with learning disabilities who were not detained could apply to be put on the electoral register. This enabled them to vote in elections.[26]

Consultant Staffing
The consultant staffing of the mental handicap hospital service became seriously depleted in many districts as consultants retired. In 1983 the Royal College of Psychiatrists recommended one consultant in mental handicap to 200 000 of the population and a 'key' worker to each family. The college recognized three modes of consultant posts: first, the whole time post; second, joint posts, 50% in mental handicap; and third, joint posts with two to four sessions in mental handicap.[27]

Community Care Strategy
The strategic objective was to provide comprehensive community-orientated district-based services where these did not exist or were inadequate and by so doing replace the services currently provided by the mental handicap hospitals, leading to their eventual closure.[28] In 1985, general managers were introduced into the NHS. The running down and closing of hospitals, and the sale of their sites, usually for housing, began to appear on their agendas. The Second Report from the Social Services Committee, published on 30 January, 1985, stated that 'any fool can close a long-stay hospital; it takes more time and trouble to do it properly and compassionately'.[29] The prolonged uncertainties before an inevitable closure could adversely affect the morale of parents, relatives, patients and staff. Darenth Park Hospital, which dated from 1878 and had served almost half of the South East Thames Region, was closed under the Darenth Park Project, reported in 1985,[30] as the earliest attempt by a regional health authority to close completely a large mental handicap hospital.

RESCARE
Many parents and relatives of mentally handicapped people in hospitals were concerned about the policy of community care, on which they felt they were not consulted. The National Society for Mentally Handicapped People in Residential Care (RESCARE) was formed in November 1984. This resulted from the initiative of Richard Jackson, Chairman, and the committee of the Parents/Relatives and Residents Welfare Society of Cranage Hall Hospital, Cheshire. RESCARE wanted to see village-style communities. Dr G.C. Kanjilal, RESCARE's medical advisor, published a critique on trends in the service.[31]

In 1985 Dr E.D. Acheson, Chief Medical Officer of the Department of Health and Social Security, expressed concern about 'that over-used word, community'. Community care was the provision of alternatives to long-term institutional care for those with long-term disabilities. Most observers agreed that there was a minority of patients for whom an adapted institutional environment had value.[32]

Service Developments

At hospital and community day centres activities broadened from industrial-type tasks to social education, rehabilitation, leisure and recreation. Occupational therapists ran sessions in cookery, self-esteem, art, music and drama; physiotherapists advised on wheelchairs, moulded seat inserts (MSI), hoists, aids to mobility and rebound therapy using trampolines; trainees went horse riding, canoeing and rock climbing. Aromatherapy and multisensory rooms with soft and soothing lights and sounds, the Snoezelen (from Dutch, for 'to sniff and doze') were introduced. In 1986 the Department of Health and Social Security issued a circular giving guidance to doctors on atlanto–axial instability in Down's syndrome; it was estimated to affect 2–3% of people with Down's syndrome.[33] Clinical psychologists held behaviour clinics. Speech therapists and dieticians advised carers in hospital and community. Dieticians used more intragastric feeding. Multiprofessional reviews of residents' progress took place, often annually, to prepare Individual Care Plans (ICPs) or Individual Programme Plans (IPPs). From the mid-1980s children with learning disability were no longer admitted for long-stay care in mental handicap hospitals.[34]

The Post-Hospital Culture

Health Care

As the traditional hospitals for mental handicap were closing, new patterns of services developed. Health Service Guidelines[35] advised 'purchasers' (health authorities) that some people with learning disabilities could need specialist assessment and treatment services in hospital, and that there was a small number of people with severe or profound learning disabilities, and physical, sensory or psychiatric conditions, who needed long-term residential care in health settings. Such NHS provision would often be 'core' or 'resource' units, and NHS group homes, and would offer assessment and treatment, short-stay care, outreach, and day services. Professional staff developed a supportive advisory and consultational role to parents, other carers, family doctors, residential and day services.

Social Care

From April 1993, local social services departments had new responsibilities for assessing people's need for social care. Social services had a unified budget for residential and nonresidential care, which would allow them to offer appropriate care to meet assessed needs. People previously admitted to residential homes had rights preserved and continued to receive funding from the social services budget. Many mental handicap hospitals were deliberately closed by 31 March, 1993, before the change in funding was applied. The number of people living in hospitals dropped from over 45 000 in 1979 to 16 000 in 1993. Social services residential places increased from 4200 in 1961 to over 11 000 in 1979, and over 15 000 in 1993 with over 24 000 people living in residential facilities provided by private and voluntary agencies.

Some health authorities as 'purchasers' used 'market testing' to obtain residential 'social care' for hospital residents by advertising for bids from caring agencies in the independent sector. NHS Trusts remained responsible for people with learning disability deemed to need 'health care'. Some authorities used a 'dowry' system which gave carers a lump sum of money. A Canadian approach, 'service brokerage', involved people with learning disability choosing and purchasing their own care. 'Voucher' systems were suggested which would enable people with learning disability or their families to buy care. For people with learning disability who could not live at home, a widening range of accommodation opened, largely in the independent sector, with some offering specialist, but expensive, services.

Further Education
In April 1993, under the Further and Higher Education Act 1992, colleges of further education became independent of local authority control, and funded by the Further Education Funding Council. A three year committee of review was formed to advise on provision for people with learning disability.

Medical Developments – Discovery and Diagnosis

The clinical study of mental retardation is usually dated from the description of mongolism, later called Down's syndrome, by J.H. Langdon Down in 1866.[36] In the 100 years that followed many more conditions in which mental retardation was associated with characteristic patterns of physical abnormalities and neuropathological findings were reported, for instance, Laurence–Moon–Bardet–Biedl syndrome (1866, retinitis pigmentosa), microcephaly (1875), Sturge–Weber syndrome (1879, facial port wine stain), tuberous sclerosis (1880, epiloia), neurofibromatosis (1882, von Recklinghausen's disease), Cornelia de Lange syndrome (1933, Amsterdam dwarfism), Prader–Willi syndrome (1956, obesity), Rubinstein–Taybi syndrome (1963, large first toes and thumbs).

Conditions were discovered as a result of astute clinical observation, serendipity, and, in later years, from the use of screening tests for biochemical, chromosomal, and dermatoglyphic anomalies. A battery of tests could be applied to a sample of patients, or one test, for example, screening urine by amino acid chromatography, applied to a large number such as a hospital population. Occasionally a condition has been discovered by two groups of workers virtually simultaneously.

In some conditions, for instance the XYY syndrome (1961), no specific clinical features have been identified. Sometimes, when a new biochemical or chromosomal abnormality was found, it was necessary to re-examine cases for any somatic features that could be correlated with the new disorder. Progress has depended on the discovery and elaboration of new techniques, for instance, nuclear sexing and human chromosomal analysis. In the 1950s and 1960s, discoveries in genetics, chromosomes and inborn errors of metabolism explained some known disorders such as

Down's syndrome, phenylketonuria (1933), Turner's syndrome (1938), Klinefelter's syndrome (1942), and revealed many other specific causes of mental retardation. Diagnosis led to the introduction of population screening programmes (phenylketonuria), prenatal detection (amniocentesis), dietary treatments (inborn errors), and prevention. More recently the fragile-X, or Martin–Bell–Renpenning, syndrome, typically a triad of sex-linked mental retardation (IQ 35–50), elongated faces and large everted ears, and macro-orchidism, in 60% of cases, has emerged as possibly the commonest cause of mental retardation, affecting one in 600 males and accounting for 20–30% of all mental retardation. In general, no clear relationships between a syndrome and intelligence level or personality type have been elucidated, only generalizations are possible.

Wahlström[37] published a gene map in 1990 based on a compilation of genetic disorders involved in mental retardation. This paper described 69 genes assigned to an autosome, 73 genes assigned to the X chromosome, and genetic disorders without any known chromosomal location. The map is testimony to the extensive advances in human genetics that aid the diagnosis and prevention of conditions associated with learning disability.

Psychological Developments

IQ

The WHO's classification of mental and behavioural disorders[38] includes categories of mental retardation, mild, moderate, severe and profound, to which are assigned ranges of intelligence quotients. The IQ is the mental age divided by the chronological age and multiplied by 100. Limitations on the value of IQ tests were recognized in the 1950s. IQ and social behaviour do not perfectly relate. The same IQ on different tests do not mean the same. The IQ is not always constant and cannot be taken as the sole criterion of mental retardation. IQ was attractive because it was measured by standardized tests that were apparently scientific and reproducible. The IQ tended to correlate with an individual's adaptive capabilities.

Clarke pointed out that a considerable degree of intellectual subnormality, measured on reputable and appropriate intelligence tests, should be a *sine qua non* of certification as a mental defective,[40] a view advanced by the Joint Committee of the WHO in 1954.[39] Clarke and Clarke[40] considered subnormality was primarily an administrative concept for the purpose of social action. IQ below 70, social incompetence, and educational retardation could occur in many conditions other than mental retardation. In combination, these criteria were highly intercorrelated in the small section of the population with IQ below 50, and above this level, suggested a need for short- or long-term special help for the individual. In clinical practice from the 1970s many psychologists ceased to apply intelligence tests. Other professionals in learning disability began to pay less attention to IQ scores. IQ continued to be justifiably determined for reports to courts, for legal purposes, and for categorization under the Mental Health Act.

Rehabilitation
H.C. Gunzburg, Consultant Psychologist and Director of Psychology
Services, Monyhull Hospital, Birmingham, UK, wrote a book on the *Social
Rehabilitation of the Subnormal* in 1960.[41] This was a landmark in its field.
He devised a series of progress assessment charts (PACs) used in Britain
and many parts of the world. The charts gave a comparison on functioning
and progress in four main areas of personal development, self-help,
communication, occupation, socialization. The charts comprised a series
of questions, the answers to which could be marked in different colours
on the record forms. He wrote with Anna Gunzburg about environmental design, preceding a growing concern about the importance of
the physical environment in shaping social learning and behaviour.
Gunzburg also completed the book *Subnormal Personalities* in 1961,[42]
after the untimely death of its author, C.J.C. Earl. Its original and pioneering approach investigated personalities by considering nine different
aspects. These were under the headings: Weakness, Simplicity, Immaturity,
Instability, Schizoidia, Viscosity, Neurosis and Reading Neurosis,
Psychopathy, and Psychosis.

Education
The Education (Handicapped Children) Act 1970 received the Royal
Assent on 23 July, 1970. It amended the Education Act 1944 so that
the education authorities became responsible for the education of children
who previously attended junior training centres in England and Wales
under the health authorities and also children living in hospital. After
the change no child was considered 'ineducable'. This acknowledged that
the learning process in mentally retarded children followed, in general,
the same basic natural patterns as in normal children. Many disabled
children needed physiotherapy, speech therapy and psychological
help. The Act was consistent with normalization in services for disabled
people.

Social Developments

Research
From 1948, thinking about mental handicap in the UK was influenced substantially by Jack Tizard and his colleagues at the Medical
Research Council Social Psychiatry Research Unit at London's Maudsley
Hospital. O'Connor and Tizard's *The Social Problem of Mental Deficiency*[43]
influenced the 1954–57 Royal Commission. Tizard and Grad prompted
thought about keeping mentally handicapped children in their own
homes.[44] Tizard later reported four studies – a study of the prevalence
of mental handicap in London and in Middlesex, a study of family
problems, and a study of ESN children and the 'Brooklands Experiment'
which showed how 16 imbecile children taken from the Fountain Hospital
into small group nursery care at Reigate improved in language and
intelligence.[45]

Responsibilities

Russell Barton[46] postulated that institutions had adverse effects on the people who lived in them; Goffman raised similar issues in 1961.[47] An initiative in advocating ordinary environments as a major factor in alleviating and even eradicating to some extent the problems of mental handicap was taken in 1962 by President Kennedy's Panel in the USA[48] which proposed a programme for national action. The Panel stated that it was society's special responsibility to persons 'with extraordinary needs' first to 'permit and actively foster the development of their maximum capacity', and second, 'to provide some accommodation or adjustment in our society for those disabilities which cannot be overcome'. It was conceded that placement in the community would not by itself be enough automatically to encourage mental and social growth.

Rights

In October 1968, a Declaration of Rights of the Mentally Retarded was made at the Congress of the International League of Societies for the Mentally Handicapped in Jerusalem. On 20 December, 1971, at its 2027 Plenary Session, the United Nations Assembly adopted a Declaration of the Rights of Mentally Retarded Persons comprising seven articles. In essence, the retarded person had the same rights as other citizens to medical care, education, work, economic security, normal family life, a qualified guardian and protection under the law.

Normalization

In the early 1970s Nirje,[49] Bank-Mikkelsen[50] and Grunewald[51] in Scandinavia, and later Wolfensberger[52] in Canada and the USA, focused attention on the benefits of 'deinstitutionalization'. 'Normalization', defined in the *Shorter Oxford English Dictionary* as 'the action or process of making normal', in relation to mental handicap was generally regarded in the UK as a concept from Scandinavia which many professionals visited on study tours in the early 1970s. They saw normalization in Denmark, 'to let the mentally handicapped obtain an existence as close as possible to the normal' (Bank-Mikkelsen)[50] and in Sweden, 'to make available to the mentally handicapped patterns and conditions of living which are as close as possible to those in the mainstream of the general community around the mentally handicapped' (Grunewald).[51] 'Integration' was a means to normalization which was a 'striving towards the normal'. In practice, the essentials were a bisexual world, small-group living, a normal day routine, work in a different environment from the living environment and staff without uniforms. The developmental principle assumed that mentally retarded people were capable of growth and development in general skills. Goals became an ordinary life with rights and choices and care in the least restrictive environment.

Social Role Valorization

In 1983, an American psychologist, Wolfensberger, who had worked in the MRC Social Psychology unit at the Maudsley Hospital, London, from 1962 to 1963, proposed 'Social Role Valorisation' as a new term for the Principle of Normalization.[52] The goal of social role valorization was the enhancement of the social role of individuals or groups at risk of social devaluation. Such a goal could be achieved only through an improvement in their social image and their social competence.

Citizen Advocacy
The idea of citizen advocacy for people with learning disability originated in 1970 with Wolfensberger and the 'Association for Retarded Citizens' in Lincoln, Nebraska, USA. It spread to Canada, Australia, Scandinavia and Britain, where it was introduced into urban areas, often with funding from local authorities. Citizen advocacy is a partnership between two people. The advocates work on their partners' behalf, representing their interests and wishes, working together to enable them to make choices and decisions that affect their lives.

The Separation of Mental Retardation from Mental Illness

Legal and Administrative Developments

In the last 100 years, by a curious quirk of history, mental health legislation has been revised at intervals of 23 years, or 2 × 23 years, in 1890, 1913, 1959 and 1982–83.

The Lunacy Act 1890

The Lunacy Act 1890, section 341, stated that 'lunatic' meant an idiot or person of unsound mind. No special distinction was made between the two states. In 1904 a British Royal Commission on the care and control of the feeble-minded was set up. It reported in 1908, giving an estimated incidence of mental defect of 4.6 per 1000.[53] Its main recommendations were embodied in the Mental Deficiency Act of 1913.[54]

The Mental Deficiency Act 1913

This Act repealed the Idiots Act 1886 which provided for the control of idiots and imbeciles only.[55] It defined mental defectiveness as a condition of arrested or incomplete development of mind existing from birth or from an early age. The Act defined subsections. *Idiots* were persons so deeply defective as to be unable to guard themselves from common physical dangers, a social criterion. *Imbeciles* were incapable of managing themselves or their affairs, or, in the case of children, of being taught to do so – an educational criterion. The *feebleminded* (or morons) needed care, supervision and control, for their own protection or for the protection of others, or, in the case of children, they appeared to be permanently incapable of receiving proper benefit from the instruction in ordinary schools. The

Education (Miscellaneous Provisions) Act 1948, Section 11, amended this to, in the case of children, involves disability of mind of such a nature and extent as to make them, for the purposes of Section 57 of the Education Act 1944, incapable of receiving education at school. *Moral imbeciles* were persons who from an early age displayed some permanent defect coupled with strong vicious or criminal propensities on which punishment had little or no deterrent effect. Bradford claimed to be the first municipality to take advantage of the Act when it opened Ashfield House in 1917 as a residence for 36 mentally defective boys.

Amendment of the Mental Deficiency Act 1927

After the occurrence of epidemic encephalitis, of which 5039 cases were notified in England and Wales in 1924, the 1913 Act was amended in 1927 to 'a condition of arrested or incomplete development of mind existing from the age of 18 years whether arising from inherent causes or induced by disease or injury'. The 1927 Act replaced 'moral imbecile' with 'moral defective'. Institutions for the mentally ill were separated from the mentally defective which later became mental handicap hospitals.

The Wood Report

The report of the 1924 Joint Committee of the Board of Education and the Board of Control, the Sir Charles Wood Report, 1929, defined a mentally defective individual as one who by reason of incomplete mental development, was incapable of independent social adaptation – a social criterion.[56] E.O. Lewis carried out a survey of the incidence of mental defect in six districts in England and Wales, two rural, two urban, two mixed, with a total population of 622 880; 8.57 persons per 1000 were found to be mentally defective, idiot, imbecile and feeble-minded, roughly in the ratio 5:20:75. The figure was nearly twice the 1908 estimate. The report recommended that the institution should no longer be a stagnant pool, but a flowing lake, always taking in and always sending out. The Committee drew attention to 10% of families in the population who were allegedly socially incompetent. The feeble-minded originated from this lowest social group.

The Royal Commission, 1954–57

After 40 years, mental deficiency legislation began to cause unease. The criteria of mental deficiency and its grades were hard to apply precisely. The definitions were not scientific. In 1954 the Royal Commission on the law relating to Mental Illness and Mental Deficiency was appointed and received written and verbal evidence on 31 days from 1954–57.[57] The Royal Commission advised a reorientation of the mental health services towards community care and away from hospital care except where the special facilities of the hospital were needed. The clinical differences between mental illness and mental deficiency were well established, but at the time it was considered that they be treated administratively as one set of problems.

The Mental Health Act 1959

The Mental Health Act 1959 replaced the Lunacy and Mental Treatment Acts of 1890 and 1930 and the Mental Deficiency Acts, 1913–38, and made fresh provision with respect to the treatment and care of mentally disordered persons. The Act received the royal assent on 29 July, 1959.[58] The Act introduced the expressions 'Severe Subnormality' and 'Subnormality' used in the detention of the patients under the Act. At the same time 'Mental Subnormality' or simply 'Subnormality' came into use for what had been previously called Mental Deficiency. This usage was open to confusion. 'Subnormal' could also carry the connotation of subhuman, although the term 'educationally subnormal' (ESN) was in use over many years for school children with intelligence below normal.

Section 4 of the Act stated in paragraph (2) that 'severe subnormality means a state of arrested or incomplete development of mind which includes subnormality of intelligence and is of such a nature or degree that the patient is incapable of living an independent life or of guarding himself against serious exploitation, or will be so incapable when of an age to do so'. Here, the criterion was one of social incapacity. In paragraph (3) 'Subnormality' means a state of arrested or incomplete development of mind (not amounting to severe subnormality) which includes subnormality of intelligence and is of a nature or degree which requires, or is susceptible to, medical treatment or other special care or training of the patient. Here, treatment was a clinical criterion. In paragraph (4) 'Psychopathic Disorder' means a persistent disorder or disability of mind (whether or not including subnormality of intelligence) which results in abnormally aggressive or seriously irresponsible conduct on the part of the patient and requires or is susceptible to medical treatment.

The Mental Health Act 1983

This Act aimed to consolidate the law relating to mentally disordered persons.[59] It introduced the term 'mental impairment' for use within the meaning of the Act. This was a purely legal expression and was not intended to replace mental handicap as the overall name for the subject. In the Act, Section 1, paragraph (2) '*Severe Mental Impairment*' means a state of arrested or incomplete development of mind which includes severe impairment of intelligence and social functioning and is associated with abnormally aggressive or seriously irresponsible conduct on the part of the person concerned and severely mentally impaired shall be construed accordingly. The 1983 Act has taken the definition of psychopathic disorder in the 1959 Act ('abnormally aggressive or seriously irresponsible conduct') and applied it to both 'Severe Mental Impairment' and 'Mental Impairment', in addition to retaining it for 'Psychopathic Disorder'. The 1983 Act deleted the 1959 Act's reference to medical treatment.

Clinical Conditions

Dual/Multiple Diagnosis/Disability/Disorder
The Manual of the ICD-10[38] points out that mentally retarded individuals can experience the full range of mental disorders and the prevalence of other mental disorders (the ICD-10 classifies mental retardation itself as a mental disorder) is at least three to four times greater in this population than in the general population. Anxiety, phobias, obsessive–compulsive disorders, affective disorders, the schizophrenias, dementias, epilepsies and psychopathic disorder all occur alone or in combination with learning disability. Dual/Multiple Diagnosis/Disability/Disorder, the presence of mental illness, sometimes combined with drug or alcohol misuse, with learning disability, has always been a difficult area for diagnosis and research especially in 'nonverbal' patients with little or no speech. The features of mental illnesses in people with learning disability differ from those in patients of normal intellect. The association of dementia, and possibly depression, with Down's syndrome, has become well-known. People with learning disability may also present challenging behaviour which can coexist with mental disorders.

Challenging Behaviour
In the 1980s the term 'challenging behaviour' came into use. Emerson *et al.*[60] define challenging behaviour as behaviour of such an intensity, frequency or duration, that the physical safety of the person or others is placed in serious jeopardy, or behaviour which is likely seriously to limit or deny access to the use of ordinary community facilities. Challenging behaviour is not a transient phenomenon. Many people show such behaviour throughout their lives. Challenging behaviour includes physical assault upon others, the most frequent example, damage to the environment, self-injury, severe noncompliance, persistent screaming, pica, public masturbation, inappropriate sexual behaviour and recurrent vomiting. Emerson *et al.* reported that the ratio of people identified as presenting challenging behaviour to the general population is 1:116 000, mostly young adults, with 87% aged 15–35 years.

Classification (Nosology) in Mental Retardation

Classification Systems

Early Classifications

Early classifications in Mental Deficiency adopted traditional dichotomies such as 'endogenous' and 'exogenous', blaming nature or nurture. Ireland

(1877) called hereditary causes 'genetous'.[5] Shuttleworth (1895) used 'congenital' and 'noncongenital'.[5] Some people with mental retardation were found to have medical diagnoses of pathology to account for their conditions. In others with no such diagnoses the mental retardation was ascribed to natural, physiological and subcultural effects. There was statistical support for these two groups if the ability on intellectual tests in a human population is assumed to have a Gaussian 'normal' distribution. Lewis (1933) suggested 'pathological' and 'subcultural' – not exclusive terms.[5] There was statistical support for this if the ability on intelligence tests in a human population is assumed to have a Gaussian 'normal' distribution. Too many people have abilities more than three or four times the standard deviation (SD) below the mean to be fitted under a Gaussian curve. In typical long-stay mental handicap hospitals clinicians could make a certain diagnosis in only 50% or less of the patients; many had short stature and physical abnormalities but did not have any known syndromes. The discovery of the fragile-X syndrome showed that cases previously seen as 'subcultural' could have a specific cause.

The Heber Classification 1961

In 1964 the Ministry of Health decided on the introduction of a classification of diagnosis in mental subnormality. It adopted the classification produced by the American Association on Mental Deficiency (AAMD), the Heber classification.[61] This stated that mental retardation referred to subaverage general intellectual functioning which had originated before the age of 16 years and was associated with impairment in adaptive behaviour manifest as: (1) delayed maturation, (2) slowness in learning, and (3) social adjustment. The whole classification had three parts, clinical, behavioural and intellectual. The clinical section was introduced into hospital practice.

The ICD-8

In 1969, as a member state of the WHO, the UK Department of Health and Social Security agreed to use the International Classification of Diseases, Injuries and Cause of Death, for recording psychiatric diagnosis. Clinicians were asked to use the eighth revision of 1965, the ICD-8, for which a later glossary of mental disorders provided an explanatory background.[62] The glossary gave prime place to recording the degree of mental retardation, but also recorded aetiological factors by using a fourth digit subdivision. This glossary cited the definition of subnormal intellectual functioning in the England and Wales Mental Health Act 1959, Section 4.[58]

The ICD-8 categories of mental retardation were based on the Stanford–Binet Form L which had an SD of about 16 points. The categories were: borderline, IQ 68–85, 1 SD; mild, IQ 52–67, 2 SDs; moderate, IQ 36–51, 3 SDs; severe, IQ 20–35, 4 SDs; profound, IQ under 20, 5 SDs; and finally, unspecified mental retardation.

The fourth digit aetiological categories were:

0 Following infection and intoxication
1 Following trauma or physical agent
2 With disorders of metabolism, growth or nutrition
3 Associated with gross brain disease (postnatal)
4 Associated with diseases and conditions due to (unknown) prenatal influence
5 With chromosomal abnormality
6 Associated with prematurity
7 Following major psychiatric disorder
8 With psycho-social (environmental) deprivation
9 Other and unspecified.

At the time the ICD-8 classification was a useful clinical tool.[63]

The Revised AAMD Classification

In 1973 a revised *Manual of Terminology and Classification* was published, the sixth such publication since 1921.[64] It used the definition that mental retardation refers to significantly subaverage general intellectual functioning existing concurrently with deficits in adaptive behaviour and manifested during the developmental period. *'Significantly subaverage'* referred to performance which was more than 2 SDs from the mean or average of the tests (Heber's classification used 1 SD). This represented IQ 67 on the Stanford–Binet Test and IQ 69 on the Wechsler Test. The *'developmental period'* had an upper limit of 18 years. *'Adaptive behaviour'* was the effectiveness or degree with which the individual meets the standards of personal independence and social responsibility expected of his/her age and cultural group. These were reflected in the following areas: during infancy and childhood in (1) sensory motor skills development, (2) communication skills (including speech and language), (3) self-help skills, and (4) socialization (development of ability to interact with others); and during childhood and early adolescence in (5) application of basic academic skills in daily living activities, (6) application of appropriate reasoning and judgement in mastery of the environment, and (7) social skills (participation in group activities and inter-personal relationships); and during late adolescence and adult life in (8) vocational and social responsibilities and performances. By using 'concurrently' Grossman emphasized the importance of adaptive behaviour, IQ alone not being a sufficient criterion of mental retardation. In a sense he changed from the notion of cause and effect to one of the two converging factors operating at the same time. Adaptive behaviour became a separate and distinct dimension of mental retardation.

The ICD-9

In 1978 the ICD-9 was adopted in the NHS to replace the ICD-8.[65] This defined mental retardation as a condition of arrested or incomplete development of mind which is especially characterized by subnormality of intelligence. The classification of a patient was based on the individual's current level of functioning without regard to its nature or cause. The ICD-9 incorporated separate codes for impairment and handicap. The category 'borderline mental retardation' of the ICD-8, opposed by the WHO Expert Committee on Mental Health (1968),[66] was omitted from the ICD-9. People with borderline intelligence, amounting to 16% of the general population, were increasingly being perceived as within the normal range of variation of IQs from 70 to 130.

The ICD-9 incorporated the categories: 'mild mental retardation', IQ 50–70, equivalent to the 'subnormality' of the Mental Health Act 1959, and 'other specified mental retardation', equivalent to 'severe subnormality' in the Act. This was subdivided into: moderate (IQ 35–49), severe (IQ 20–34), and profound (IQ under 20) mental retardation. The IQs were based on a test with a mean of 100 and an SD of 15, such as the Wechsler scales.

The ICD-10

The ICD-10, 1992, was introduced into the NHS from April 1995 to replace the ICD-9. The ICD-10 has 60% more codes to provide greater detail than the ICD-9. It adopted an alphanumeric code, one letter followed by three numbers plus a possible further numeric subdivision. In the ICD-10 classification of mental and behavioural disorders[38] mental retardation is defined as a condition of arrested or incomplete development of the mind, which is especially characterized by impairment of skills manifested during the developmental period, which contribute to the overall level of intelligence, that is, cognitive, motor and social abilities. The ICD-10 diagnostic guidelines advise that IQ should be determined from standardized individually administered tests for which local cultural norms have been determined. Scales of social maturity and adaptation, locally standardized, should be completed if possible, by interview with a parent, relative or carer. The diagnosis should be based on the current level of functioning.

The DSM III

The *Diagnostic and Statistical Manual of Mental Disorders III-R* (DSM III-R), published in 1987, defined the criteria for the diagnosis of mental retardation as (a) significantly subaverage general intellectual functioning, (b) a significant deficit or impairment in adaptive functioning, and (c) onset before 18 years.[67]

The DSM-IV

The fourth edition of *The Diagnostic and Statistical Manual of Mental Disorders*, published in 1994,[68] states that the essential feature of mental retardation is significantly subaverage general intellectual functioning (Criterion A) that is accompanied by significant limitations in adaptive functioning in at least two of the following skill areas: communication, self-care, home living, social/interpersonal skills, use of community resources, self-direction, functional academic skills, work, leisure, health, and safety (Criterion B). The onset must occur before age 18 years (Criterion C).

General intellectual functioning is defined by the IQ assessed on one or more standardized individually administered intelligence tests, for example, the Wechsler Intelligence Scales for Children – Revised, Stanford–Binet, and Kaufman Assessment Battery for Children. *Significantly subaverage intellectual functioning* is defined as IQ of about 70 or below, approximately 2 SD below the mean. The DSM-IV manual acknowledges a measurement error of approximately five points in assessing IQ. Mental retardation could be diagnosed on this basis in people with IQ 70–75 who show significant deficits in their adaptive behaviour.

The American Association on Mental Retardation Classification

The classification system of the American Association on Mental Retardation (AAMR) 1992, includes the same three criteria as the DSM-IV, but instead of levels of severity, it specifies 'Patterns and Intensity of Support Needed', graded as 'Intermittent', 'Limited', 'Extensive', and 'Pervasive'. Table 2.1 compares the definitions and diagnostic classifications of various systems that have been introduced in the twentieth century.

Categories of Mental Retardation

The ICD-10, AAMD and DSM-IV classifications include the categories of mental retardation, mild, moderate, severe and profound. These form a continuum of recognizable groupings of people about whom generalizations are possible. These generalizations can extend to the range of support and help needed by people in the different categories. The DSM categories of severity: mild, moderate, severe, profound, are not directly comparable with the AAMR Classification, 1992, approach of 'Patterns and Intensity of Support Needed' (intermittent, limited, extensive, pervasive). Table 2.2 presents the categories of mental retardation with their characteristics and diagnostic features.

Multidimensional Initiatives – Converging Dimensions in Mental Retardation/Learning Disability

The ICD-10 classification of mental and behavioural disorders states that it has always dealt with mental retardation briefly, acknowledging that justice to this topic required a comprehensive, possibly multiaxial, system.[38] A multiprofessional working party, including co-opted members from various disciplines, was coordinated by the Royal College of Psychiatrists and proposed seven aspects or axes.[69] This work recognized

Table 2.1. A comparison of definitions and diagnostic classifications in mental retardation.

Instrument	Categorization	State of arrested or incomplete development of mind	Significantly subaverage general intellectual functioning	Impairment of adaptive functioning	Age limit	Abnormally aggressive or seriously irresponsible conduct
Mental Deficiency Acts 1913–38	Idiot, imbecile, feeble-minded	+	–	–	18 years	Moral imbecile/defective
Mental Health Act 1959	Subnormality, severe subnormality	+	Subnormality of intelligence	–	–	Psychopathic disorder susceptible to medical treatment
Heber classification (1964)	Borderline, mild, moderate, severe, profound	–	+	+	–	–
ICD-8 glossary 1968	Borderline, mild, moderate, severe, profound	–	Subnormality of intelligence	+	Originated before 16 years	–
Grossman revised AAMD classification (1973)	Borderline, mild, moderate, severe, profound	–	+	+	Manifested during the developmental period, upper limit 18 years	–
ICD-9 glossary (1978)	Mild, moderate, severe, profound	+	Subnormality of intelligence	–	–	–
Grossman revised AAMD classification (1983)	Mild, moderate, severe, profound	–	+	+	Developmental period conception to 18 years	–
Mental Health Act 1983	Mental impairment, severe mental impairment	+	–	–	–	Mental impairment, severe mental impairment, psycho-pathic disorder
DSM-III (1987)	Mild, moderate, severe, profound	–	+	+	Before 18 years	–
AAMR classification (1992)	Patterns and intensity of support needed: Intermittent, Limited, Extensive, Pervasive	–	+	+	Before 18 years	–
ICD-10 Manual (1992)	Mild, moderate, severe, profound	+	–	+	Developmental period	–
DSM-IV (1994)	Mild, moderate, severe, profound	–	+	+	Before age 18 years	–

Table 2.2 Categories of mental retardation/learning disability.

Categories	Mild	Moderate	Severe	Profound
% Of total population	1.2–1.5	0.3–0.5 (moderate and severe)		0.05
% Of people with mental retardation	75	20	3–4	1–2
IQ: Wechsler adult Intelligence scale	55–69	40–54	25–39	Below 25
Stanford–Binet	52–67	36–51	20–35	Below 20
Mental age	9 to under 12	6 to 9 years	3–6 year	Below 3 years
Former categories	'Educable'	'Trainable'	'Imbecile'	'Idiot'
Infancy, childhood	Should develop social self-help and communication skills. Minimal impairment in sensory-motor areas. Indistinguishable from normal children until a later age	Should acquire communication, self-help, motor skills and speech. Most are fully mobile, physically active. Able to join in social activities	Little or no speech. In school years may learn to talk and can be trained in self-care	Limited in use and understanding of language and in self-help skills. Many are immobile or have restricted mobility and are incontinent. May acquire simple visuo-spatial skills – sorting and matching

Adult years	Should be literate, able to work, maintain good social relationships. Contribute to society by doing practical unskilled or semi-skilled jobs. Majority are part of mainstream community. Work in open employment. Work skills centres or sheltered employment schemes. May marry and have own homes	Able to look after themselves. Do practical work under structured and sheltered conditions. Benefit from educational programmes. Travel independently. May live in minimally staffed group homes	Capable of simple tasks in sheltered conditions. May live in group homes with care staff	Need much or total help in daily living. May need specially adapted wheelchairs, physical aids to bathing, physiotherapy, massage, aromatherapy snoezelen. May be highly dependent needing accommodation to mobility standards with 24-h care.
Medical impairments	Emotional social immaturity, psychopathic traits, severe epilepsy, aggressive or violent propensities			Specific neurological conditions: cerebral palsy, ataxia, athetosis. One third or more have epilepsy, visual hearing impairments. Risks: infections, choking. Organic pathology of brain, and specific syndromes, often present
	Organic pathology infrequent			

that standard assessment and screening techniques covering all aspects of the lives of people with learning disability and their interactions with the environment could provide databases for professionals for resettlement and community care. The Education Act 1981, the Disabled Person's Act 1986 and, from April 1993, changes in the funding of residential care gave education and social services new statutory responsibilities to assess individuals' needs. The many disciplines involved in learning disability, nursing, psychology, and social work, have devised their own assessment methods and profile systems.

In March 1995 the Department of Health published a strategy document in the 'Health of the Nation' series.[70] This stated that learning disability meant a reduced ability to understand new and complex information, to learn new skills (impaired intelligence), and reduced ability to cope independently (impaired social functioning), which started before adulthood with a lasting effect on development. This amounts to a restatement of three cardinal points accepted as the *sine qua non* of learning disability. The document lists the health problems and disabilities which are common in people with learning disability. These points all represent measures of disabilities, their occurrences, range and degree varying with each person. Hence, they reflect a multidimensional appraisal of the person with learning disability. There are parallels between previous definitions and classifications, the multi-aspect model from the Royal College of Psychiatrists, and the practical issues presented in the Health of the Nation Strategy. Table 2.3 illustrates the inter-relations of the converging dimensions of various initiatives.

Evolution and Process in the Concept of Learning Disability

History shows that the concept of learning disability is not rigid, fixed or immutable, but is an evolving process, an interaction and an amalgam of numerous influences. The concept has components that are constants and variables. Constants are the occurrence and nature of learning disability as a biological phenomenon in human societies; variables are the reactions, attitudes and responses to it, the terminology used, the knowledge that is accumulating, the possibilities of treating and preventing conditions associated with it. Other constants are the everyday needs and rights of people with learning disability to have care, education, occupation, leisure, recreation, respect and appropriate help, and variables are the ways in which these needs are met. Constants are also the special needs of a significant minority of people with learning disability who have high dependency, behavioural disorders or mental illness, and the variables are the therapies for these people who need the time and expertise of professionals and specialized services. Variables determine that as the wisdom and convention of one generation are questioned and threatened they become virtually the opposite of the principles, practices, insights and ideologies of the next generation.

Table 2.3 Converging dimensions in mental retardation/learning disability.

WHO-ICD AAMR, DSM-IV, Mental Health Act 1983	Royal College of Psychiatrists multi-aspect assessment, seven aspects/axes	Health of the Nation: A strategy for people with learning disabilities, social/health issues	
Onset before age 18 years	Current life context: Family and living circumstances, services contracts	Self-care and home-making, making friends, holding a job, sport and leisure, practising religion, making choices	Key principles: Normalization Participation Integration Choice Advocacy Contribution Development Least-restrictive environment Disability etiquette
Significantly subaverage general intellectual functioning, IQ 70 or below	Intellectual: Level of general learning and reasoning ability	Education, training, employment, school, college, libraries	
Arrested or incomplete development of mind	Developmental: Developmental impairments of specific functions, e.g. language Physical illness: Possible causation, e.g. Down's syndrome	Communication, hearing, eyesight problems; orthopaedic problems, other problems of mobility Obesity, poor cardiovascular fitness, respiratory problems, epilepsy, dental care, congenital heart disease	Five key areas for priority and specific targets. 1. Coronary heart disease and strokes 2. Cancers: smoking, breast and cervical screening
Mental impairment: Associated with abnormally aggressive or seriously irresponsible conduct	Psychiatric and behaviour disorders: Depression, self-injury	Multidisciplinary skills. Care programme approach. Supervision Registers, Mental Health Act Guardianship. Aftercare. Dual disability	3. Mental illness
Significant deficit or impairment in adaptive functioning	Psychological factors: Family relationships, residential care Functional adaptation: Level of overall personal and social functioning in everyday life	Sex education, contraception, family planning, sexual abuse. Alcohol/drug abuse Information and counselling. Respite and shared care. Welfare rights advice. Family/citizen advocacy	4. HIV/AIDS and sexual health 5. Accidents. Atlanto-axial instability. Epilepsy drugs. Vision

Much in the field of learning disability awaits scientific evidence and a research base. Therefore, approaches tend to be empirical, experimental, expedient or cosmetic. As it finds its way this multifaceted specialism calls for a broad flexible eclectic ethos to solve the continuing problems learning disability presents. If preventable how far should it be prevented? How can people with learning disability have the best quality of life? Such issues depend inevitably on the resources a society is able and willing to make available. This will in turn reflect the society's concept of learning disability.

References

1. *The Shorter Oxford English Dictionary of Historical Principles*, Volume 1, 1987, Oxford: Clarendon Press.
2. Royal College of Psychiatrists (1995) *Section for the Psychiatry of Learning Disability Newsletter*, August. London: Royal College of Psychiatrists.
3. Tredgold RF & Soddy K (1963) *Tredgold's Textbook of Mental Deficiency*, 10th Edn. London: Baillière, Tindall and Cox.
4. Hilliard LT & Kirman BH (1965) *Mental Deficiency*, 2nd Edn. London: J & A Churchill.
5. Penrose LS (1972) *The Biology of Mental Defect*, 4th Edn. London: Sidgwick and Jackson.
6. James FE & Cooper MA (1989) *The Neuropsychiatry of Mental Handicap*. Birmingham: The British Society for Developmental Disabilities.
7. Waitman A & Conboy-Hill S (1992) *Psychotherapy and Mental Handicap*. London: Sage Publications.
8. Penrose LS (1963) *The Biology of Mental Defect*, 3rd Edn. London: Sidgwick and Jackson.
9. Clarke AM & Clarke ADB (1974) *Mental Deficiency – The Changing Outlook*, 3rd Edn. London: Methuen.
10. Itard JMG (1798) *The Wild Boy of Averyon*. (Translated by G & M Humphrey 1932). New York: The Century Co.
11. Ministry of Health (1952) Circular 5/52. *Short Term Care of Mental Defectives in Cases of Emergency*. London: HMSO.
12. National Health Service (1965) HM(65)104. *Improving the Effectiveness of the Hospital Service for the Mentally Subnormal*. London: HMSO.
13. Ministry of Health (1962) HM(62)29. *Voluntary Help in Hospitals*. London: HMSO.
14. Morris P (1969) *Put Away: A Sociological Study of Institutions for the Mentally Retarded*. London: Routledge & Kegan Paul.
15. National Health Service (1969) CMND 3975. *Report of the Committee of Inquiry into the Allegations of Ill-Treatment of Patients and Other Irregularities at the Ely Hospital, Cardiff*. London: HMSO.
16. Department of Health and Social Security/Welsh Office (1971) CMND 4683. *Better Services for the Mentally Handicapped*. London: HMSO.
17. Report of the Tripartite Committee (1972) *The Mental Health Service After Unification*. Tripartite Committee with authorization of the Royal College of Psychiatrists, the Society of Medical Officers of Health and The British Medical Association. London: British Medical Association (Journals Department).
18. Jones K (1975) *Opening the Door*. London: Routledge and Kegan Paul.
19. Department of Health and Social Security (1971) CMND 4557. *Report of the Farleigh Committee of Inquiry*. London: HMSO.
20. Department of Health and Social Security (1974) *Report of the Care of Patients at South Ockenden Hospital*. London: HMSO.
21. National Development Group for the Mentally Handicapped. (1978) *Helping Mentally Handicapped People in Hospital*. London: DHSS.
22. Creating a Learning Environment (1979) Chapters 5 & 6 of *Helping Mentally Handicapped People in Hospital* (DHSS 1978). London: DHSS.
23. Spain B & Wigley G (1975) 'Right from the Start'. A service for families with a young handicapped child. National Society for Mentally Handicapped Children.
24. CMND 7468 I & II (1979) *Report of the Committee of Enquiry into Mental Handicap Nursing and Care*. London: HMSO.

25. Care in the Community (1981) HC(81)9. *A Consultative Document on Moving Resources for Care in England*. London: DHSS.
26. DHSS (1983) Health Circular HC(83)14. *Voting in Elections – A Leaflet for Patients in Mental Handicap Hospitals. ER(MH)1*. Heywood, Lancashire: Health Publications Unit.
27. Royal College of Psychiatrists (1983) Mental Handicap Services – The Future. *Bulletin of the Royal College of Psychiatrists* **7**, 131–134.
28. Yorkshire Regional Health Authority (1984) *Outline Regional Strategy*, p. 13. Harrogate: Yorkshire Regional Health Authority Headquarters.
29. House of Commons, Second Report from the Social Services Committee, Session 1984–85 (30 January 1985) *Community Care with Special Reference to Adult Mentally Ill and Mentally Handicapped People*, Vol. 1, p. xxii, para. 40. London: HMSO.
30. Korman N & Glennerster H (1985) *Closing a Hospital, The Darenth Park Project. Occasional Papers on Social Administration*, No. 78. London: Bedford Square Press.
31. Community Care for the Mentally Handicapped: a Consultant Psychiatrist's Point of View (1986) *The British Society for the Study of Mental Subnormality* Newsletter, **12**, Nos. 1 & 2.
32. Acheson ED (1985) *Health Trends* Vol **17**(1), 3.
33. Acheson ED (1986) CMO(86)9. *Atlanto-axial Instability in People with Down's Syndrome*. London: DHSS.
34. Mental Health Division (1983) DA(83)2, HC(83), LAC(83). *Helping to Get Mentally Handicapped Children Out of Mental Handicap Hospitals*. London: DHSS.
35. NHS Management Executive (1992) HSG(92)42. *Health Services for People with Learning Disabilities (Mental Handicap)*. London: Department of Health.
36. Down JH Langdon (1866) Observations on the ethnic classification of idiots. *London Hospital Clinical Lectures and Reports* **3**, 259–262.
37. Wahlström J (1990) A gene map of mental retardation. *Journal of Mental Deficiency Research* **34**, 11–27.
38. World Health Organisation (1992) ICD-10 *The ICD-10 Classification of Mental and Behavioural Disorders: Clinical Descriptions and Diagnostic Guidelines*. Geneva: WHO.
39. World Health Organisation (1954) *Report of Expert Committee on the Mentally Subnormal Child*. Geneva: WHO.
40. Clarke AM & Clarke ADB (1974) *Mental Deficiency: The Changing Outlook*, 3rd Edn, p. 28. London: Methuen.
41. Gunzburg HC (1960) *Social Rehabilitation of the Subnormal*. London: Baillière, Tindall & Cox.
42. Earl CJC (1961) *Subnormal Personalities*. London: Baillière, Tindall and Cox.
43. O'Connor N & Tizard J (1956) *The Social Problem of Mental Deficiency*. London: Pergamon Press.
44. Tizard J & Grad JC (1961) *The Mentally Handicapped and their Families*. London: Oxford University Press.
45. Tizard J (1964) *Community Services for the Mentally Handicapped*. London: Oxford University Press.
46. Barton R (1959) *Institutional Neurosis*, 2nd Edn. Bristol: Wright.
47. Goffman E (1961) *Asylums*. New York: Anchor Books. (1971, London, Pelican Books.)
48. President's Panel on Mental Retardation (1962) *A Proposed Program for National Action to Combat Mental Retardation*. Washington, DC: Government Printing Office.
49. Nirje B (1969) The normalisation principle and its human management implications. In Kugel RB and Wolfensberger W (eds) *Changing Patterns in Residential Services for the Mentally Retarded*, pp. 181–194. Washington, DC: President's Committee on Mental Retardation.
50. Bank-Mikkelsen N (1969) A metropolitan area in Denmark; Copenhagen. In Kugel RB and Wolfensberger W (eds) *Changing Patterns in Residential Services for the Mentally Retarded*, pp. 227–254: Washington, DC: President's Committee on Mental Retardation.
51. Grunewald K (1974) *The Mentally Retarded in Sweden*. Stockholm: The Swedish Institute.
52. Wolfensberger W (1983) Social role valorisation: a proposed new term for the principle of normalisation. *Mental Retardation* **21**, 234–239.
53. CMND 4202 (1908) *Report of the Royal Commission on the Care and Control of the Feebleminded*, Vols I–VIII. London: HMSO.
54. The Mental Deficiency Act, 1913. (3 x 4 Geo, 5, Ch. 28) 15 August 1913.
55. Greig JW & Gattie WH (1915) *Archbold's Lunacy and Mental Deficiency*, 5th Edn. London: Butterworth and Shaw & Sons.

56. Report of the Mental Deficiency Committee (1929) Wood Report Parts I–IV. London: HMSO.
57. Report of the Royal Commission on the Law Relating to Mental Illness and Mental Deficiency (1957) 1954–57 Cmnd. 169. London: HMSO.
58. Mental Health Act, 1959 (7 & 8 Eliz 2. Ch. 72). London: HMSO.
59. Mental Health Act, 1983 (Ch. 20). London: HMSO.
60. Emerson E, Cummings R, Barrett S, Hughes H, McCool C, & Toogood A (1988) Challenging behaviour and community services. 2. Who are the people who challenge services? *Mental Handicap* **16**, 16–19.
61. Heber R (1961) A Manual on Terminology and Classification in Mental Retardation Monograph Supplement. *American Journal of Mental Deficiency*, 2nd Edn.
62. General Register Office, London (1968) Studies in Medical and Population Subjects, No. 22: *A Glossary of Mental Disorders*. London: HMSO.
63. Spencer DA (1974) The use of the WHO International Classification of Diseases (Mental Retardation) in a hospital for mentally handicapped. *British Journal of Psychiatry* **125**, 333–335.
64. Grossman HJ (1973) *Manual on Terminology and Classification in Mental Retardation*. American Association on Mental Deficiency. Special Publication No. 2.
65. WHO (1978) *Mental Disorders: Glossary and Guide to their Classification in Accordance with the Ninth Revision of the International Classification of Diseases*. Geneva: WHO.
66. WHO (1968) *Organisation of Services for the Mentally Retarded. Fifteenth Report of the WHO Expert Committee on Mental Health, WHO, Technical Report Series*, 392. Geneva: WHO.
67. American Psychiatric Association (1987) *Diagnostic and Statistical Manual of Mental Disorders (DSM-III-R)*. Washington DC: American Psychiatric Association.
68. American Psychiatric Association (1994) *Diagnostic and Statistical Manual of Mental Disorders*, 4th Edn. Washington DC: American Psychiatric Association.
69. Royal College of Psychiatrists (1991) A multi-aspect assessment for people with mental handicap. *Psychiatric Bulletin* **15**, 146.
70. Department of Health (1995) *The Health of the Nation, A Strategy for People with Learning Disabilities*. London: HMSO.

3

Communication and Learning Disability

Margaret Walker

Introduction

'Doctors and Lawyers have common responsibilities to ensure the protection of people who are incapable of deciding matters for themselves and to promote the choices for those who can and should regulate their own lives. The careful assessment of whether individuals have or lack capacity is essential to the protection of their rights. Effective communication both between professionals involved and with the person being assessed is vital'.[1]

This statement, although relating specifically to mental capacity can equally be applied to all interactions that health care professionals have with people with learning disability whether it be medical, educational, therapeutic or social.

Over many years, various studies have confirmed that a significant proportion of people with learning disability have severe communication difficulties. The exact figures vary according to the criteria set by different researchers.[2-4] It is generally agreed that the presence of learning disability makes people more vulnerable to communication problems and that the more severe the learning disability the more complex and limiting the communication difficulty.

The Communication Development of People with Learning Disabilities

It will be necessary first of all, to review the development of communication in children and adults without learning disability and then against this background to consider the precise communication difficulties of people with learning disability. It will also be essential to define the meanings of communication, nonverbal communication and language according to the manner in which they will be used in this discussion.

Communication is the transmission and reception of human messages which convey our thoughts, needs, feelings and events via any human modality, e.g. speech, writing, signing, use of symbols, body language, gestures, touch, facial expression, etc. Nonverbal communication will refer to all those elements described above which have no speech component. Language is the highest level of human communication in which our thoughts, needs, feelings and events are coded in a standardized lexicon/ vocabulary of words/signs/symbols. These are then used individually or combined, recombined and modified according to specific and precise grammatical and syntactic rules. Language provides an immense facility which can be used at all levels of communication, both concrete and abstract.

Human Communication

In Figure 3.1, the entire repertoire of communication skills is shown. By the age of 5 years, the average child will be a skilled user of most of these components, with the exception of reading and writing, which is normally mastered over the next two years at school (excluding the specific skills of sign language and symbol language use).

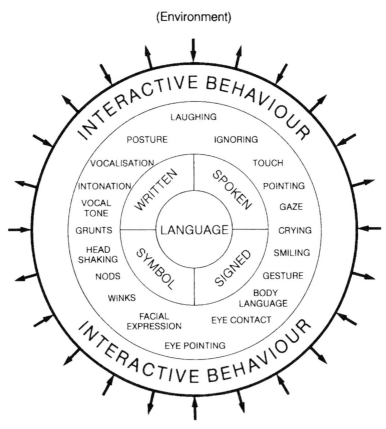

Figure 3.1. Human communication represented by four concentric circles; the innermost circle represents the individual's language ability, which is manifest through one or more of the four modalities in the next layer out. For interactive behaviour and effective communication to occur, a vast array of nonverbal techniques are employed which enhance and enrich the quality of the communication. Effective communication can be seen to comprise of language ability, a linguistic system, nonverbal skills, and motivation to communicate. Reproduced with permission of the Makaton Vocabulary Development Project.

Essential to this whole development is the motivation on the part of the individual to want to communicate with others and the availability of responsive communication partners in an environment who offer relevant and broad opportunities for interactive experience. Communication begins immediately after birth. There is now a large accumulation of literature supporting and providing detailed information on how the infant and mother communicate.[5] From birth, an infant and mother will engage in two-way reciprocal communication, where one initiates the communication, the other responds and so on. In the first few weeks after birth, these interactions revolve around the patterns of care during the baby's waking hours. Together, they use a variety of nonverbal behaviours. In addition, the mother uses speech, although the baby only recognizes it as vocalization at this early stage. Initially, the infant's cries will be purely reactive in response to physical comfort or discomfort states – hunger, tiredness, contentment. They do not carry any communication intent. As the mother gradually interprets these cries, attaching to them the baby's needs and responding consistently to them, she helps the young baby to associate a particular response on her part to its different cries. From about 4–6 weeks onwards, the baby slowly begins to associate these connected events and gradually over the next few months attaches intention to some of his communicative cries and nonverbal behaviours. In the first few weeks after birth, this shared communicative interaction occurs at very close physical proximity. The nonverbal behaviours used by both, involve a great deal of physical contact: touch, stroking, patting, cuddling, rocking; with vocalization, cooing, crying, intonation and gaze and eye contact.

Gradually, as the baby matures and his attention can be attracted and held when not in such close proximity with the mother, for example, when the baby is reclining in a baby chair or propped against cushions, then the mother spontaneously adds gestures to the range of nonverbal communication she uses and soon after the baby does the same. Gesture linked with vocalization now takes on a significant role in the communicative interaction between the two of them and the baby's enlarging social experience with others and events in the environment. The combination of gesture with vocalization appears to be a significant precursor to prespeech development.

During the second half of the baby's first year, the average baby masters many of the interactive behaviours which are part of the conversational dialogue, which he will use later when speech develops. Nonverbally he will be able to request, to indicate, to greet, to protest, to play anticipatory games, to understand simple statements, instructions and questions, e.g. 'where's daddy?', 'all gone!', 'do it again', 'give it to mummy'.

Studies have shown that between 8 and 12 months there are clear indications that the baby uses particular forms of gesture with different types of vocalization patterns to distinguish when he/she wishes to use an adult as a means to an object goal – 'I want. . . .' (protoimperative) – or the use of an object as a means of attracting an adult's attention – 'look at this. . . .' (protodeclarative).[6]

During the same period the baby is beginning to engage on a much broader basis with people and happenings in the environment. Not only is the young baby practising all the speech sounds in strings of babbling, but it is also producing a type of jargon speech with intonated speech patterns which resembles the phrasing and cadence of many of the familiar spoken utterances of the mother and other close family members.

Any time between 12 and 15 months, the average baby says his or her first recognizable word. Before this the baby will have shown that he has understood spoken words for at least 10–15 familiar objects and phrases that are frequently used, e.g. 'wave goodbye', 'where's the car?', etc.

The first words and phrases that the baby utters are always accompanied and supported by gesture and it appears that the need for these to be used in combination continues into early childhood. Mothers and workers with preschool children continue to use gesture spontaneously in combination with speech and to promote it through activities and rhymes, although the child is beginning to talk.

After the first words appear, others follow quickly and by 15 months the average child has an expressive vocabulary of approximately 20 words.[7,8]

The Development of Intention and Nonverbal Communication in People with Learning Disability

Studies of communication development in children with learning disability suggest that they follow the same sequence of development, but at a slower rate depending on the degree of disability.[9] Their behaviour in communication interactions may also be different in that they do not initiate as many or as often as the normal child.

Children and Adults with Profound Learning Disability

The degree of learning disability is crucial (reference to Figure 3.1 may be helpful). Some children and adults with profound learning disability and certain children and adults with autism, may lack either the motivation to communicate or an understanding of the purpose of the communication process. Their behaviour lacks communicative intent and most often the signals they give, which utilize many of the nonverbal components shown in Figure 3.1, often tend to be produced as a reaction to their personal physical needs for self-stimulation, e.g. rocking movements, or as a basic reaction to the effect another person or event has on them. It is often very difficult to identify the beginnings of intentional nonverbal communication in people with this degree of learning disability. Frequently, they will be multiply-handicapped, possibly having additional sensory and physical disabilities which further complicate the issue. As a result, their attempts to attract an interactor's attention and their responses to other people are often extremely delayed and laboured and may be difficult to identify as conventional nonverbal communicative behaviour. Their attempts frequently go unnoticed, which in turn leads them to lose motivation to try again. Carers and professionals are aware of this difficulty but strangers may not be. It is important that sufficient time is available to observe children and adults with these profound learning disabilities so as not to miss any attempts they make. Often, these occur during periods of routine care, when carers are busy. Even if there are only suggestions of an attempt or response, this will provide the signal that the person has the potential to develop some intentional nonverbal communication, although it may only be particular to the individual and limited in range.

Children and Adults with Severe Learning Disability

People with this degree of learning disability will have the capacity to understand the intention and purpose of communication. Within this group of people are a large number who will understand and use a variety of nonverbal behaviours with basic speech at one-, two- and three-word sentence levels. Many will be effective functional communicators although the level of their communication will be simple and concrete and some nonverbal behaviour could be idiosyncratic. In order to achieve effective functional communication they must be provided with the relevant social opportunities, stimulation and training. The amount they learn and the rate at which they progress will depend on the individual's degree of learning difficulties.

For some people, their development may be erratic and at certain times the person may appear to have reached a plateau which continues for a longer period than expected. When this occurs, it is necessary to investigate if there are other contributory factors which have gone undetected. For example, a hearing loss or unrewarding experiences in cases where the person's attempts have been ignored, or conversely where every need of the person is anticipated and met, thus reducing motivation to communicate.

Some people with severe learning disability may misuse or persist in using nonverbal communication inappropriately. For example, the person who uses nonspecific gestures/mannerisms may be attempting to engage another's attention without being able to communicate anything specific. Often a person with learning disability will do this as a form of interactive behaviour, but because of a lack of communication skills cannot develop the communication any further. Other people may exhibit nonspecific repetitive gestures/mannerisms when agitated, excited or bored.

An example of inappropriate use of nonverbal behaviour would be where an adult enthusiastically greets a visitor arriving at his Centre with either an enthusiastic hug or arm placed around the shoulders, instead of a conventional greeting. This is a clear indication that social skills training is required.

Children and Adults with Challenging Behaviours

Within the group of children and adults with severe learning disability, there will be a smaller proportion who display extremely challenging behaviours. Often, these tend to be negative behaviours with a high level of aggression and violence which may be directed by the person at themselves or at others or at the environment in general. Frequently, people with challenging behaviour lack an effective conventional communication system,[10,11] although it could be argued that their negative behaviour is extremely effective in that it achieves a particular personal goal. Their difficulties often reflect a lower level of understanding of other people's speech which may not have been appreciated. There are many causes for these challenging behaviours which are reviewed in depth elsewhere in this book.

Frequently, the establishment of an acceptable communication system is fundamental to their progress and an essential part of their remediation and rehabilitation.[12]

Additional Sensory Deficits

The serious effect of a sensory deficit on the development of communication for people with learning disability must not be overlooked. A hearing loss will exacerbate the learning difficulties with particular relevance to the development and monitoring of speech and language. Certain people with Down's syndrome and cerebral palsy will have a greater tendency to high frequency hearing losses. Anyone who has repeated respiratory tract infections whether treated with antibiotics or not should be monitored for possible undetected otitis media.

Visual deficits may restrict all forms of visual stimulation, the exploration of the environment and observation of others' communication behaviour which in turn could slow down development of communication.

Additional Physical Disability

The adverse effects from a dual disability such as severe physical and a learning disability will depend on the degree and type of impairment caused by the physical limitations. If the physical disability is specific, for example, affecting only the lower limbs with mild involvement of upper limbs, then all nonverbal components, speech and language will develop in proportion to the degree of the learning difficulties. If the physical impairment is severe, then nonverbal and probably verbal output will be seriously limited, especially if the physical disability affects the chest and speech muscles.

Expressive communication is often most seriously affected. The physically disabled person is very likely to be able to receive and process the communication of others, both nonverbal and verbal, and to develop a level of appropriate internalized language but owing to physical limitations may not be able to produce intelligible speech or signs/gestures. Unfortunately, many interactive partners often find it difficult to sustain natural conversation with people who are severely physically disabled and the interactors' communication may degrade in terms of quantity and quality unless a concerted effort is made to redress these difficulties, which results in the disabled person having limited opportunities for normal speech and language experiences.[13,14]

Communication devices such as computerized speech synthesizers, symbols boards and access switches to computers, are available and have been designed and personalized to provide an alternative form of communication output for people with severe physical disability. Whether a person with this dual disability can effectively operate these devices will depend on their overall level of ability and degree of physical impairment, coupled with their motivation level to participate in what can only be described as an effortful form of communication. Quite often, in common with some people with severe physical disability within the average range, those with learning disabilities tend to adopt a 'learned helplessness' role, unless positively supported and encouraged.

Autism

A severe communication and language impairment is one of the major diagnostic criteria for the identification of autism.

Coupled with this, are the findings that approximately 85% of people diagnosed as having severe autistic behaviours will have a learning disability, with about 50% being in the severe–profound range.

Mention was made earlier in this chapter about people with autism having a fundamental difficulty in understanding the purpose and function of communication. The severity of this problem will depend on the degree of autism. The range is from moderate in Asperberger's syndrome to profound. Those who do develop communication and language skills, often have difficulty interpreting nonverbal communication and will have a limited range of purposeful nonverbal behaviours though they may use many discreet personalized and ritualistic behaviours for self-stimulation and/or as a distraction/blocking device.

Children and Adults with Moderate and Mild Learning Disabilities

People with this level of learning disability will usually have a good understanding of communication intention and the whole communication process. They will also combine a wide range of nonverbal communication with spoken language and have the potential for becoming effective communicators. Their repertoire of language skills will be discussed in greater detail under the section concerned with language development.

Speech Development

The development of speech presents yet another challenge to the average child, let alone the child with the learning disability. Speech comprises a code of sounds, combined in specific ways and influenced by the position of a word or utterance. Children have to master rules of production, sequencing and performance which make demands on auditory perception, auditory memory, discrimination, imitation, sequencing and production skills.[15-17]

Speech sounds comprise consonants and vowels. In English, there are voiced and voiceless consonants. For example, the plosives (p) + (b) are made with exactly the same lip closure and release; for (p) the vocal cords in the larynx remain apart when air is expelled from the lungs, whereas for (b), the vocal cords are together and vibrate as the air passes through them. The same occurs for many other paired voiceless and voiced consonants (t) + (d), (c/k) + (g), (f) + (v), etc.

Vowel sounds are produced by air from the lungs passing through vibrating vocal cords and then through the mouth cavity which assumes specific shapes characteristic of different vowels, e.g. ee (i) and oo (u).

Speech sounds develop from early feeding patterns, the baby's vocalizations in comfort and discomfort states and then experimentation and expansion during the babbling periods. Numerous studies have confirmed a definite sequence in sound acquisition:[18] the significant period for speech sound acquisition and mastery in the average child is between $3^1/_2$ and $7^1/_2$ years.

There is a high incidence of speech or phonological disorders in children with learning disabilities, which is not surprising if mental age is equated with the ages of speech sound acquisition above. Statistics vary according to the particular disorders studied, but more complex problems appear to arise as the intellectual level falls.[9] Children who suffer brain damage may have articulatory dysarthria or dyspraxia and have more problems. Children with Down's syndrome have notably more speech disorders, but show considerable improvement after intervention and training,[15] as do many other children and adults with learning disability.

Often, the speech difficulties of people with Down's syndrome are assumed to result from differences in speech musculature, e.g. size of tongue/oral cavity. Although this is a popular view, there is no evidence suggesting that people with learning disability have larger tongues than those of the normal population. The tongue may appear larger because it sometimes protrudes but this is due to low motor tone not size.[15]

Voice Production

A person's voice, as heard by the listener, will have originated in the larynx when air under pressure from the lungs is passed through the vibrating vocal cords. The pitch or frequency of the note will have been achieved by tensing or relaxing the vocal cords and the volume adjusted by the force and amount of air expelled from the lungs. From the larynx the voice passes through the resonating cavities of the upper chest, nose and mouth. This enriches the original sound, giving the voice its characteristic quality. Speech sound patterns are applied with different types of pressure by the speech muscles so that the resulting vocalized speech has stress and intonation, which increases meaning. The majority of people with learning disability develop normal voices. Sometimes, help is required with voice production techniques for social interaction, e.g. correcting volume, intonation, etc., but essentially the vocal mechanism is normal.

Certain people with Down's syndrome have a characteristically deeper voice because of low motor tone affecting not only the vocal cords but also the tone in the resonating cavities. People with severe autism sometimes have unusually high-pitched voices, which lack intonation and are contextually and socially inappropriate. Often, people who are extremely nervous, anxious, disturbed or confused may reflect these states in their voice.

Fluency of Speech

The prevalence of stammering and disfluency in the general population is estimated as 1 in 100.[19] In considering the complex skills required to master speech sound and voice synchronization and the greater chance of brain damage or neurological conditions, e.g. epilepsy, in people with learning disability, it is surprising that the frequency of stammering is not noticeably greater than in the general population.

The Development of Spoken Language

Most readers will be familiar with the normal development of language which has been presented in depth in numerous studies. The scope of this chapter only allows a few to be mentioned.[20, 21] These describe and discuss the development of language in the child from the prelinguistic period through the emergence of first words, pivotal phrases to complex sentences.

The processing and production of language is dependent on a range of critical cognitive processes. These include attention, association, organization, recall or memory and generalization.

Attaching Meaning to Words

The child first has to collect a store of words to represent objects, people, places, events, etc. Meaning has to be attached to this vocabulary/lexicon. The storage of the vocabulary has to be flexible to allow for expansion and for some words to be discarded and replaced by others as new life experiences change from childhood to adulthood. Collective results of 23 studies of the lexical development in children with moderate learning disability, carried out between 1960 and 1987,[22] suggest that the majority of children with moderate learning difficulty, learn the meaning of words at the same mental age as normal children. At first, they appear to have the same size vocabulary, but their development becomes slower as the quantity and complexity of the lexicon increases. In certain cases the development is uneven.

There is a strong suggestion that people with severe–mild learning difficulties will go on acquiring vocabulary over a longer period of time, even into adulthood.[23] This may mean that with more normalized lifestyles, people with learning disability are more likely to achieve an average-size functional vocabulary equivalent to a non-learning disabled person. There appear to be some differences in the manner in which people with learning disability attach meanings to words. Findings from one particular study[24] suggest that concrete references were attached more often to word meanings by people with learning disability when compared with non-learning disabled.

It is appreciated that words related to abstract concepts, e.g. time, values, etc., will be more difficult for people with learning disabilities to understand. The person may use familiar expressions such as 'see you next week', but not fully understand the value of that period of time.

It is important not to assume that words related to unfamiliar routines or specialized functions cannot be understood completely and used appropriately by someone with a learning disability. Comprehension depends on the frequency and exposure that a child or adult has to the use of these words in a functional context. Crystal[25] describes a very young child who suffered frequent respiratory infections, who had a thoroughly good understanding of detailed vocabulary related to his respiratory condition and treatment. Adults with learning disability who work in specialized jobs, for example horticulture, may have a broad functioning understanding of specifically related vocabulary.

Cognition and Language Development

An efficient short-term memory facility is vital for language production/expression. In the process of speaking, as we utter the first word of a phrase, it goes into short-term memory, which services as a cueing device for the subsequent words we will string together in that utterance.

Attention is vital for all learning situations. In communication development a person needs to attend to become aware of communicative interaction. Associations are then formed between the word and the object, person, experience, event that it represents. It is also needed to monitor the different styles of language for comprehension and production. This information must be stored in long-term memory, in an easy to access organized manner: it is usually organized by category or 'chunked', to speed retrieval. When information is required, memory and recall come into play.

Generalization represents the ability to apply information stored to new novel situations and to combine previously stored information with new. This is a very important process in expanding communication skills.

Problems of Cognitive Processing in People with Learning Disability

It is thought that people with learning disability and non-learning disabled people go through the same stages of cognitive development.[24] There is a relationship between measured intelligence and the speed of information processing.[26] People with learning disability have slower short-term memory and slower retrieval of information from long-term memory.[27] This affects not only what can be retrieved, but also the availability of information for retrieval.[28] The differences tend to be qualitative and related to operational and processing deficits.

Attention

People with moderate to mild learning disability have poorer attention. They are more easily distracted and some may have poor scanning ability and find it difficult to focus attention. Their reaction time is often slower and they need a longer period for inspection.[29,30] By projection, we can therefore assume that people with severe learning difficulty will be proportionately less efficient. Findings from a variety of studies have confirmed that people with learning disability learn best through visual rather than auditory channels and that this is also the case for autistic people.[31–34] This has particular significance with reference to the development of spoken language. It also offers support for the current widespread use of signing and symbols with individuals who have communication and learning disabilities.

Organization

Sensory information has to be stored. Poor organization can overload the storage capacity of the brain.[35] Generally, people with learning difficulties have more problems in developing categorizing strategies. They use mediational strategies less, i.e. linking one symbol form to some other information to categorize it. If information is provided in pre-organized forms, this has been shown to aid recall and retrieval.[36,37]

Memory

Short-term memory is more limited and most adults with mild learning difficulties can hold fewer than 10 items simultaneously. Information can be retained effectively in long-term memory if pre-organized as suggested above. Organizational deficits may result in an over-reliance on rote memory.[38]

Visual memory has been found to be more effective than auditory memory in people with autism and learning disability in retaining and accessing information.

Generalization

People with learning disabilities find it easier to generalize information the greater the similarity of that information. The teaching of learning strategies to people with mild learning disability can enhance performance, but training must include specific practice in detecting similarities and differences as these are not easily apparent to many people with learning disability.

Operational Language

Language operates at three distinct levels.[39-41] These are:

- *Syntax*, which is the relationship between words (linguistic symbols). Rules of syntax establish the unique grammars of individual languages;
- *Semantics*, which is the relationship of meaning between words and the objects, people, events, experiences they represent;
- *Pragmatics*, which is concerned with the relationship between words and their interpretation; in other words, the rules governing the use of language in context.[7]

To give an example, consider this sentence and imagine the context is where a mother is entertaining a friend in the living room and her young children are playing in the adjoining hall. She calls out to them: 'I can hear you in the hall'. At a syntactic level this sentence is correct and appropriate. At a semantic level the meaning is expressed correctly, but had she said instead 'I you hear in hall', it would have still been semantically correct because the same meaning would have been conveyed. At the pragmatic level of operation, we would have had to know what the mother intended to convey. The same sentence 'I can hear you in the hall', could simply be a descriptive comment or if said with particular intonation and stress could be spoken as a warning/admonishment to the children letting them know that they are becoming noisy and are distracting her and her friend.

Children and adults with severe to mild learning disability understand the application of these relationships even at a simple more concrete level of language and can be very efficient communicators. In order to gain an understanding of the correct use of syntax and semantic relationships, formal training will be required.

An understanding of the pragmatic relationships can only be gained from having opportunities to socialize in normal, naturalistic settings and to be exposed to and offered opportunities to participate in conversational dialogue with non-learning disabled people. This is not the case with children and adults with severe autistic behaviour. They will have particular difficulty with the semantic and pragmatic functions of language. Studies of the 'Theory of Mind' have been applied to people with autism to account for their inability to relate to others. This helps to account for their lack of social empathy which makes them unaware of how other people may feel, think and act.[42,42]

There are characteristic problems in the speech and language used by autistic people. Their language proceeds to develop in a nonconversational way.[44] When they are gaining vocabulary they seem to collect nouns almost in an obsessive manner and not for functional use. Among those who do develop speech, there may be a variation of echolalia where the child/adult repeats exactly what is said to him or her or with a small variation. Self differentiation is a problem and this is demonstrated in their confusion over pronouns related to themselves and others. Frequently they use 'I' when they mean 'You'. Formulating questions is another area which is very difficult for them; often, they make a statement when a question should have been used. On the whole, people with severe autistic behaviours and severe learning disabilities have very poor conversational skills, which in turn limits social interaction.

At the upper end of the autistic spectrum will be specific syndromes such as Asperger's syndrome.[45] Whilst these children and adults have some of the specific language and communication problems associated with autism, which may be severely handicapping, usually they only have a mild learning difficulty.

Conversational Language

All too often the emphasis when measuring a person's communication skills, is on formal language use and understanding. While this produces valuable information about a person's ability to process and generate forms of language, it still gives us no idea about how the person copes in real-life interactions where there is less formal language usage. In ordinary everyday conversation, a much more relaxed and incomplete form of language is used which depends on the interactive partners having shared knowledge of the topic that is being discussed. Listening in to a typical conversation of two competent language users, one might hear for example:

A. *'Sorry I'm late, the traffic...'*
B. *'Dreadful, yes I know, I couldn't cross the road at the corner where they're building...'*
A. *'Oh yes! Those builders have no idea of the trouble they're causing with their lorries on the pavement.'*
B. *'Very difficult for pedestrians and old people.'*

There are some people with learning difficulty who may score fairly low results on a formal language assessment, yet their carers will report that they are very effective communicators. This may be because in a typical conversation like the one above, the demand to generate long syntactically correct phrases is reduced, the semantic rules are easier to apply and the intention is clearly shared, thus reducing the overall effort and cognitive load.

There are not many studies on the type and quality of conversational language used by people with learning difficulty. From the few there are, while many people cope effectively, it is suggested that in certain cases people with learning difficulty may not always perform quite as efficiently and at times may increase their own handicap. Accounts of the social inter-action of several people with mild learning difficulties, as reported by Kiernan and Sabsay,[46] illustrate that confusion may be created on the part of the person with the mild learning difficulty in the following ways: changing the topic midsentence, referring to people as he/she without defining them first and introducing irrelevant information in midflow. All these result in the person not making him/herself clear and being mis-understood. When the listener indicates that he or she is confused, this adds to the speaker's confusion.

Without any specific training, the average person without a learning disability seems to be able to adjust his style of language to suit situations where we are face-to-face with the listener or separated from them, as in a telephone call. The first situation involves speech supported with a variety of nonverbal communication behaviours and instant feedback from the listener; the latter requires the speaker to set the scene and define, and describe, the unseen. This is what seems difficult for the otherwise able communicator with mild learning difficulty.

Confidence and knowledge about the acceptable style of language to use to initiate conversations, to engage others' attention, to maintain a conver-sational topic once started, to state a different opinion from another's and to assert one's rights is essential for people with learning disabilities living in the community. Appropriate programmes are available which provide experiential training to teach these skills.

Training can also help modify behaviours which some people display during spoken conversation. These are the tendency some people with learning disabilities have to exaggerate their reactions or descriptions of events, in a manner which draws attention to themselves as being different. For example, overuse of nonverbal communication to the point of almost acting out events or descriptions of events, e.g. feigning shock, disap-pointment, alarm, sadness, etc. Possibly, these behaviours were initially encouraged to help the understanding of abstract concepts and have remained as part of the current communication style.

Written Language Development

When average children are taught to read and write they will already be competent communicators; they will understand a wide variety of conver-sational language styles and, from having stories read to them, they will have an idea about written word patterns representing the spoken word. Therefore, when they start learning to read, they will be acquiring another coding system with written language rules for the language they already use and understand.

There are many different styles of written language from extremely formal and abstract to functional writing where one writes exactly what one says. This is often encouraged, to capture the interest and motivation of young children learning to read and write and to help them understand the basic function of reading and writing.

People with moderate–mild learning disability often can read and write at a functional level. Recognition of social sight vocabularies of essential words providing important public and safety information is encouraged, e.g. push, pull, private, toilet, etc., and can be taught successfully to people with severe learning disabilities.

In the last 10 years, a significant breakthrough has occurred for people with learning disability who were unable to read. Symbol systems have been developed to provide a pictorial code for spoken and written language. Some of these systems are sufficiently sophisticated and developed to provide an equivalent in symbols to match the grammatical elements of English and other languages (see section below on Graphic Symbols).

Sign Language

Sign languages are visual languages with unique grammar and syntax which are completely different from spoken language. Sign language is the cultural language of prelingually deaf people and is a rich, living language, which, like speech, has evolved over centuries. New signs are generated constantly to cover new emerging life experiences and events, in the same way that new words are generated.

Sign language is not the same across the world. Each country has its own sign language reflecting unique cultural differences. In the UK, there is British Sign Language (BSL);[47] in France, French Sign Language (FSL) and so on. Although culturally different, there are strong similarities between the grammars of the different sign languages and it has been suggested that approximately 35% of signs may be the same or similar.[47] Sign language therefore is not a visual representation of spoken language which once was mistakenly thought to be the case. For example, the order in which signs are presented in a sentence when compared with the spoken version would be completely different. For some deaf children and adults for whom sign language may be their first language, they have to approach the learning of English as if it is a second language.

Sign Systems

Sign systems are artificial systems which have been devised by educators and others to provide a visual representation of spoken/written languages. They have been specifically created to assist deaf school children learn spoken/written English or other spoken/written languages. Sign systems are different in each country in which they have been developed: not all countries have sign systems. Most utilize relevant signs from the sign language with which the children will already be familiar and then sign markers are specifically devised for the unique grammatical elements of spoken/written language which are not present in sign language. Examples of sign systems used in the UK are the Paget–Gorman Sign System (PGSS)[48] which is mostly used for children with specific language disorders, and Signed English, which is used widely with deaf children in schools throughout the UK.

Graphic Symbols

Symbols are graphic representations of language incorporating logical strategies of varying sophistication to classify linguistic groups. For example, in the Makaton Symbol System symbols concerned with possession employ a circle, and all symbols concerned with quantity are contained within a triangle. Graphic symbol systems in common usage in the UK at present include Makaton symbols, Blissymbolics[49] and Learning with Rebus. Some symbols and symbol systems are more abstract in nature than others which have a more pictorial or manual sign reference incorporated into their design. This improves recognition and dovetails into other modalities of communication.[50–52] Symbols can offer people with severe physical and learning disability a primary method of communication to enable them to express their thoughts and needs (Figure 3.2). The use of symbols is by no means reserved for people with physical disability and they are in widespread use throughout Special Education, schools and the community as a whole. Makaton symbols are now used to provide public information for people with learning difficulties to enable more independent living (Figure 3.3) and also in more focused applications such as the teaching of national curriculum key stages in Special Schools.[53–56]

The advent of computer databases of symbols allows for flexible manipulation of this medium. The potential for using graphic symbols to develop prereading and literacy skills is also being recognized and widely developed. However, this is an area where practice is currently leading research.

It has been proposed that the iconicity of signs and symbols may explain why language acquisition is improved when taught through these means.[57,58] It is possible that existing comprehension is unmasked by the use of a more referential and less abstract mode of communication.

Clients who exhibit challenging behaviours frequently have extremely poor communication skills,[59] adding both to their distress and to the complexity of their management. Signs and symbols have been used to mediate behavioural training and to give greater insight into the client's mood and mood changes (Figure 3.4).[60–62]

Total Communication

Total communication has been increasingly used over the last 20 years to attempt to facilitate the teaching of language to children and adults with learning disability.[63] In essence, language is taught through a combination of media (signs/symbols/speech) which reinforce each other.[53,64,65] The choice and sequence of concepts taught is obviously very important in individuals whose retention and organization of information and speed of recall may be limited; for this reason, nuclear or core vocabularies were devised.

The most widely used core vocabulary in the UK and internationally is the Makaton Vocabulary[53,64] which comprises a small structured vocabulary of essential concepts for functional everyday needs and an open-ended Resource Vocabulary of over 7000 concepts to allow a high degree of personalization and breadth of usage. This contrasts strongly with many other alternative and augmentative language systems, such as PGSS, Blis-symbolics and Rebus. These systems provide an iconic language, but are not inherently structured in such a way that the cognitive processes in the acquisition and use of communication and language are facilitated.[31,32,36,37] More recently, variants of the Makaton Vocabulary have become available and it is interesting that these retain a very similar structure and utilize the same core vocabulary.

Communication and Mental State

'It has been estimated that of the 2–3 million people in the UK who have some form of speech and language disorder, 800 000 have severe disorders and are unable to speak or are intelligible only to their family and 1.5 million have moderate disorders, i.e. recognized impaired speech.'[66] 'The prevalence of speech and language difficulties in psychiatric problems is unclear'.[67]

The number of people with learning disability with a major psychiatric problem is extremely difficult to obtain because the problem is often blurred by the degree of the learning disability itself and by poorly developed or immature communication and social skills. Psychiatrists tend to agree that it is not possible to establish the presence of major psychiatric pathology, e.g. schizophrenia, in people with IQs below 40–45.[51]

History taking and the mental state examination depends on the patient's ability to convey his/her thoughts, feelings, mood and emotions, through a recognizable form of communication. Clearly, great flexibility and adaptation will be required in assessing the psychiatric history and mental state of people with learning disability. The use of open questions is recommended, e.g. 'when did you last feel well?' 'what can we do to help you?' so as not to influence the person's response. For someone with learning disability, this form of questioning would be too abstract and unfocused. A more direct style of questioning would be appropriate, although it carries the risk of leading the person's replies, e.g. 'are you feeling well?', 'do you sleep badly?', 'do you want us to help you?'.

Obtaining the family and personal history from the patient can be attempted with some people who have a sense and ability to relate past events, although the sequence may not always be correct and memory for more recent events may be better. Understanding of family relationships can vary: some people can clearly define family members, others are more confused. Despite this, the individual's perception of these relationships will be significant. Social history for recent past and current events may be good and provide a vehicle for discussion and assessment. Although

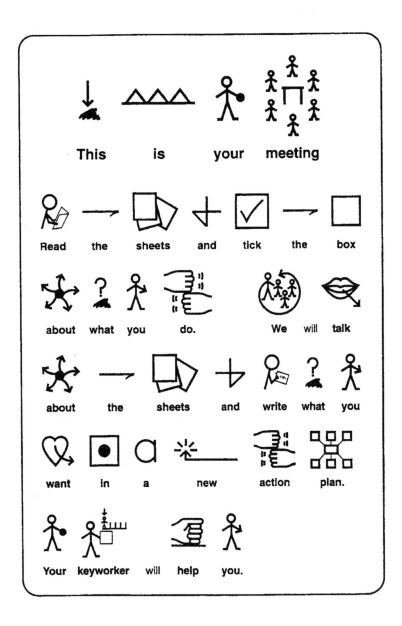

This is your meeting

Read the sheets and tick the box

about what you do. We will talk

about the sheets and write what you

want in a new action plan.

Your keyworker will help you.

Figure 3.2. Written and symbolled Individual Programme Plan (IPP) used by Lincolnshire County Council (Makaton symbols). Plans are constructed in consultation with clients whose views and wishes are discussed through any effective medium. Reproduced with permission of Lincoln County Council Social Services Directorate.

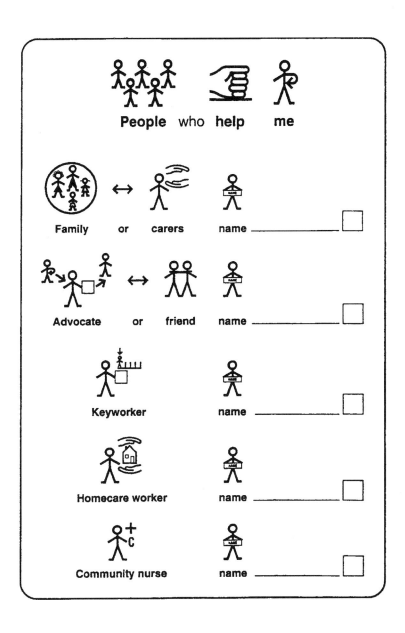

Figure 3.2. *Continued*

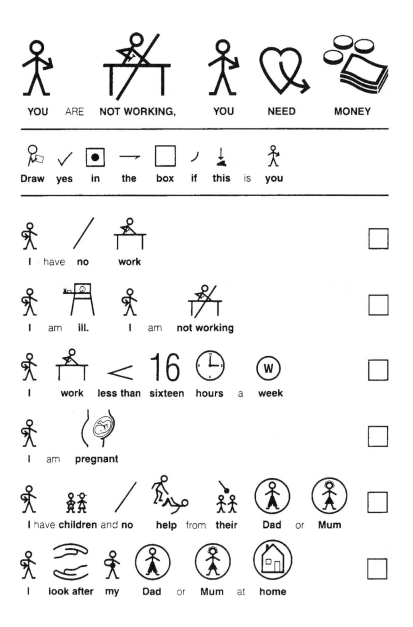

Figure 3.3. Written and symbolled Benefit Agency Leaflet (Makaton symbols). Public information in this form is essential if client independence and autonomy is to be achieved living in the community. Reproduced with permission of the Benefits Agency (BA).

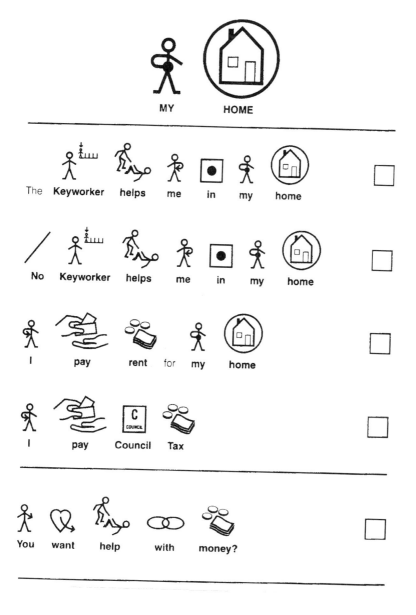

MY   HOME

The Keyworker helps me in my home

No Keyworker helps me in my home

I pay rent for my home

I pay Council Tax

You want help with money?

Figure 3.3. *Continued*

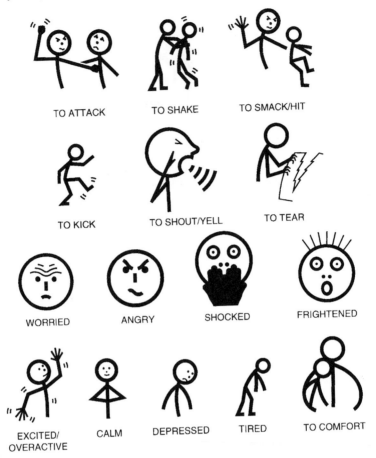

TO ATTACK   TO SHAKE   TO SMACK/HIT

TO KICK   TO SHOUT/YELL   TO TEAR

WORRIED   ANGRY   SHOCKED   FRIGHTENED

EXCITED/   CALM   DEPRESSED   TIRED   TO COMFORT
OVERACTIVE

Figure 3.4. Some examples of Makaton symbols representing feelings and emotions. The use of these symbols facilitates discussion, training and assessment of clients with challenging behaviour. Reproduced with permission of the Makaton Vocabulary Development Project.

premorbid personality and past medical history can be gained from other professionals' records and reports and from close informants, the individual's perception of these events may be disproportionate. Current mood may be fairly easy to assess at the interview, but what is more significant will be to discuss with close informants whether there have been noticeable changes in mood and behaviour.

The Mental State Examination will be similarly difficult to apply. Various parameters are routinely assessed – appearance and behaviour, including speech, mood, thought, illusions and hallucinations, obsessive–compulsive phenomena, cognitive assessment, insight and rapport. Clearly, assessment under these criteria will be difficult to apply and fraught with possible problems.

Those people with learning disability who present social conversational language, which habitually includes behaviour similar to derailment (changing topics in midflow), over-literal thought processes and atypical nonverbal behaviour, can make assessment of appearance and behaviour difficult. Special attention must be placed on discriminating between unusual behaviours which are usual for the client and new behaviours which, in themselves, are unusual for that person. This second group may result from organic pathology which cannot be adequately expressed to others, or may stem from a psychiatric problem, that is, pathology of thought. Since many non-drug-based therapies are inappropriate or impracticable for these individuals, prescribed psychotropic medication may itself cloud the nature of communication. Discussion with other professionals and psychiatrists experienced in learning disability can often help, as there does appear to be a qualitative difference between the way a person with severe psychiatric pathology displays these symptoms compared with a person with learning disability who uses this style of communication habitually.

Video-taped interviews would provide a reference library of individual idiosyncrasies; however, this is problematic with regard to patient consent and may distract from the purpose of the interview.

Psychiatrists work as part of a multidisciplinary team comprising other professionals with significant experience in learning disability (e.g. clinical psychologists, social workers, nurses, speech and language therapists). All members contribute their skills in the examination of the patient and share results of their assessments and findings in order to make a diagnosis and recommendations for treatment. Information from immediate family and carers is crucial at all stages of this process.

The difficulties of diagnosing mental health problems in people with learning disability and the need to gather information from different sources, i.e. professionals, care staff, families and the individual, has attracted the interest of researchers over recent years and, as a result, specifically designed assessment instruments, such as the Psychiatric Assessment Schedule for Adults with a Developmental Disability (PAS-ADD) have been developed by the Hester Adrian Research Centre.[68] This assessment instrument is a multilevel system consisting of three components: (1) a PAS-ADD, which comprises a semistructured clinical interview with respondents who have intellectual disability and for key informants; (2) the PAS-ADD check list, which is a psychiatric symptom checklist for use by direct care staff and families; and (3) the Mini PAS-ADD for use by staff who do not necessarily have a professional background in psychopathology, but who are in regular contact and can use this to recognize unfolding pathology.

The Communication and Behaviour of the Nondisabled Person

Communication clearly is a two-way process. The quality of interaction will depend as much on the interviewer as the interviewee. Factors that would improve interviewer performance are:

1. Use clear and appropriate level of language;
2. Pace, adjusting speed to allow for slow response by client;
3. Using concrete terms of reference to frame the questions;
4. Using augmentative communication as appropriate;
5. Monitoring one's own nonverbal behaviour so as not to send mixed messages.

Speech and language therapists make detailed assessments of individuals' communication skills and need. Some assessments have been standardized on a population of people with learning disability such as the Communication Assessment Profile (learning disabled adults),[69] the Bristol Scales for use with learning disabled children[4] and Tests for the Reception of Grammar.[70] Other assessments use normal individuals as a control population, e.g. Living Language[71] and the Derbyshire Language Scheme.[72] While these assessments allow a detailed breakdown of language skills into component parts clearly delineating areas of difficulty, communication of these results to other professionals is difficult because of the specialized nature of the information. A particular strength of the Derbyshire Language Scheme, which is widely used in the UK, is the description of language in terms of the number of information-carrying words that a person can either use or process. The significance of a one- or two-word level is that the individual is able to process one or two words embedded in a sentence, where those words carry the essential information. For example, if a client with a one-word level were asked to 'pass me a sandwich' when we were alone, and there were only sandwiches on the table, they would be likely to respond appropriately, as there is only one information-carrying word in the sentence (sandwich). Similarly, if the same request were made but both sandwiches and cake were on the table, there would still only be one information-carrying word (sandwich). However, if several people were sitting at the table and cake and sandwiches were available, the same request, to pass a sandwich, would have two information-carrying words (me, sandwich). This would be beyond the ability of a client with only one-word level understanding.

Clearly the complexity of any question is related to its content and context. This particular assessment is easy to assimilate and to apply to one's own communication and helps in the understanding of how at times people with learning difficulties appear to understand something in one situation but not in another.

Conclusion

Learning disability has a reciprocal relationship with communication: poor communicative ability exacerbates poor cognitive function, which in turn slows or prevents improvement in communication skills. However, it is at the communication skills level that this negative cycle can be broken most easily, and the degree of handicap from the underlying disability reduced.

Psychiatry of disability by necessity draws on a broad range of skills from a multidisciplinary team, and influences many aspects of the lives of learning disabled people. Effective communication with clients is essential in the diagnosis, assessment and management of learning disability. Because no two clients are alike, many of the accepted norms of behaviour and communication cannot be assumed to be constant. In effect, each case must be considered from first principles, weighing the impact of the disability and its attendant handicap on linguistic development as well as emotional, social and broader cognitive aspects of development.

Use of interventions at a communication level such as total communication language programmes are now widely accepted in their own right as having therapeutic benefits. The psychiatrist in learning disability must be aware of these interventions, and in some cases may need a working knowledge in order to communicate with and assess the individual effectively.

Despite some excellent attempts to adapt the mental state examination to make it more applicable in learning disability, inherent problems remain. It is difficult to devise a system with a very simplified interaction that yields subtle and reliable information. Communication strategies such as the use of concrete terms of reference, etc., can be employed to break down sophisticated questions into manageable components; in effect the answer will only be as good as the communication.

With the continuing changes in the way learning disability is provided for in the UK, community-based resources and government agencies are having to become aware of the particular communication needs of learning disabled people, and provide them with access to new communication media.[73]

Communication is central to daily living, adding richness and colour by facilitating interaction with others at every level of usage. Only by maximizing an individual's ability to communicate through any means that is available can we hope to minimize handicap and fulfil whatever potential exists.[74]

References

1. The British Medical Association and the Law Society (1995) *The Assessment of Mental Capacity: Guidance for Doctors and Lawyers*, December. London.
2. CMND 1971. *Better Services for the Mentally Handicapped*. London: HMSO.
3. DHSS (1979) *Development Team for Mentally Handicapped*, 2nd Report.
4. Johnson CR (1995) Specific development disorders. In Hersen M & Ammerman RT (eds) *Advanced Abnormal Child Psychology*, Hillsdale: Laurence Erlbaum.
5. Grove N & Walker M (1984) Communication before language. In Walker M (ed) *The MVDP Research Information Service*, Vol 2: issues 2, 3 & 4. Camberley, Surrey: MVDP.
6. Bullowa M (1980) *Before Speech; The Beginning of Interpersonal Communication,* 2nd edn. London: Cambridge University Press.
7. Bates E (1976) *Language and Context: The Acquisition of Pragmatics*. London: Academic Press.
8. Brown R (1973) *A First Language: The Early Stages*. London: George Allen & Unwin.
9. Schiefelbusch R (1972) Language and disabilities of cognitively involved children. In Irwin JV & Marge M (eds) *Principles of Childhood Language Disabilities*. New York: Apple-Century Crofts.
10. Donnellan AM, Mirenda PL, Mesaros RA & Bassbender LL (1984) Analysing the communicative functions of aberrant behaviour. *Journal of the Association for Persons with Severe Handicaps* **9**, 201–12.

11. Axelrod S (1987) Functional and structural analyses of behaviour: approaches leading to reduced use of punishment procedures. *Research in Developmental Disabilities* **8**, 165–78.

12. Durand VM (1990) *Severe Behaviour Problems: A Functional Communication Training Approach*. New York: Guilford Press.

13. Light J, Collier B & Parnes P (1985) *Communicative Interactions Between Young Non-speaking Physically Disabled Children and Their Primary Caregivers*. Part 1 Discourse patterns; Part 2 Communicative functions; Part 3 Modes of communication. AAC. Baltimore: Williams and Wilkins.

14. Benkelman DR & Mirenda P (1993) *Augmentative and Alternative Communication: Management of Severe Communications Disorders in Children and Adults*, 2nd edn. Baltimore: Paul Brookes Publishing Co.

15. Dodd B & Leahy J (1989) Phonological disorders and mental handicap. In Beveridge M, Conti-Ramsden G & Leudar I (eds) *Language and Communication in Mentally Handicapped People*, pp. 31–53. London: Chapman and Hall.

16. Menyuk P & Menn L (1981) Early strategies for the perception and production of words and sounds. In Fletcher P & Gorman M (eds) *Language Acquisition Studies in First Language Development*, pp. 49–70. Cambridge: Cambridge University Press.

17. Grunwell P (1981) *The Nature of Phonological Disability in Children*. London: Academic Press.

18. Berry MF & Eisenson J (1964) *Speech Disorders: Principles and Practices of Therapy*, 2nd edn, p. 36. London: Peter Owen.

19. Enderby P & Phillipp R (1986) Speech and language handicap: towards knowing the size of the problem. *British Journal of Communication Disorders* **21**, 151–65.

20. Fletcher P & Gorman M (1981) *Language Acquisition: Studies in First Language Development*, 2nd edn. Cambridge: Cambridge University Press.

21. Cromer RF. (1991) *Language and thought in Normal and Handicapped Children*. Oxford: Basil Blackwell.

22. Barratt DB & Diniz FA (1989) Lexical development in mentally handicapped children. In Beveridge M, Conti-Ramsden G & Leudar I (eds) *Language and Communication in Mentally Handicapped People*. London: Chapman and Hall.

23. Mein R & O'Connor N (1960). A study of the oral vocabularies of severely subnormal patients. *Journal of Mental Deficiency Research* **4**, 130–43.

24. Owens R (1989) Cognition and language in the mentally retarded population. In Beveridge M, Conti-Ramsden G & Leudar I (eds) *Language and Communication in Mentally Handicapped People*. London: Chapman and Hall.

25. Crystal D (1987) Teaching vocabulary: the case for a semantic curriculum. *Child Language Teaching and Therapy*, March, 40–56.

26. Sperber R & McCauley C (1984). Semantic processing efficiency in the mentally retarded. In Brooks R, Sperber R & McCauley C (eds) *Learning and Cognition in Mentally Retarded*, pp. 141–63. Hillsdale: Lawrence Erlbaum.

27. Maisto A & Jerome M (1977) Encoding and high speed memory scanning of retarded and non-retarded adolescents. *American Journal of Mental Deficiency* **82**, 282–6.

28. Winters J & Semchuk M (1986) Retrieval from long-term store as a function of mental age and intelligence. *American Journal of Mental Deficiency* **90**, 440–8.

29. Mercer C & Snell M (1977) *Learning Theory in Mental Retardation*. Columbus, Ohio: Charles E. Merrill.

30. Zeaman D & House B (1979) A review of attention theory. In Ellis N (ed) *Handbook of Mental Deficiency: Psychological Theory and Research*, pp. 63–120. Hillsdale: Lawrence Erlbaum.

31. O'Connor N & Hermalin B (1978) *Seeing and Hearing in Space and Time*. London: Academic Press.

32. Bonvillian JD & Nelson KE (1982) Exceptional cases of language acquisition. In Nelson KE (ed) *Child Language*, Vol. 3. Hillsdale: Gardner Press.

33. Kiernan CC (1983) The use of non-vocal communication techniques with autistic individuals. *Journal of Child Psychiatry and Psychology* **24(3)**, 339–75.

34. Anwar F (1983) In Hogg J and Mittler P (eds) *Advances in Mental Handicap Research*, Vol. II, pp. 203–31. Chichester: John Wiley.

35. Case R (1978). Intellectual development from birth to adulthood. A neo-Piagetian interpretation. In Siegler R (ed). *Children's Thinking: What Develops?*, pp. 37–71. Hillsdale, NJ: Lawrence Erlbaum.

36. Harris D (1981) Children's understanding of time. *Topics in Language Disorders* **2**, 51–66.

37. MacMillan D (1972) Paired-associate learning as a function of explicitness of mediational set by EMR and non retarded children. *American Journal of Mental Deficiency* 76, 686–91.
38. Spitz H (1966) The role of input organisation in the learning and memory of mental retardates. In Ellis N (ed) *International Review of Research in MR*, Vol 2. New York: Academic Press.
39. Oldfield RC & Marshall JC (1968) *Language: Penguin Modern Psychology Readings*. Harmondsworth: Penguin.
40. Brown R (1972) *Psycholinguistics: Selected Papers*. New York: The Free Press/Macmillan.
41. Herriot P (1971) *An Introduction to the Psychology of Language*, Methuen's Manuals of Modern Psychology. London: Methuen.
42. Frith U (1989) A new look at language and communication in autism. *British Journal of Communication Disorders* 24, 123–50.
43. Boucher J (1989) The theory of mind hypothesis of autism: explanation, evidence and assessment. *British Journal of Communication Disorders* 24, 181–99.
44. Fay WH & Schuler AL (1980) *Emerging Language in Autistic Children*. London: Edward Arnold.
45. Bishop DVM (1989) Autism, Asperger's syndrome and semantic pragmatic disorder: Where are the boundaries? *British Journal of Communication Disorders* 24, 107–21.
46. Kiernan KT & Sabsay S (1989) Communication in social interactions: aspects of an ethnography of communication of mildly mentally handicapped adults. In Beveridge M, Conti-Ramsden G & Leudar I (eds) *Language and Communication in Mentally Handicapped People*, pp. 229–53. London: Chapman and Hall.
47. *A Dictionary of British Sign Language/English*. (1992) British Deaf Association, David Brian (ed). London: Faber and Faber.
48. Newey R (1992). A useful tool to support language development. Personal communication. London. May 1992.
49. McNaughton S (1985) *Communicating with Blissymbolics*. Blissymbolics Communication Institute, 350 Rumsey Road, Toronto, Ontario, Canada.
50. Harbutt BI, Iwata BA & Green JD (1982) Nonvocal language acquisition in adolescents with severe physical disabilities; Blissymbol versus iconic stimulus formats. *Journal of Applied Behavioural Analysis* 15, 241–58.
51. Clark C (1981) Learning words using traditional orthography and the symbols of Rebus. Bliss and Carrier. *Journal of Speech and Hearing Disorders* 46, 191–96.
52. Goosens CA (1984) The Relative Iconicity and Learnability of Verb Referents Differentially Represented by Manual Signs, Blissymbols and Rebus Symbols. An Investigation With Moderately Retarded Individuals. *AAC Conference Proceedings*. Baltimore: Williams and Wilkins.
53. Grove N & Walker M (1990) *The Makaton Vocabulary: Using Manual Signs and Graphic Symbols to Develop Interpersonal Communication*, pp. 15–28. AAC, Augmentative and Alternative Communication. Baltimore: Williams and Wilkins.
54. Andrews G (1989) Which therapy is best? The role of research design. In Davidson K & Kerr A (eds) *Contemporary Themes in Psychiatry*. London: Royal College of Psychiatrists.
55. National Curriculum Council (1989) *Curriculum Guidance 2: A Curriculum for All*. York: NCC.
56. National Curriculum Council (1992) *Curriculum Guidance 9: The National Curriculum and Pupils with Learning Difficulties*. York: NCC.
57. Grifith P & Robinson J (1980) Influence of iconicity and phonological similarity on sign learning by mentally retarded children. *American Journal of Mental Deficiency* 85, 291–8.
58. Luftig R (1983) Translucency of sign and concreteness of gloss in the manual sign learning of moderately/severely retarded students. *American Journal of Mental Deficiency* 88, 279–86.
59. Lindsey M, O'Brien G, Baker R, Regan A & Berney T (1994) *Consensus Protocols for the Assessment, Investigation and Treatment of Aggression in People with Learning Disabilities*. London: Medical Audit Working Party of The Royal College of Psychiatry.
60. Carr EG & Durand VM (1985) Reducing behaviour problems through functional communication training. *Journal of Applied Behaviour Analysis* 18, 111–26.
61. Horner RH & Budd CM (1985) Acquisition of manual sign use: collateral reduction of maladaptive behaviour, and factors limiting generalisation. *Ed Train MR* 20, 39–47.
62. Lowrey MA (1995) Anger: A root of problem behaviours in the depressed. *The Habilitative Mental Health Care Newsletter* 14(6), 101–13.
63. Kiernan CC, Reid B & Jones L (1982) Signs and symbols: Use of non-vocal communication systems. *Studies in Education*, No. 11. London University Institute of Education.

64. Walker M (1977) Teaching sign language to deaf mentally handicapped adults. In *Language and the Mentally Handicapped*. Conference proceedings 3. Kidderminster: BIMH (now BILD).
65. Barera R & Sulzer-Azaroff B (1983) An alternating treatment comparison of oral and total communication programs with echolalic autistic children. *Journal of Applied Behaviour Analysis* **16**, 379–94.
66. Emerson J & Enderby P (1996) Prevalence of speech and language disorders in a mental illness unit. *European Journal of Disorders of Communication* **3**, 221–36.
67. Reid A (1985) Psychiatry and mental handicap. In Craft M, Bicknell J & Hollins S (eds) *Mental Handicap*. London: Baillière Tindall.
68. Moss SC, Patel P, Prosser H, Goldberg DP, Simpson N, Rowe S & Lucchino R (1993) Psychiatric morbidity in older people with moderate and severe learning disability (mental retardation). Part I: Development and reliability of the patient interview (the PAS ADD). *British Journal of Psychiatry* **163**, 471–80.
69. van der Gaag (1988). A *CASP (The Communication Assessment Profile)*. London: Speech Profiles Ltd in association with Speech Therapy In Practice.
70. Bishop DVM (1989). *TROG (Test for the Reception Of Grammar)*. The Age and Cognitive Performance Research Centre, Department of Psychology, University of Manchester.
71. Locke A (1985) *Living Language*. Windsor: NFER Nelson.
72. Masidlover M & Knowles M (1982) *The Derbyshire Language Scheme 1982*. Ripley: Derbyshire County Council.
73. Bouras N & Drummond K (1992) Behaviour and psychiatric disorders of people with mental handicaps living in the community. *Journal of Intellectual Disability Research* **36**, 349–57.
74. Disability Discrimination Act, November 1995. London: National Disability Council.

4
Behavioural Phenotypes

Shoumitro Deb

Introduction

Recent advances in molecular genetics have made it possible to identify specific genetic loci for conditions associated with learning disability. It has been known for some time that many of these genetically determined conditions associated with learning disability manifest specific physical phenotypes. The concept of a behavioural phenotype (a constellation of specific behaviours associated with a genetic disorder) is, however, a recent one. It is important to make the readers of this chapter aware at the outset of the possible methodological problems ingrained in the design of many studies of behavioural phenotypes. Many of these reports consist of single case studies; thus they do not exclude the possibility of chance association. It is also well known that papers with positive findings find their way to a journal much more easily than the papers which show no association between two conditions. Once a paper reporting a possible behavioural phenotype is published, others tend to become biased in observing that phenotype in their patients and report them for their newsworthiness. Some who reported more than one case often had a small number of a cohort in their study which caused statistical bias. Most importantly, authors often failed to include a properly matched control group in their studies.

Another bias lies in the variability of the definitions used. Different studies have used different definitions for the same condition. Autism is a classical example of this. Some studied nuclear autism, whereas others used a broader definition of autism. Some also clustered autism and autistic-like conditions together. Some studied Asperger's syndrome and autism separately, whereas others grouped them together in the same sample. Similar difficulties arose in diagnosing fragile-X syndrome. In the studies reported before the discovery of the gene for the fragile-X syndrome, different authors used different cut-off points for the percentage of cells expressing fragile X. Problems are also encountered because of the use of nonvalidated and nonstandardized rating scales for behaviours where reliability had not been properly tested. It is important to warn readers of these methodological shortcomings so that they are able to interpret the data presented in this chapter with appropriate caution.

So, how does one rectify these methodological shortcomings? Rosen[1] argued that at first a check-list of behaviours should be drawn up. This list should be drawn from the commonly observed behaviours in many people with both idiopathic and nonidiopathic learning disability. In the second stage all these behaviours should be rated among people with a learning disability with or without an underlying genetic cause by raters who are familiar with the behaviours of these people. The ratings should be blind, without the knowledge of the genetic conditions. Similarly, genetic analysis should be blind to the ratings of behaviours. In the final stage a cluster analysis of these behaviours should be carried out to identify possible behavioural syndromes associated with each genetic disorder. A multitrait–multimethod approach would utilize diverse measurements for a broad range of traits in order to establish construct validity for the underlying constellation of behaviours being measured. It is likely that many of the behaviours rated will be found across different genetic conditions. It is the group of behaviours occurring most frequently in each syndrome which will constitute the behavioural phenotype for that particular genetic disorder. Rosen's proposed approach would create a working hypothesis for each behavioural syndrome to be tested.[1] This process, however, should be taken a step further to establish its scientific validity. In this second step case-control studies should be included. Samples of individuals with specific genetic disorders should be drawn from a community-based general population. In some studies selection bias was caused because of the selection of cases from either institutions or a clinic-based population. A properly matched control group of subjects without a specific genetic disorder should be drawn from the same general population base. Matching should be done not only on the basis of gender and chronological age but also on the basis of level of intellectual functioning. If possible, another control group of an age- and sex-matched sample of individuals with average intelligence should be included. It is often said that many behaviours associated with genetic conditions are nonspecific manifestations of underlying brain damage and associated intellectual disability. The size of the cohort in all these groups should be large enough to give adequate statistical power to the study. The behavioural syndrome to be tested should then be rated by the same raters and informants for each group who are familiar with their clients' behaviours. The rating should be blind to the genetic conditions and vice versa. The behavioural rating scale should be properly validated for the study group and tested for inter-rater, inter-informant and test–retest reliability. In a cross-sectional study behaviour should be rated for a reasonable time as behaviours tend to vary among these individuals over time. Where possible prospective studies should also be undertaken. Internationally accepted commonly used definitions should be used for each condition.

After such rigorous hypothesis testing one should be able to establish an association (if it exists) between a genetic condition and a behavioural syndrome. Even if one finds such an association, the exact mechanism by which a genetic abnormality causes the manifestation of a behavioural syndrome will remain an enigma for some time to come. To complicate the situation, many genetic conditions are now shown to be associated not with a single gene defect but with a quantitative trait loci (QTL). A behavioural phenotype includes both absence of adaptive behaviours (e.g. intellectual disability, language disorders, specific learning disability, etc.) and the presence of maladaptive 'problem' behaviour. Maladaptive behaviours may sometimes involve personality traits but should never include specific psychiatric syndromes; this could cause confusion. This chapter describes those learning disability syndromes which are reported to be associated with a specific behavioural phenotype, although in some conditions the precise genetic defect has yet to be discovered.

Prader–Willi Syndrome (PWS)

Prader, Labhart and Willi[2] first described their syndrome in 1956: it was characterized by neonatal hypotonia, mental retardation, short stature, obesity and cryptorchidism affecting both genders. This is a rare condition affecting between 1 in 25 000 and 10 000 live births. The estimated population prevalence is approximately 1.2 to 1.3 per 10 000 with a boy:girl ratio of 1.6 to 1.2.[3] In the initial pre-obesity phase, babies with PWS are limp, sleepy, nonresponsive and typically present with a narrowed bifrontal diameter, a triangular-shaped mouth, strabismus and acromicria.[4] Feeding difficulties in the form of absence of swallowing and sucking reflex are common at this stage. Between age 1 and 4 years the children with PWS gradually develop hyperphagia owing to either persistent hunger or a decreased perception of satiety. This eventually causes gross obesity. They show developmental delay and limited sexual function owing to hypogenitalism. Appearance of few secondary sex characteristics is manifested as micropenis and cryptorchidism in males and amenorrhoea and irregular menstrual cycle in females. This syndrome has been found in different ethnic groups.

Other associated features include small hands and feet, cleft palate, almond-shaped eyes, incurved foot, club foot, congenital hip dislocation, scoliosis, unspecified abnormalities of hips, knees and ankles, squint. Other systemic involvement causes diabetes, bowel obstruction, asthma, eczema, duodenal ulcer, rectal prolapse, heart disease, cor pulmonale, boils, deafness, renal stones, gallstones and hypothermia. In around 40% of PWS the IQ score will fall between 70 and 90, the remainder are mildly and moderately learning disabled. PWS subjects may also show a specific pattern of cognitive impairment. Whereas their visuo-spatial skills remain particularly strong they show reduced short-term memory and a greater loss of information from memory over time.

In approximately 50–70% of cases of PWS cytogenetic tests reveal deletion of chromosome 15 which is of paternal origin. PWS, however, appears to be genetically heterogeneous. In some cases this is caused by inheritance of two chromosomes 15 from their mothers (maternal disomy); in others, PWS with normal chromosomes may be caused by a paternal gene mutation. Except for possible differences in pigmentation, the PWS group with chromosome deletion is clinically identical to the PWS group without such chromosomal abnormality. Greenswag[4] found that fathers of PWS children with normal chromosomes were significantly older when their PWS child was born than fathers of PWS children with abnormal chromosomes. He described similar genetic heterogeneity in retinoblastoma, which can be caused by an autosomal dominant mutation and by the deletion of the long arm of chromosome 13.

A behavioural phenotype associated with PWS has been described.[5] This consists of abnormalities in speech, sleep and behaviour and also a specific pattern of cognitive deficit, as described earlier. Although speech abnormalities in PWS have often been mentioned in the literature, they are poorly defined. Around 23% showed articulation disorder in a series,[5] along with echolalia or abnormal syntax in 17% of cases and other speech abnormality in 18% of cases. A higher proportion of males than females showed these speech abnormalities. Some individuals showed more than one type of speech abnormality. Various types of sleep abnormalities have been reported among individuals with PWS. Excessive daytime sleepiness (EDS) was found in over 90% of cases, frequent EDS in over 60% of cases, 8 h nocturnal sleep in over 50% of cases and over 10 h nocturnal sleep in around 23% of cases. The mean duration of daytime sleep ranged between 5 and 180 min with a mean around 68 min. Other sleep abnormalities found in PWS subjects include initial insomnia, sleep onset REM (rapid eye movement) and hyperventilation during REM sleep but not sleep apnoea. Conversely, some reported a strong association between sleep apnoea and obesity. The sleep abnormality does not appear to be related to the degree of obesity. EDS often occurs when the subjects are unoccupied, watching television or travelling by car. Hypothalamic dysfunction and chronic REM sleep deprivation due to REM sleep-related hyperventilation are the two proposed explanations for sleep abnormalities observed in PWS.

Although PWS subjects have often been described as 'pleasant', 'good tempered' and 'cheerful', they can manifest severe behavioural problems associated with hyperphagia, self-injurious behaviour, particularly in the form of incessant spot-picking, and temper tantrums. A behavioural syndrome of motor slowness, skin-picking, sleepiness, ritualistic behaviour, impulsive talk and stubbornness has been described in PWS. Other behavioural problems include belligerence (both food related and non-related), irritability, impulsivity, laziness, antisocial actions with peers and family, moodiness and physical aggression directed to other persons and property. Behavioural problems tend to appear as PWS children grow older, particularly after the age of 4 years. These are often the manifestation of the combined effects of organic aspects of the syndrome, such as central nervous system anomalies, metabolic defects etc., and the relentless hunger and psychosocial pressure of being obese, learning disabled and sexually immature. Hyperphagia can lead to stealing of food and similar antisocial behaviour and eventual aggression due to confrontation. Deliberate picking of spots is another common behavioural problem in PWS and causes persistent sores and cellulitis. It is not clear whether or not PWS subjects have a higher pain threshold which predisposes to the picking behaviour. No association is found between the increased weight in PWS people and their behavioural problem; however, some families reported a worsening of behaviour if the person with PWS had less than usual sleep. These severe behaviour problems have a serious impact on family lives and subsequently on the wider community.

Brachmann–de Lange Syndrome (BDLS)

In 1933, de Lange[6] described this multisystem syndrome which includes congenital malformation, growth retardation and developmental delay. Earlier, Brachmann (1916) had reported a similar syndrome in a child with an additional finding of upper limb deficiency.[7] The characteristic features of this syndrome are hypertricosis (hirsutism, low posterior hair line, synophrys, long eyelashes), facial abnormalities (depressed nasal bridge, ocular anomalies, prominent philtrum, thin lips, anteverted nostrils, down-turned angles of mouth, bluish tinge around eyes, nose and/or mouth, widely spaced teeth, high arched palate, low set ears, micrognathia, short neck), limb deformities (grossly malformed upper limb(s); oligodactyly; phocomelia in 27% of cases, small hands and feet with short digits, limitation of extension of elbow(s), proximally placed thumbs, clinodactyly of fifth finger(s), single transverse palmar crease in 51% of cases, webbing of second and third toes), other anomalies include cryptorchidism, hypoplastic genitalia in males (57% of cases), cutis murmorata (60% of cases), small umbilicus (53% of cases), low-pitched cry and small nipples in 55% of cases.[8]

BDLS is found in different ethnic groups. As neonates they have feeding difficulties and respiratory problems and fail to thrive. Severe gastrointestinal problems such as pyloric stenosis, severe gastrointestinal reflux or malrotation of the bowel and intestinal obstruction, as well as congenital heart disease, are common accompaniments of this syndrome. Many children are diagnosed at birth or within a few days after birth. Approximately 87% of BDLS subjects have an IQ below 60. The prevalence of this condition is estimated with a wide variation between 1 per 100 000 and 1 per 50 000 general population. Other clinical features of BDLS include a low-pitched cry frequently noted in the newborn period or early infancy, eye problems such as myopia, ptosis and nystagmus, severe hearing loss due to stenotic external auditory canal, skin problems and seizures reported in a minority of cases. A small proportion of BDLS subjects develop language skills within normal to low-normal levels. Language deficit affects expressive speech more than comprehension. The level of speech abnormality does not seem to be directly related to the level of cognitive deficit whereas factors such as birth weight, social relatedness, hearing impairment, upper limb malformation, and developmental ages for sitting and walking show a relationship to the acquisition of language skills.

Clinical variability within BDLS, particularly a mild form, has been described in the literature.[9] Most cases of BDLS are single sporadic occurrences within families. Although many familial cases have been reported, the exact mode of inheritance still remains unknown. Most of the recent reports suggested dominant transmission on the basis of the finding of one or more affected children in families where a parent has had mild features of the syndrome. No gene has been identified for this condition but speculation suggests the possibility of more than one aetiology. There are phenotypic similarities between BDLS and the duplication 3q (26.3) syndrome.[10] This rearrangement provides access to a limited sequence of nucleotides surrounding the breakpoint where a search for duplication or deletion is feasible.

A behavioural phenotype for BDLS has been suggested. This consists of feeding difficulty in infancy and childhood, sleep disturbance, self-injurious behaviour, temper tantrums, cyclical mood change and some autistic features, the degree of which is related to the degree of cognitive disability. Other commonly associated behaviours are diminished ability to relate socially, repetitive and stereotyped behaviour, infrequent facial expression of emotion and severe delay in language development. As children they show a preference for rigid routine and rigid thinking, ritualistic obsession, and hyperactivity. As they grow old they show explosive aggressive outbursts and self-injurious behaviour (e.g. hit, throw things, bite themselves and other children, destroy clothing by chewing). These behaviours occur most frequently during conditions of low adult attention and are often maintained by the carer's attention to the maladaptive behaviour. BDLS children and adults show many behaviours similar to those of autistic children or those with Pervasive Developmental Disorder Not Otherwise Specified (PDD-NOS).[9] These behaviours include restricted repertoire of activities and interests, which can be stereotyped and repetitive. Both verbal and nonverbal communications are impaired. Children often exhibit echolalia, pronoun reversal, and occasionally language regression. Nonverbal communication such as facial expression and gesture may be absent or minimal. Abnormalities of posture and movement, such as hand flapping, odd responses to sensory input, abnormal patterns of eating, drinking or sleeping associated with delays or distortions in development in cognitive skills are common.

Phenylketonuria (PKU)

PKU is an autosomal recessive inborn error of amino acid metabolism associated with learning disability occurring in approximately 1 in 12 000 live births. Cognitive deficit is often severe and occasionally mild in untreated cases. Owing to lack of the skin pigment precursor tyrosine, PKU subjects are characteristically fair-haired, fair skinned and blue-eyed and have lower than normal birth weight and microcephaly. Nonspecific neurological signs include stooped posture, rigid, broad-based gait, some degree of muscular hypertonicity, hyperreflexia involving the deep tendon reflexes, tremor of the outstretched hands, stereotyped motor movements such as rocking of the body, digital mannerisms such as flicking, twiddling, pill-rolling and habitual manipulation of objects such as wheels of toys. A small proportion show evidence of pyramidal or extrapyramidal tract involvement. Epilepsy could be present in around 26% of cases.

Abnormal electroencephalogram (EEG) activities such as fast wave and excessive slow background wave are common in PKU subjects both with and without epilepsy, and in a proportion of parents of PKU children. However, excessive slow background activity in EEG is shown to be a nonspecific common finding in people with learning disability.[11]

In PKU there exists a considerable amount of both genotypic and phenotypic heterogeneity. The metabolic disorder in PKU results from a deficiency of the hepatic enzyme phenylalanine hydroxylase causing hyperphenylalaninaemia and phenylketonuria. The known phenotypes include absent (PH°) or deficient (PH⁻) phenylalanine hydroxylase activity, absent (DHPR°) or deficient (DHPR⁻) pteridin reductase activity, and deficient (BH₂) biopterin synthesis.[12] PH phenotypes affect phenylalanine hydroxylation alone, whereas DHPR⁻ and BH₂ phenotypes also involve tryptophan and tyrosine hydroxylation. Phenylalanine level in serum is usually above 1 mmol l⁻¹ (more than eight times normal) and phenylalanine hydroxylase levels less than 1% of mean normal activity. Routine neonatal screening through the Guthrie test detects PKU during the neonatal period. A corrective diet of low phenylalanine during the developmental period prevents learning disability and maladaptive behaviour in later life. Even after treatment with corrective diet, PKU subjects as a group show lower than average IQ. In DHPR⁻ and BH₂ phenotypes (which affect about 10% of cases), in addition to restriction of phenylalanine intake, administration of carbidopa, L-3,4-dihydroxyphenylalanine and 5-hydroxytryptophan has been shown to be partly effective. In malignant hyperphenylalaninaemia, despite restoration of *in vivo* phenylalanine homeostasis, progressive neurological deterioration takes place. Persistent maternal hyperphenylalanin-aemia during pregnancy can cause cardiac anomalies, intrauterine growth retardation, microcephaly and learning disability in the surviving obligate heterozygous offspring. However, prognoses for the offspring of heterozygous mothers are relatively better.

PKU shows considerable genotypic heterogeneity. The human phenylalanine hydroxylase gene has been located on the long arm of chromosome 12. It includes 13 exons and extends up to 90 000 base pairs of the DNA. More than 50 restriction fragment length polymorphism (RFLP) haplotypes and 31 different mutations have been documented in the human phenylalanine hydroxylase locus. Most patients who have any combination of mutant phenylalanine hydroxylase alleles of RFLP haplotype 2 or 3 have a severe form of the disease, whereas patients who have mutant phenylalanine hydroxylase alleles of RFLP haplotype 1 or 4 have a variety of phenotypes, suggesting that mutant haplotype 1 and 4 phenylalanine hydroxylase alleles bear multiple independent mutations.[13] Because of the likelihood that there are several alleles for each phenotype, patients can be either homozygous or compound heterozygous.

Older literature on PKU describes a behavioural phenotype associated with this condition.[14] Behaviours described were hyperactivity, irritability, episodes of screaming, noisiness and uncontrollable temper tantrums. Individuals were also described as having dull, expressionless faces, negativistic behaviour, emotional outbursts and speech disturbances such as difficulty in pronouncing consonants, labile mood and 'nervous prances'. Self-injurious behaviours such as biting and head banging along with clumsiness and poor motor coordination were also reported. Other behaviours described were short attention span, distractibility, low tolerance of frustration, perseveration, echolalia, continuous crying and abnormal locomotor activities. Relative absence of reports of behavioural problems in PKU subjects in the current literature suggests that corrective diet not only prevents developmental delay but also prevents development of maladaptive behaviour. This hypothesis has recently been tested by using phenylalanine-restricted diet in adult subjects with both treated and untreated PKU who developed behavioural problem, but the outcome of this treatment is not encouraging. To exclude the influence of corrective diet some groups studied psychopathology among patients, particularly mothers of people with PKU. The findings in this field are equivocal in that whereas some showed an increased psychopathology among mothers, others have failed to do so. However, it is worth keeping in mind that among the mothers studied some were obligate heterozygote carriers and the others were not.

Williams Syndrome (WS)

WS, otherwise known as hypercalcaemia, with supravalvular aortic stenosis and unusual facies occurs in approximately 1 in 55 000 live births and is inherited in an autosomal dominant fashion. Although the precise aetiology and genetic cause of WS are unknown, some have been related to excessive maternal vitamin D intake. The risk for siblings of an isolated case is probably 10% at most. Infants with WS are usually irritable, have feeding problems and fail to thrive, and as a result become developmentally delayed and have retarded growth. The majority of subjects with WS have moderate to severe learning disability. Other characteristic features of WS include a distinctive 'elfin-like' face, renal and cardiovascular abnormalities, such as supravalvular aortic stenosis and peripheral pulmonary artery stenosis. Because of incomplete genetic penetration in some cases there is a variable expression of phenotype. In over half the cases serum calcium level is raised. These cases are also known as idiopathic infantile hypercalcaemia (IIH) and are treated with low-calcium and vitamin D-restricted diet.

There have been a few reports of a possible behavioural phenotype being associated with WS. Of these, three were case–control studies.[15] WS children show a distinctive pattern of cognitive deficit in that their verbal abilities are markedly superior to their visuo-spatial and motor skills. In a case–control study Udwin and Yule[15] found that WS children (*n* = 19) scored significantly lower than the control group of children (*n* = 19) on four of the five subtests of performance scale of Wechsler Intelligence Scale for Children-Revised (WISC-R).[16] These subtests were picture completion, block design, object assembly and coding. These tests assess a variety of visuo-spatial abilities and fine motor skills, including sequencing, eye–hand

co-ordination and copying visual patterns. There was no significant difference observed between the groups on the scores of the picture rearrangement subtest on the performance scale of WISC-R. However, on three other
tests for visuo-spatial skills, namely nonverbal card sorting task, total recall
score for visuo-spatial items on the Rivermead Behavioural Memory Test
(RBMT)[17] and Memory for Spatial Location Test (MSLT;[15] as a personal communication with Wykem, 1986) (significant for two out of five trials) the
two groups did not differ significantly, although there was a tendency for
the WS group to perform more poorly than the control group. Verbal comprehension tasks did not reveal any inter-group difference. WS children
performed better on face-recognition tasks. Although the authors should be
congratulated for using an appropriately matched control group, the number in each group remains too small to achieve an optimal statistical power
and thus the study is vulnerable to type 2 error. It is also not clear whether
or not WS children in their study were selected from a general population-
based sample or a clinic-based sample. There is always a tendency on the
part of the tertiary referral centres to accumulate the most difficult and
abnormal cases. The large number of univariate analyses used in the study
in the absence of Bonferroni correction or expression of confidence interval
increased the scope of type 1 error and chance association.

WS infants show abnormal attachment behaviour in the form of indiscriminate affection and anxiety. As they grow old, children with WS
develop higher rates of emotional and behavioural disturbance in the form
of over-activity, poor concentration, eating and sleeping difficulties, excessive anxiety, and poor relationship with peers. They sometimes show excessive friendliness to adults including strangers owing to social disinhibition.
After an initial delay in the preschool age their speech develops normally
at a superficial level but subtle abnormalities could be detected at careful
listening. A very high proportion of WS children show 'hyperacusis' in
that they tend to be highly sensitive to a variety of noises, including noises
from vacuum cleaners, washing machines and thunder, etc., in the absence
of any auditory abnormality. WS children are fussy, fearful, over-anxious
and show more mannerisms both at school and at home. Udwin and Yule[15]
argued that the behavioural disturbance in the WS children could be
explained by their poorer visuo-spatial skills, their lack of attention,
distractibility and over-activity or by the frustration they experience
because of the marked discrepancy between their verbal and nonverbal/
visuo-spatial and motor abilities.

Rett Syndrome (RS)

This is a syndrome of unknown aetiology which affects girls exclusively
because it is fatal for male foetuses. The estimated prevalence rate varies
between 1 in 15 000 and 10 000. Associated learning disability is of severe
to profound degree. No gene has been discovered for RS, although some
suspect a dominant gene on the X chromosome. In the absence of detectable
genetic abnormality the diagnosis depends on clinical features. Girls

affected by the condition tend to develop normally up to 18 months to 2 years. At around that age they develop stereotyped motor movements, particularly involving hands and fingers in the form of hand flapping and wringing movements. Their development starts to slow down and they manifest many features of autistic disorder and could be misdiagnosed as autistic at this stage. By age 4 or 5 years a high proportion of them (59–72%) develop epilepsy. Later, they develop spasticity of limbs and at the same time become generally more sociable. Their deterioration reaches a plateau at this stage, although the overall prognosis for this condition remains poor.

Many have suggested a behavioural phenotype associated with RS. Sansom and colleagues[18] carried out a postal questionnaire survey of 107 families who rated the behaviour of their children with RS. Thirty of these families were directly interviewed by the authors. Episodes of low mood were reported in 70% of children along with brief episodes of mood changes in 67% and sustained mood change in only 9% of cases. Episodes of anxiety characterized by hyperventilation, screaming, self-injury, a frightened expression and general distress occurred in 75% of children. Sudden noises, some types of music, strange people or places, change of routine and excessive activity in proximity to the child all seemed to precipitate episodes of anxiety. Self-injurious behaviours particularly affecting hands can occur in 39–49% cases. Milder forms of these involve biting and chewing of fingers and hands and more severe forms involve hand-to-hand banging, hand-to-object banging, hair pulling, scratching and head banging may also occur. Up to 74% of the children can have sleep problems particularly involving laughing at night. About one-third of children were described as having brief 'attacks', often associated with hyperventilation and alteration in consciousness. These attacks were thought to be of nonepileptic origin. Sansom and colleagues[18] found that the families used various strategies to cope with the behavioural problem in their children. These strategies included distraction, reinforcement of alternative, incompatible behaviours together with confrontation. Other methods were hydrotherapy, massage, music therapy and in some instances avoidance of certain foods and excessive stimulation. There was a tendency for behavioural problems to improve with age.

Joubert Syndrome

Episodic hyperpnoea, abnormal eye movements, ataxia, mental and motor retardation are key clinical features of Joubert syndrome.[19] The diagnosis is confirmed by the demonstration of the partial or complete agenesis of the cerebellar vermis. Intermittent hyperpnoea is characterized by a baseline respiratory rate followed by a 10–20 s apnoeic episode and then a 20–90 s episode of hyperpnoea and extreme tachypnoea, usually over 120 breaths per minute. These episodes of rapid, deep breathing resemble the panting of a dog. Children are often not cyanosed and their blood gases remain within the normal range. Children show gross neurological delay characterized by generalized hypotonia, poor head control, no social smile, bilateral ptosis, abnormal ocular movement such as rotatory nystagmus and large saccades at birth and ataxia. Other occasional clinical features include rhythmic tongue protrusion, polydactyly, chorioretinal coloboma, gastroesophageal reflux, facial spasms, syndactyly and cystic kidney. To date, 65 cases have been reported; most had severe to profound learning disability. Prognosis of this condition remains poor and mode of inheritance is possibly autosomal recessive. Neuro-imaging findings include a dilated and abnormally shaped fourth ventricle sometimes communicating with a larger posterior fossa cyst, abnormal position of superior cerebellar peduncles and a smaller brainstem. Neuropathology also showed dysplasia of cerebellar nuclei, narrow pons, absence of pyramidal decussation and abnormality of the solitary and trigeminal tracts. One MRI report showed abnormal white matter signal in parietal lobes.[20]

Holroyd and colleagues[20] reported two cases of Joubert syndrome (a 6-year-old white female and her $3^1/_2$-year-old brother of normal parents) who showed features of autistic disorder. Both had either normal (IQ>85) or near-normal abilities (IQ 64). The sister showed marked perseveration, displayed minimal initiative behaviour, played by herself, never liked being held, and if hurt did not seek or accept parental comfort. She showed no self-injurious behaviour but displayed repetitive finger and hand movements. She was preoccupied with lining-up objects and became extremely upset if the objects were moved. Although she was generally a happy child she had cycles every 1–2 months, each lasting for 4–5 days, of irritability, temper tantrums and decreased sleep but no other evidence of psychiatric illness. Conversely, her brother was overly sensitive to noise, developed a fascination to touch smooth textures, showed perseveration but played with parents and other children, sought parental comfort when distressed and was not upset when routine was changed. Both children showed developmental delay in motor and expressive language rather than global cognitive disability. The sister met DSM3-R criteria for autistic disorder. The brother showed some features of autism such as language abnormality in the form of perseveration, persistent preoccupation with sounds and textures, but displayed no abnormalities in social interaction. Previous neuro-imaging studies have shown cerebellar abnormality in both autism and fragile-X syndrome.[21] Holroyd and colleagues thus hypothesized that cerebellar abnormality is the possible cause of autistic features in Joubert syndrome.[20]

Down's Syndrome (DS)

DS is the most common cause of learning disability which affects approximately 1 in 1000 live births (previously quoted incidence of DS was 1 in 600 live births). The incidence rises with advancing maternal age at the time of conception. Approximately 95% of cases of DS are caused by trisomy 21, 4% by translocation and 1% by mosaicism. The cause of trisomy 21 is not known. Individuals with DS have characteristic clinical features. They have short stature with a round skull and brachycephaly. The eye signs include typical 'mongoloid slope' of the palpebral fissures, the 'epicanthic fold' in which the upper eyelid overlaps the lower at the inner canthus, the 'Brushfield spots' (a fine white speckling of the iris). They are also prone to develop cataract prematurely, whereas some develop strabismus or nystagmus. Some have high arched palate and protruded tongue.

In a proportion of cases of DS transverse palmar crease (simian crease) could be observed. Other hand abnormalities include syndactyly (webbed finger) or clinodactyly (incurving of the finger). Syndactyly of the toes with a 'sandal gap' is observed in some cases of DS. People with DS tend to suffer from some congenital abnormalities of the internal organs. These include atrial or ventricular septal defect, oesophagial atresia, congenital dilatation of the colon (Hirschprung's disease), umbilical and inguinal hernia.

Other commonly observed medical conditions among people with DS include biochemical hypothyroidism when TSH level is raised just over the normal reference range and the total T4 level remains at a lower normal range. This is possibly caused by an autoimmune thyroiditis. Transient leukaemoid reaction may be slightly more common among the children with DS. Individuals with DS are likely to suffer from sleep apnoea and a repeated chest infection. The full blood count of many people with DS shows macrocytosis with a normal level of haemoglobin. Epilepsy can affect 10–20% of people with DS; this is more prevalent over age 40 when almost all tend to develop Alzheimer's neuropathology, although only a proportion manifest clinical dementia.[22]

Individuals with DS have been described as cheerful, affectionate, humorous, good at 'mimicry', amiable, music-loving and easily amused. Earlier studies on the characteristics of the DS children found that although when compared with non-learning disabled children they tend to show a higher rate of behaviour problems, this trend tends to disappear when their behaviour is compared with that of the other non-DS learning disabled children. In most of these studies data was collected from the case-notes or in some cases information regarding the children's behaviour was gathered from the carers and often no structured, validated behaviour rating scale was used. When the behaviours of the DS children were compared with those of a control group of non-DS learning disabled children some observed a difference whereas others did not. In studies where a difference in the rate of behaviour between DS and non-DS children was observed, the DS children often had a higher rate of good behaviour as opposed to bad (maladaptive) behaviour.

The previous studies of behaviour of adults with DS revealed similar equivocal findings. In a recent study Collacott and colleagues (R. A. Collacott, personal communication, 1996) analysed the data on behaviours of DS and non-DS adults with learning disability from the information gathered by the Leicestershire Information Co-ordination Centre for people with a learning disability. They used the Disability Assessment Schedule to rate adaptive and maladaptive behaviours among 360 adults with DS and 1829 non-DS adults with a learning disability. They reported a significantly lower rate of maladaptive behaviour in the DS adults compared with the non-DS group. Subsequent cluster analysis of the behaviours showed DS adults to display lower prevalence of most clusters containing maladaptive behaviours and higher prevalence of one cluster without significant behavioural difficulties. Because DS adults are known to develop Alzheimer's neuropathology at an early age, which could be demonstrated by neuro-imaging findings,[22] Collacott and colleagues further divided the DS group according to their age. The behaviour characteristic of younger (age less than 35 years) and older (age 35 years and over) adults with DS remained remarkably constant, although there was a tendency for the older DS adults to show more maladaptive behaviour. On the basis of their findings Collacott and colleagues concluded that a behavioural phenotype exists among DS adults. However, a relative absence of maladaptive behaviour when compared with the non-DS adults with learning disability does not provide sufficient evidence to support a specific behavioural phenotype in DS adults. This area requires further careful exploration before we can confidently conclude that a specific behavioural phenotype exists in people with DS.

Fragile-X Syndrome (FRAX)

Fragile-X syndrome is the most common inherited cause of learning disability. In 1938, Penrose found an excess of males among people with learning disability.[23] Despite being a geneticist Penrose sought a sociocultural explanation for this excess rather than a genetic one. He thought that society's demand from males exposes their disability more easily than that of females. Martin and Bell, in 1943, described a family from England which contained 11 learning disabled males in two generations.[24] Although no physical anomalies were reported at that time, Richards and Webb later (1982) found macro-orchidism and a fragile-X chromosome in those males.[25] In 1962, Renpenning and colleagues described a Canadian Mennonite family with 20 learning disabled males with microcephaly.[26] Subsequent study by Fox and colleagues in 1980 did not reveal fragile-X in the affected males in Renpenning's reported family.[27] While geneticists such as Penrose and Reed failed to perceive a sex-linked genetic contribution to learning disability, Lehrke, an educational psychologist from Wisconsin, suggested the connection after studying several families with X-linked learning disability.[28] At that time his views were challenged and he was asked to provide evidence for his hypothesis.

It was Lubs' pioneering work in 1969 that provided the first evidence in support of Lehrke's hypothesis.[29] His cytogenetic investigation demonstrated an area of constriction near the end of the long arm of the X chromosome in four males in three generations of a family. Lubs called this constriction in the X chromosome, 'the marker x chromosome', which is now known as fragile-X. Turner and colleagues' study in 1971 and 1972 from New South Wales, Australia provided further support for Lehrke's hypothesis.[30] For a few years research in this area remained dormant until

1977 when Harvey and colleagues[31] described in eight families clinical and cytogenetic findings similar to those reported by Lubs. Coincidentally, in the same year, Sutherland showed that the fragile-X chromosome can only be demonstrated when the lymphocytes are cultured in media deficient in folate and thymidine.[32] This observation explained the apparent failure of others to replicate Lubs' finding, because in 1969 most laboratories had stopped using medium 199, which is deficient in folate and thymidine. The abnormality in the X chromosome is situated at the region of Xq 27.3 which is expressed on average as between 10% and 40% of cells (range between less than 5% to greater than 60%) when cultured in media deficient in folate and thymidine with additional cytotoxic agents such as methotrexate and 2-deoxy-5-fluorouridine (Fudr). Currently accepted practice is to examine between 50 and 200 cells using a threshold of 4% expressivity as evidence of the syndrome. However, recent discovery of the gene for this condition has made cytogenetic testing almost obsolete.

Fragile-X syndrome affects approximately 1 in 1200 males and 1 in 2000–2500 females. However, almost all the prevalence studies have included children with learning disability alone. Some have questioned these prevalence figures and claimed that the actual prevalence is much lower than believed and might vary from one region to another. The syndrome is reported among various ethnic groups. The syndrome accounts for 50% of all X-linked cases and between 2% and 5% of learning disabled population. Previous studies quoted slightly higher figures. Mosaicism of fragile-X with other X chromosome disorders such as XXY have been reported.[33] About 100 different fragile sites have been reported of which *FRAXA* and *FRAXE* have been shown to be associated with specific phenotypes. *FRAXF* in Xq27-q28 distal to both *FRAXA* and *FRAXE* has also been described. The gene for fragile-X syndrome called fragile-X mental retardation-1 (*FMR-1*) was discovered simultaneously in 1991 by three groups.[34-36] The *FMR-1* gene consists of abnormal trinucleotide repeat of CGG at the fragile site of the X chromosome consisting of 17 exons spanning 38 kb. In normal individuals the CGG repeat ranges between 6 and 54 with an average of 30 repeats. In phenotypically normal male carriers and a proportion of female carriers a pre-mutation stage of between 43 and 200 CGG repeats are found. In clinically affected individuals CGG repeats are always over 200 (range 230 to over 1000) and this is associated with an adjacent cluster of hypermethylated sites. Both blood and salivary epithelial cells can now be used for molecular genetic studies. Pre-mutation often expands to a full mutation when transmitted by female carriers.

Dysmorphoses associated with the syndrome are subtle and often not visible until the subjects reach their adulthood. Fragile-X children have above average birthweight and height but on growing to adulthood become shorter, whereas their head circumference remains larger than normal. In adults macro-orchidism can be found in a proportion of cases; however, macro-orchidism could also be associated with other X-linked learning disabilities. The characteristic facial appearance, such as large forehead with supraorbital fullness, long nose, prominent chin and large ears can only be observed in some adult males. The length of the ear is increased, the helix is frequently unfolded and a bat-eared or loop-eared appearance is not uncommon. Abnormality of the eye includes pale irises, which is a subtle finding and difficult to detect. Genital anomalies, such as hypospadias and cryptorelvidism, have been reported in fragile-X males, although their semen analysis is normal and they are able to father children. Hyperextensible joints, flat feet, inguinal and hiatus hernia, enlarged aortic root and mitral valve prolapse detected in some cases of fragile-X syndrome point towards connective tissue dysplasia. Certain dermatoglyphic abnormalities have also been described. Occasional features include high arched palate, torticollis and/or kyphoscoliosis, pectus excavatum, epilepsy, hyperreflexia and nystagmus. A proportion of adult males have a hypogonadal appearance with decreased body hair, gynaecomastia and striae. Some reported a high incidence of foot abnormalities, including flat feet, a sandal gap and long, broad toes with recurrent paronychia of the first toes. No abnormality in the endocrine system has been reported except for abnormal thyroid stimulating hormone (TSH) release in response to administration of thyrotropin releasing hormone (TRH) in some cases. Intellectually normal females show no physical phenotype and only a proportion of intellectually retarded females show a phenotype similar to that found in adult males. In females X-inactivation may be responsible for variability of phenotypic expression in certain cases. A number of sets of twins and one set of triplets with fragile X have been reported.

Although fragile-X syndrome is now recognized as a common genetic cause of learning disability inherited in an X-linked dominant manner with reduced penetrance, the level of cognitive deficit varies considerably. Intellectually normal as well as profoundly learning disabled individuals with fragile-X syndrome have been reported. Older studies suggested a range of mean IQ of 27–36 among adult males, more recent studies, however, point towards a milder range of mean IQ between 50 and 70. Among female carriers, between 30% and 50% show cognitive deficit (on average one-third). There appears to be a decline of mean IQ score in fragile-X males as they grow old. There is an interesting parallel here between individuals with fragile-X syndrome and Down's syndrome. The explanation for this apparent drop in IQ score with age may lie in either a biological or a sociocultural reason or a combination of both. Whether or not the family has an influence on the IQ among fragile-X male relatives has not been determined. No consistent correlation between the level of intelligence and the proportion of fragile-X-positive cells in males has been shown. A curvilinear relationship between the length of CGG repeat (and also the level of methylation) and level of intelligence among fragile-X males has recently been reported.[37] A comparison of IQ between female carriers with either pre-mutation or full mutation showed the mean IQ in the full mutation group to be significantly lower. However, no significant relationship was found between IQ score and the number of CGG repeats or percentage methylation of the mutant allele within each mutation category.[38] In addition, no significant relationship was found between IQ score and the proportion of normal FMR-1 alleles on the active chromosome in the carrier female group as a whole or in either mutation.

There have been attempts to analyse various aspects of cognitive and neuropsychological profile, and to establish an overall estimate of IQ among fragile-X subjects. Theobold and colleagues (1984) reported an 8-year-old boy of normal IQ who did miserably on some of the subtests of the WISC-R, namely similarities, immediate memory and delayed memory, yet scored in the normal range on the Peabody picture vocabulary test (PPVT),[39] digit span and block design subtests.[40] Current neuropsychological studies of fragile-X males showed a slightly different cognitive profile than that reported by Theobold and colleagues in that the fragile-X males have relatively better verbal skills, despite their language problem, than performance and visuo-spatial skills; overall they do well on vocabulary and comprehension tests and poorly on arithmetic, digit span, block design and object assembly. In other words, the fragile-X males show weakness in sequential processing (thus are poor at arithmetic skills) rather than in simultaneous processing of information, as often demonstrated by the Kaufman Assessment Battery of children (K-ABC).[41]

Although hearing has been reported to be normal in fragile-X males, either delay in language development or development of abnormalities of language is very common. The delay in language development is proportional to the intellectual development. Various characteristic speech abnormalities have been described in subjects with fragile-X syndrome. Perseveration of words and phrases is more commonly found than echolalia. 'Litany-like speech' associated with swings in pitch, jocular (characterized by compulsive garrulous speech), echolalia, palilalia (repetition of words with increasing speed and descrescendo of volume), 'cluttering' or 'tackyphemia', narrative speech (language which is often devoid of content yet the language structure remains intact); their speech sound substitution difficulties are the main descriptions of speech abnormalities commonly associated with fragile X. Some suggested syntactic competency (ability to put words together to form a sentence) and semantic concept (knowledge of word meanings) remain intact in fragile-X males but they show problems in comprehending sentences with high associate compounds, and show productive semantic error and pragmatic competence (normal social behaviour associated with language). Hyperarousal is proposed as being the main contributory factor in the production of deviant language by fragile-X males.

The behaviour of fragile-X males is highly variable. Some are friendly, amiable and attractive and others are behaviourally disordered. In one study a behaviour problem was noted among 74% of 27 fragile-X males. Hyperactivity, restlessness and lack of concentration were most common (56%), followed by excessive shyness and anxiety (52%), aggression and frequent 'mood spells' (33%), psychotic features including paranoia and hallucinations, ritualistic behaviour and other autistic features. Another small cohort study ($n = 18$) of behaviours among fragile-X males revealed similar findings. Stereotyped behaviour and mannerisms were most commonly reported (44%), followed by hyperactivity (33%), inappropriate interpersonal behaviour (33%), withdrawal (28%), unacceptable vocal habits (28%), unacceptable eccentric habits, and antisocial behaviour (22%).

Rebellious, untrustworthy, violent, destructive, self-abusive, psychologically disturbed are other descriptions but none show sexually aberrant behaviour.

Much interest and also controversy has been generated regarding the suggestion that autism and fragile-X syndrome may be associated. Case reports and many studies have been published in the literature addressing this particular issue, and this has become a battlefield where the conceptual debate regarding the existence of behavioural phenotype is currently being fought. Turk, in a review, summarized the studies that addressed the relationship between autism and fragile-X syndrome.[42] The prevalence of fragile-X syndrome among subjects with autism was estimated in 16 studies. The number of cohorts in these studies varied between 18 and 144; only two included population-based samples. The prevalence figures varied between 0% (in three studies) and 22.7%, the recent figures ranging between 2% and 3%. Four studies estimated prevalence of autism among patients with fragile-X syndrome. The number of cohorts ranged between 14 and 50 and the prevalence ranged between 7% and 69.2% with a mean of 34.8%. It is worth keeping in mind that 14.3% of learning disabled children also have autism according to DSM3-R.[43] Therefore, it is unclear whether the association between autism and fragile-X syndrome is a reflection of an association between autism and learning disability. These above-mentioned studies are riddled with methodological problems, the main one being the lack of appropriately matched control groups. Three studies used a control group; the number of cohorts being 15, 17 and 45, respectively. In two studies no significant difference was found in the prevalence of autism in fragile-X syndrome and the control group. In the third study, however, there was a significantly higher prevalence of autism found among the fragile-X group ($n = 17$) when compared with the controls.

The types of autistic features described among the fragile-X subjects are as follows: echolalia, perseverative speech, self-injurious behaviour (most notably hand-biting, hand flapping and scratching), poor eye contact (active gaze avoidance), profound delays in initiative and symbolic play, stereotyped and repetitive behaviour, social anxiety, pervasive lack of ability to relate to others, and perseverative preoccupations and interests. Another area of controversy is the suggested association between fragile-X syndrome and attention deficit hyperactivity disorder (ADHD). Most reports showed lack of hyperactivity and concentration being the two most important behavioural correlates of fragile-X syndrome which are present even in intellectually normal subjects with fragile-X syndrome. Turk and Hill suggested that while boys with fragile-X syndrome are not generally more overactive than other children with similar learning disabilities, they show impaired concentration with more restlessness and fidgetiness.[44]

Subtle social and psychological disabilities have been reported in intellectually normal female carriers.[45] Psychotic problems, shyness, anxiety, schizotypal features and intermittent depressive disorder have all been shown to be significantly higher among female carriers than the control group. However, Reiss and Freund recently suggested a behavioural phenotype for fragile-X syndrome which is distinct from both autism and ADHD yet incorporates behaviours from both syndromes.[46] The suggested syndrome includes the following behaviours: dysfunction in social play, verbal communication (e.g. rate, volume, word/phrase perseveration, etc.), nonverbal communication (e.g. gaze aversion, gesturing, etc.), repetitive motor behaviours (e.g. hand flapping, hand biting, rocking), attention deficit, hyperactivity, poor mathematical skills, abnormal sensitivity to external stimuli (including hyperacusis) and increased mouthing or smelling of objects. The neurobiological explanation for this behavioural phenotype remains unknown, although recent neuro-imaging studies showed cerebellar vermis dystrophy with associated dilatation of fourth ventricle and other abnormalities in the brains of individuals with fragile-X syndrome.[21]

Other Possible Behavioural Phenotypes

Nyhan possibly described the term behavioural phenotype first when he proposed an association between excessive self-injurious behaviour and Lesch–Nyhan syndrome which is caused by an inborn error of purine metabolism.[47] Some observed autistic features like delayed social and communicatory skills, difficulties in using gestural or sign systems, and possibly sleep problems in subjects with Angelman syndrome even when learning disability is taken into account.[44] Smith–Magenis syndrome causes moderate learning disability and is associated with an interstitial deletion of 17p11.2. Common physical features include brachycephaly, midfacial hypoplasia, ear malformation and brachydactyly. A characteristic behavioural phenotype including aggression, self-injurious behaviour such as head-banging and head-biting, onychotillomania (pulling out of fingernails and toenails), polyembolokilamania (insertion of foreign objects into various bodily orifices) and severe sleep disturbance has been described.[48] Finucane and colleagues recently reported a behaviour which they called 'self-hugging' and described as the 'spasmodic upper-body squeeze' which they claimed to be characteristic of the syndrome.[48]

FG syndrome is an X-linked, incompletely recessive complexly pliotrophic syndrome with considerably variable expressivity.[49] The syndrome is associated with moderate learning disability, hypotonia, cleft palate, congenital contractures, rare nystagmus, occasional seizure and sensorineural deafness. People with FG syndrome are described as 'busy', mischievous, impulsive, hyperactive, impatient, gregarious and some show maladaptive behaviours such as biting, crying, throwing tantrums, being aggressive, hyperresponsive, and overaroused; they show moderate to severe sensory hypersensitivity and tend to touch everything indiscriminately. Many children with tuberous sclerosis (TS) tend to show autistic features in the form of social aloofness, noncommunicativeness and obsessive behaviours. Overactivity, aggression and destructive outbursts have also been observed among TS children. As epilepsy, particularly infantile spasm, is quite common in TS, some of the behavioural problems may originate directly from ictal disturbance.[50] Sleep problems, such as difficulty in settling and waking, are often associated with the seizures. It is worth emphasizing, however, that learning disabled adults with epilepsy do not show significantly increased psychopathology when compared with learning disabled adults who do not suffer from epilepsy.[51]

It has been hypothesized that sex hormones have a specific effect on the development of the brain areas subserving particular cognitive skills. The brains of the children with Turner syndrome (45 XO) develop in the absence of sex hormones. These children show poorer performance than verbal skills (difference between 11% and 14.5%), although the overall intellectual deficit, if any, is very subtle.[52] Some reported hyperactivity, difficulty in social interaction and emotional problems in subjects with Turner's syndrome. In contrast, subjects with Klinefelter's syndrome (47 XXY) show poor verbal skill but relatively intact nonverbal skill. Their intellectual ability is often at the average or low-average end. Other behavioural characteristics such as lack of assertiveness, introversion, tendency to have low levels of activity and withdrawal from group activities, and apprehension and feelings of insecurity in peer relationships have been reported among these subjects.[44] Subjects with XYY syndrome tend to have dull normal intelligence, show excessive problem with temper tantrums, impaired social relationships and have language and reading difficulties. Violent crime does not appear to be a characteristic feature of this syndrome.

Noonan's syndrome (NS) is an autosomal dominant genetic disorder featuring cardiac anomaly, facial abnormality, short stature and learning disability. A behavioural phenotype has been described in this syndrome. Subjects with NS can be clumsy, stubborn, irritable, faddy eaters, show communication problems, have problematic peer relationships, show mood swings, echolalia, sleep difficulty, anxiety, severe aggression, autistic features and inappropriate sexual behaviour.[53] The oculocerebrorenal syndrome of Lowe (OCRL) is an X-linked disorder characterized by congenital cataract, learning disability and renal tubular dysfunction. The subjects have moderate learning disability, some show temper tantrums, stubbornness, stereotyped movement disorder (especially repetitive shaking of limbs), irritability, a high-pitched scream, impaired socialization skills and self-injurious behaviour. There have been reports of behaviours such as hyperactivity, clumsiness, poor coordination, articulation problems, social difficulties, sleep problems, tantrums and attention deficit in subjects with Soto's syndrome. However, when a controlled group of learning disabled subjects without the syndrome had been studied no significant excess of these behaviours was shown to exist among subjects with this syndrome.[44] Brunner and colleagues described borderline learning disability, impulsive aggressive behaviour, arson, attempted rape, exhibitionism associated with complete and selective deficiency of monoamine oxidase A (MAOA) activity caused by a point mutation in the structural gene for MAOA.[54]

Discussion

In this chapter I have described no less than 20 different learning disability syndromes in which some type of behavioural phenotype had been reported, although not in all cases has the genetic abnormality yet been detected. There have also been reports of possible behavioural phenotype being associated with another 12 or 13 syndromes of learning disability, namely Aicardi syndrome, Cri-du-chat syndrome, Duchenne muscular dystrophy, 15q-marker chromosome syndrome, classical galactosaemia, hypomelanosis of Ito, Marfan syndrome, mucopolysaccharide disorder (Hunter, Hurler and Sanfilippo syndrome), neurofibromatosis type 1, Ring chromosome 15 syndrome, Rubinstein–Taybi syndrome, 47 XXX syndrome and trisomy 8.[47] Of these 33 syndromes, there are only half a dozen or so conditions in which the genuine possibility of an association with a behavioural phenotype is gaining ground. These are fragile-X syndrome, Rett syndrome, Lesch–Nyhan syndrome, Prader–Willi syndrome, Williams syndrome, Brachmann–de Lange syndrome and possibly Angelman syndrome. And of these, fragile-X syndrome is the one where most research has been concentrated.

A pattern is emerging from the behaviours which have been described under many behavioural phenotypes. These often involve cognition, speech and language, social anxiety and problem with social interaction, lack of concentration and hyperactivity, sleep problems, an abnormal response to external stimulus, such as hyperacusis, and maladaptive behaviours such as temper tantrum, aggression and self-injurious behaviour. Cognitive deficits revealed two patterns. First, the wide distribution of IQ which is shown to be a feature of almost all the learning disability syndromes. Second, a discrepancy between the score in IQ tests of verbal and performance subscales. In some syndromes the score on verbal subscales tends to be much lower than performance subscales. This is apparent in Cri-du-chat syndrome, Ring chromosome 15 syndrome, Prader–Willi syndrome, Joubert syndrome, XXY or Klinefelter's syndrome and possibly XYY syndrome. Conversely, in fragile-X syndrome, Williams syndrome, Turner's syndrome (XO), Marfan syndrome and neurofibromatosis type 1 the score on verbal subscales in general tends to supersede that of performance subscales. This trend is also seen in autism and Asperger's syndrome and is associated with nonverbal learning disability (NLD) described by Rourke.[55]

A commonly described behaviour in many learning disability syndromes is social anxiety and a lack of two-way social interaction sometimes amounting to a full syndrome of autism. Autism and autistic behaviours have been described in fragile-X syndrome, Brachman de Lange syndrome, Rett syndrome, Joubert syndrome, Angelman syndrome, tuberous sclerosis, Noonan's syndrome, 15q-marker chromosome syndrome, hypomelanosis of Ito and possibly in untreated phenylketonuria, Williams syndrome, Turner's syndrome, oculocerebrorenal syndrome of Lowe and Soto's syndrome. It is becoming clear that autism and autistic features are caused by many conditions and there is a strong genetic predisposition for this disorder. Another commonly described behaviour among people with learning disability is a lack of concentration and hyperactivity which has been found in at least 12 different learning disability syndromes. A hypothesis that minimal brain damage causes hyperactivity was postulated in the past. Language problems usually take two different forms: either lack of proper language development or the development of an abnormal language, usually in the form of echolalia or other disorders commonly found in autism. Sleep problems, such as sleep apnoea, are often due to organic cause, such as abnormal palate, epileptic seizure, cardiopulmonary disorders, adverse drug reaction, etc. There are many causes of maladaptive behaviours such as aggression and self-injurious behaviour in individuals with a learning disability. Some of the other behaviours described under behavioural phenotypes, such as lack of concentration, hyperactivity, language problems and verbal-performance cognitive discrepancy, could cause maladaptive behaviour. It is well known that the frequency of maladaptive behaviour increases with the severity of cognitive damage, which points towards underlying brain damage being the cause of maladaptive behaviour.

Many of the behaviours described under various behavioural phenotypes have also been commonly found among people with idiopathic learning disability. Many of these behaviours are also found across various genetic disorders. The full constellation of behaviour described within each behavioural phenotype is not found in all cases of a particular syndrome; not even the individual behaviours described under a behavioural phenotype could be found in all or even in a majority of cases of a particular syndrome. The same neuropsychological hypotheses, such as white matter disturbance, inter-hemispheric connection defect or disturbance in attentional system and information processing have been used repeatedly to explain many different behavioural phenotypes. Regardless of how a genetic disorder may give rise to a constellation of behaviour, it is conceivable that the common pathway must be either structural and/or functional disturbance of the brain.

Summary

The concept that a constellation of specific behaviours is associated with a specific genetic disorder is gaining ground. There are at least 33 syndromes of learning disabilities where a behavioural phenotype has been reported. Of these, fragile-X syndrome, Rett syndrome, Lesch–Nyhan syndrome, Prader–Willi syndrome, Williams syndrome and Brachman de Lange syndrome are the important ones. A proposed association between fragile-X syndrome and autism created most interest and at the same time provoked intense controversy. A pattern of behaviour affecting cognition (mainly verbal-performance discrepancy), language (often autistic type), lack of concentration and hyperactivity, sleep difficulties including sleep apnoea (often from an organic cause), social anxiety and problem with two-way social interaction, autism and autistic features, maladaptive behaviours, such as aggression and self-injurious behaviour, is emerging from the behaviours described under many behavioural phenotypes. Within-syndrome variation and inter-syndrome overlap of behaviours are commonly observed. Many of these behaviours are also reported in people with idiopathic learning disability. Most studies are riddled with methodological flaws, thus data presented here should be interpreted with caution. Although the mechanism by which a genetic disorder could cause the manifestation of a set of specific behaviours is largely unknown, the ultimate pathway must be the structure and the function of the brain. Most of these behaviours are not curable but could be remedied with appropriate educational and management programmes. Maladaptive behaviours could be managed by using behavioural programmes along with the judicious use of pharmacotherapy.[56]

References

1. Rosen M (1993) In search of the behavioral phenotype: a methodological note. *Mental Retardation* **31(3)**, 177–8.
2. Prader A, Labhart A & Willi H (1956) Ein Syndrom von Adipositas, Kleinwuchs, Kryptorchismus und Oligophrenic nach myatonieartigem Zustand im Neugeborenalter. *Schweizer Medizinische Wochenschrift* **86**, 1260–1.
3. Åkefeldt A, Gillberg C & Larsson C (1991) Prader–Willi syndrome in a Swedish rural county: epidemiological aspects. *Developmental Medicine and Child Neurology* **33**, 715–21.
4. Greenswag LR (1987) Adults with Prader–Willi syndrome: a survey of 232 cases. *Developmental Medicine and Child Neurology* **29**, 145–52.
5. Clarke DJ, Wates J & Corbett JA (1989) Adults with Prader–Willi syndrome: abnormalities of sleep and behaviour. *Journal of the Royal Society of Medicine* **82**, 21–4.
6. de Lange C (1933) Sur un type nouveau de dégénération (Typus Amstelodamensis). *Archives Médicin des Enfants* **36**, 713–9.
7. Brachmann W (1916) Ein Fall von symmetrischer Monodaktylie durch Ulnadefeckt mit symmetrischer Flughautbildung in den Ellenbeugen, sowie anderen Abnormalitaten. *Jahrbuch für Kinderheilkunde und Physische Eriehung* **84**, 224–35.
8. Jackson L, Kline AD & Barr MA et al. (1993) de Lange syndrome: a clinical review of 310 individuals. *American Journal of Medical Genetics* **47**, 940–6.
9. Ireland M, English C & Cross I et al. (1991) A *de novo* translocation t(3:17) (Q26.3;q23.1) in a child with Cornelia de Lange syndrome. *Journal of Medical Genetics* **28**, 639–40.
10. Bay C, Mauk J & Radcliffe J et al. (1993) Mild Brachmann–de Lange syndrome: delineation of the clinical phenotype and characteristic behaviours in a six-year old boy. *American Journal of Medical Genetics* **47**, 965–8.
11. Deb S (1995) Electrophysiological correlates of psychopathology in individuals with mental retardation and epilepsy. *Journal of Intellectual Disability Research* **39(2)**, 129–35.
12. Scriver CR & Clow CL (1980) Phenylketonuria: epitome of human biochemical genetics. *New England Journal of Medicine* **303(23)**, 1336–42.
13. Okano Y, Eisensmith RC & Güttler F et al. (1991) Molecular basis of phenotypic heterogeneity in phenylketonuria. *New England Journal of Medicine* **324**, 1232–8.
14. Cowie V (1971) Neurological and psychiatric aspects of phenylketonuria. In Bickel H, Hudson FP & Woolf LI (eds) *Phenylketonuria and Some other Inborn Errors of Amino Acid Metabolism.* Stuttgart: Georg Thieme Verlag.
15. Udwin O & Yule W (1991) A cognitive and behavioural phenotype in Williams syndrome. *Journal of Clinical and Experimental Neuropsychology* **13(2)**, 232–44.
16. Wechsler D (1974) Wechsler Intelligence Scale for Children – Revised. New York: Psychological Corporation.
17. Wilson B, Cockburn J & Baddeley A (1985) Rivermead Behavioural Memory Test. Reading: Thames Valley Test Company.
18. Sansom D, Krishnan VHR & Corbett J et al. (1993) Emotional and behavioural aspects of Rett syndrome. *Developmental Medicine and Child Neurology* **35**, 340–5.

19. Edwards BO, Fischer AQ & Flannery DB (1988) Joubert syndrome: early diagnosis by recognition of the behavioural phenotype and confirmation by cranial sonography. *Journal of Child Neurology* **3(4)**, 247–9.

20. Holroyd S, Reiss AL & Bryan N (1991) Autistic features in Joubert syndrome: a genetic disorder with agenesis of the cerebellar vermis. *Biological Psychiatry* **29**, 287–94.

21. Deb S (1995) Brain imaging in mental retardation. *Current Opinion in Psychiatry* **8**, 280–5.

22. Deb S, de Silva PN & Gemmell HG et al. (1992) Alzheimer's disease in adults with Down's syndrome: the relationship between cerebral blood flow equivalents and dementia. *Acta Psychiatrica Scandinavica* **86**, 340–5.

23. Penrose LS (1938) *A Clinical and Genetic Study of 1280 Cases of Mental Defect. Special Report, Number 229*. London: Medical Research Council.

24. Martin JP & Bell J (1943) A pedigree of mental defect showing sex-linkage. *Journal of Neurology and Psychiatry* **6**, 154–7.

25. Richards BW & Webb T (1982) The Martin–Bell–Renpenning syndrome. *Journal of Medical Genetics* **19**, 79.

26. Renpenning H, Gerrard JW & Zaleski WA et al. (1962) Familial sex-linked mental retardation. *Canadian Medical Association Journal* **87**, 954–6.

27. Fox P, Fox D & Gerrard JW (1980) X-linked mental retardation: Renpenning revisited. *American Journal of Medical Genetics* **7**, 491–5.

28. Lehrke R (1972) A theory of X-linkage of major intellectual traits. *American Journal of Mental Deficiency* **76**, 611–9.

29. Lubs HA (1969) A marker X chromosome. *American Journal of Human Genetics* **21**, 231–44.

30. Turner G, Engisch B & Lindsay DG et al. (1972) X-linked mental retardation without physical abnormality (Renpenning's syndrome) in sibs in an institution. *Journal of Medical Genetics* **9**, 324–30.

31. Harvey J, Judge C & Weiner S (1977) Familial X-linked mental retardation with an X chromosome abnormality. *Journal of Medical Genetics* **14**, 46–50.

32. Sutherland GR (1977) Fragile sites on human chromosomes; demonstration of their dependence on the type of tissue culture medium. *Science* **197**, 265–6.

33. Deb S & Cowie VA (1987) A case of mosaicism with fragile X and XXY components. *British Journal of Psychiatry* **150**, 700–2.

34. Verkerk AJMH, Pieretti M & Sutcliffe JS et al. (1991) Identification of a gene (*FMR-1*) containing a CGG repeat coincident with a breakpoint cluster region exhibiting length variation in fragile X syndrome. *Cell* **252**, 1179–81.

35. Yu S, Prichard M & Kremer E et al. (1991) Fragile X genotype characterised by an unstable region of DNA. *Science* **252**, 1179–81.

36. Oberlé I, Rousseau F & Heitz D et al. (1991) Instability of a 550-base pair DNA segment and abnormal methylation in fragile X syndrome. *Science* **252**, 1097–102.

37. Loesch DZ, Huggins R & Hay DA et al. (1993) Genotype–phenotype relationship in fragile X syndrome: a family study. *American Journal of Human Genetics* **53**, 1064–73.

38. Taylor AK, Safanda JF & Fall MZ et al. (1994) Molecular predictors of cognitive involvement in female carriers of fragile X syndrome. *Journal of American Medical Association* **271(7)**, 507–14.

39. Dunn LM (1965) Peabody Picture Vocabulary Test. Circle Pines, MN: American Guidance Service.

40. Theobold TM, Hay DA & Judge C (1987) Individual variation and specific cognitive deficits in the fragile X syndrome. *American Journal of Medical Genetics* **28**, 1–11.

41. Kaufman AS & Kaufman NL. Kaufman Assessment Battery for Children. Circle Pines, MN: American Guidance Service.

42. Turk J (1992) The fragile-X syndrome: on the way to a behavioural phenotype. *British Journal of Psychiatry* **160**, 24–35.

43. Deb S & Prasad KBG (1994) The prevalence of DSM3-R autistic disorder among the children with a learning disability in north-east of Scotland. *British Journal of Psychiatry* **165**, 395–9.

44. Turk J & Hill P (1995) Behavioural phenotypes in dysmorphic syndromes. *Clinical Dysmorphology* **4**, 105–15.

45. Freund LS, Reiss AL & Hagerman R et al. (1992) Chromosome fragility and psychopathology in obligate female carriers of the fragile X chromosome. *Archives of General Psychiatry* **49**, 54–60.

46. Reiss AL & Freund L (1992) Behavioural phenotype of fragile X syndrome: DSM-III-R autistic behaviour in male children. *American Journal of Medical Genetics* **43**, 35–46.

47. Udwin O & Dennis J (1995) Psychological and behavioural phenotypes in genetically determined syndromes: a review of research findings. In O'Brien G & Yule W (eds) *Behavioural Phenotypes*, pp. 90–208. London: MacKeith Press.
48. Finucane BM, Konar D & Haas-Gilver B *et al.* (1994) The spasmodic upper-body squeeze: a characteristic behaviour in Smith–Magenis syndrome. *Developmental Medicine and Child Neurology* **36(1)**, 78–83.
49. Opitz JM, Richieri-Costa A & Aase JM *et al.* (1988) FG syndrome update 1988: note of 5 new patients and bibliography. *American Journal of Medical Genetics* **30**, 309–28.
50. Hunt A & Dennis J (1987) Psychiatric disorder among children with tuberous sclerosis. *Developmental Medicine and Child Neurology* **29**, 190–8.
51. Deb S & Hunter D (1991) Psychopathology of people with mental handicap and epilepsy. *British Journal of Psychiatry* **159**, 822–34.
52. Temple CM & Carney RA (1993) Intellectual functioning of children with Turner syndrome: a comparison of behavioural phenotypes. *Developmental Medicine and Child Neurology* **35**, 691–8.
53. Wood A, Massarono A & Super M *et al.* (1995) Behavioural aspects and psychiatric findings in Noonan's syndrome. *Archives of Diseases in Childhood* **72**, 153–5.
54. Brunner HG, Nelen M & Breakfield XO *et al.* (1993) Abnormal behaviour associated with a point mutation in the structural gene for monoamine oxidase A. *Science* **262(5133)**, 578–80.
55. Ellis HD, Ellis DM & Deb S *et al.* (1994) A preliminary study of right hemisphere cognitive deficits and impaired social judgements among young people with Asperger syndrome. *European Child and Adolescent Psychiatry* **3(4)**, 255–66.
56. Deb S & Fraser W (1994) The use of psychotropic medication in people with learning disability: towards rational prescribing. *Human Psychopharmacology* **9**, 259–72.

5

Personality Disorders

Andrew H. Reid

Introduction

Personality and personality disorder are elusive concepts which have not been well-researched by psychiatrists. All too often the term 'personality disorder' becomes a pejorative label with no implications for treatment or services. If it is no more than that it would be better abandoned. That is not an option because, however imperfect our knowledge, we know that personality is one of the key issues in determining the success or otherwise of community living for adults with learning disability, and is equally important as physical dependency needs and frank psychiatric illness. We do, therefore, need to extend and consolidate our knowledge in this area, with a view to formulating practical treatment and management programmes.

To the layman, personality probably consists of characteristics which have been present since adolescence, are stable over time despite fluctuations in mood, are manifest in different environments and are clearly recognizable to friends and acquaintances.[1] Various conceptual models of personality have been elaborated over the years in an attempt to measure and classify these characteristics. Cattell's 16 Personality Factor Questionnaire[2] constructs a personality profile through a 100-question yes/no test. Eysenck developed a dimensional classification of personality into: Extroversion–Introversion, Neuroticism–Stability, Psychoticism–Stability, and Intelligence.

Various inventories have been devised to measure personality traits including the Maudsley Personality Inventory, the Eysenck Personality Inventory and, more recently, the Eysenck Personality Questionnaire. The Minnesota Multiphasic Personality Inventory (MMPI) is a lengthy inventory of some 550 subject-driven statements about attitudes, emotional reactions, physical and psychological symptoms, which is designed to identify people with serious personality disorders. There are also psychodynamic and social learning theories of personality which have never been validated or shown to be reliable and which are of little direct use in clinical practice. Tyrer[3] carried out a systematic series of studies into the classification, diagnosis, management and course of personality disorders using the Personality Assessment Schedule (PAS).

Most of these personality assessment schedules do, however, involve a component of self-report and subject participation and this is beyond the competence of people with any significant degree of learning disability.

Hence, personality disorder has been one of the least researched areas of learning disability psychiatry, and the few studies there are tend to be idiosyncratic and unscientific.

Personality Disorder in the Learning Disability Literature

Earl was a particularly sensitive and perceptive observer of people with learning disability and in his book *Subnormal Personalities*[4] he gives many vignettes which illustrate the range and significance of temperament and personality issues in adults with learning disability. He arbitrarily selects certain aspects of personality which he names 'weakness, simplicity, immaturity, irritability, schizoidia, viscosity, neurosis, psychopathy and psychosis'. He goes on to describe a 'moron battery' comprising two verbal and two nonverbal tests for diagnostic purposes.[4] Earl's language and the underlying theory now seems very dated and inappropriate but there is a shrewdness of observation and he was correct in attributing such primacy to issues of personality.

There was a component of Earl's clinical categories in the Camberwell study in 1979.[5] In this study 402 adults with learning disability resident in Camberwell were screened and a prevalence rate of personality disorder of 25.4% more or less evenly distributed across the adult age range from 15 years upwards was reported. The researcher considered he was able to use the then current ICD classification of personality disorder for many patients, although 'by far the largest number did not meet these criteria and could be subdivided between two additional categories which might be termed "impulsive behaviour " and "immature behaviour" '. Impulsive behaviour was defined as 'unpredictable and ill-directed actions without apparent regard to consequences and often with irritability, rapid mood changes and violent behaviour'. Immature behaviour was also defined in terms of impulsiveness but associated with 'a particular sensitivity to frustration with less adequate interpersonal relationships and marked tension and agitation. This latter group shows many of the characteristics of adolescence persisting into adult life.' The percentage classification of personality disorders in this study is given in Table 5.1.

Thereafter, Reid drew attention to the range of personality and temperamental characteristics in people with learning disability and commented that

Table 5.1. Personality disorder in adults with mental retardation.

	n	%
Anxious	23	22.5
Explosive	9	9.0
Immature/irritable	48	47.5
Impulsive	15	15.0
Paranoid	4	4.0
Schizoid	2	2.0
Total	101	

'a rational form of classification would be helpful but only if it could be shown to be based on objective, measurable and reproducible parameters and to have treatment and prognostic implications'.[6] A comprehensive Swedish population study found that there were major difficulties in establishing diagnostic criteria for personality disorders, particularly in adults with severe learning disability, and did not really address the issue.[7] A UK study of psychiatric disorder in middle-aged and elderly people with learning disability, noted that behaviour and personality disorders were the commonest disorders among both the long-stay and admission groups, with a male:female ratio of 2:1. However, personality disorders were not clearly separated or distinguished from behaviour disorders in this study.[8]

Meanwhile, investigators in the USA were carrying out a study of psychiatric disorders in a community-based sample of 115 retarded persons and reported that 27.1% suffered from a personality disorder.[9] They suggested that these personality disorders were based on extrinsic factors with no relationship to the intellectual impairment and hypothesized that normalizing humane approaches could somehow alleviate these traits. In parallel with this study, Zigler and his colleagues at Yale University were rightly emphasizing the critical importance of personality issues in learning disability. They drew attention to the need to take cognisance of psychopathology and dual diagnosis and were critical of excessive deference to concerns about stigma, pointing out that 'labels can often have positive consequences, particularly since they are often a necessary precondition to the receipt of services'.[10] They concluded that 'the personality make-up of mentally retarded persons is characterized by dependency upon others, approval-seeking behaviour, wariness of strangers, "outer-directed" problem-solving styles, low expectancy of success, low aspiration level and a low ideal self-image'. They commented that 'it is likely that these personality characteristics are responsible for the high rate of mental unhealth in mentally retarded persons'.

An interesting series of studies over the last decade has drawn on the Standardized Assessment of Personality (SAP) developed at the Institute of Psychiatry.[11] The SAP is an informant-based schedule designed to reflect the clinical approach of a psychiatrist interviewing a patient's informant. After a general introduction there is an exploratory section where the description of personality is ascertained, followed by seven standard questions if necessary. If certain 'key words' have been used, a series of questions appropriate to one or more personality types is used. The result of this Standard Assessment is the classification of the patient into either normal or one of the following abnormal personality types: self-conscious, schizoid, paranoid, cyclothymic, obsessional, anxious, sociopathic, explosive or hysterical (i.e. the categories in Section 301 of ICD-9 with the addition of anxious and self-conscious personality types[12]). The interviewer then establishes the grading of personality. A Grade 1 indicates that the personality can be matched by one of the types, and a Grade 2 that the patient is very unusual or handicapped by reason of this personality, i.e. they have a personality disorder. Features of more than one type may be present but the interviewer should establish which is the more dominant.

The SAP was subsequently shown to be a useful and substantially reliable instrument for rating personality in adults with learning disability, and was utilized in a study of 100 mildly (IQ 50–70) or moderately (IQ 35–49) retarded adults over the age of 16 years living in hospital.[13,14] The investigators did not consider that the SAP was applicable to adults with severer degrees of learning disability, in whom it can be very difficult to disentangle personality factors from the long-term sequelae of childhood psychiatric disorders, and suggested that a personality typology rooted more in developmental concepts might be more appropriate with them.[15] Using the questionnaire, 56% of the sample were rated as having an abnormal personality, and in 22% the abnormality was marked, suggesting the presence of frank personality disorder. The distribution and severity of the dominant personality abnormality in these 56 patients is shown in Table 5.2. The bulk of the abnormalities fell into the categories of affective, explosive and hysterical personality types, with smaller numbers of self-conscious, schizoid, sociopathic, paranoid and obsessional personality types. Since then the interview schedule has been modified to accord with ICD-10 but this modification has not been explored in the learning disability field.[16]

Finally, in an intriguing paper, personality and trait disturbances have been studied in a sample of 384 adults with learning disability in both community and institutional settings in south-western Ontario, Canada. The high prevalence of personality disorders was confirmed and a relationship postulated between specific clusters of personality disorders and the onset of frank psychiatric illness in later life. Treatment and prevention possibilities were considered, the need for a consensus on nomenclature was highlighted, and the use of the SAP as an appropriate interview schedule for future studies was endorsed.[17]

Table 5.2. Distribution of personality types in 100 mentally retarded adults.

| | Grading | | Total (sum of Grades 1 and 2) | Male | Female | Epilepsy |
	1	2				
Anxious	0	0	0	0	0	0
Cyclothymic	7	4	11	3	8	3
Explosive	12	5	17	13	4	7
Hysterical	5	7	12	5	7	2
Neurasthenic	0	1	1	1	0	0
Obsessional	2	0	2	1	1	1
Paranoid	0	2	2	1	1	1
Schizoid	4	0	4	4	0	0
Self-conscious	3	0	3	2	1	1
Sociopathic	1	3	4	2	2	0
Total						
Abnormal	34	22	56	32	24	15
Normal	–	–	44	19	25	10

Current Classifications

The two classifications of mental disorder currently in use are DSM-IV published by the American Psychiatric Association[18] and ICD-10 published by WHO.[19] The latter is in more general use in the UK.

DSM-IV codes personality disorders on Axis II and defines and recognizes the following categories:

- 301.0   Paranoid personality disorder (276)
- 301.20   Schizoid personality disorder (277)
- 301.22   Schizotypal personality disorder (278)
- 301.7   Antisocial personality disorder (279)
- 301.83   Borderline personality disorder (280)
- 301.50   Histrionic personality disorder (281)
- 301.81   Narcissistic personality disorder (282)
- 301.82   Avoidant personality disorder (283)
- 301.6   Dependent personality disorder (284)
- 301.4   Obsessive–compulsive personality disorder (285)
- 301.9   Personality disorder NOS (286)

ICD-10 differentiates personality disorders from enduring personality changes as follows. 'These types of condition comprise deeply ingrained and enduring behaviour patterns, manifesting themselves as inflexible responses to a broad range of personal and social situations. They represent either extreme or significant deviations from the way the average individual in a given culture perceives, thinks, feels and, in particular, relates to others. Such behaviour patterns tend to be stable and to encompass multiple domains of behaviour and psychological functioning. They are frequently, but not always, associated with various degrees of subjective distress and problems in social functioning and performance.

'Personality disorders differ from personality change in their timing and the mode of their emergence: they are developmental conditions, which appear in childhood or adolescence and continue into adulthood. They are not secondary to another mental disorder or brain disease, although they may precede and co-exist with other disorders. In contrast, personality change is acquired, usually during adult life, following severe or prolonged stress, extreme environmental deprivation, serious psychiatric disorder, or brain disease or injury.'

ICD-10 defines and recognizes the following categories of specific personality disorder:

- F60.0   Paranoid personality disorder
- F60.1   Schizoid personality disorder
- F60.2   Dissocial personality disorder
- F60.3   Emotionally unstable personality disorder
          .30 Impulsive type
          .31 Borderline type
- F60.4   Histrionic personality disorder
- F60.5   Anancastic personality disorder

- F60.6   Anxious (avoidant) personality disorder
- F60.7   Dependent personality disorder
- F60.8   Other specific personality disorders
- F60.9   Personality disorder, unspecified

Cyclothymia and schizotypal disorders are now classified with the affective disorders and schizophrenia, respectively. Enduring personality change following catastrophic experience and after psychiatric illness are classified separately (F62.0 and F62.1). There is also a code for personality and behavioural disorders caused by brain disease, damage and dysfunction – 'organic personality disorder' (FO7.0).

Both the DSM-IV and ICD-10 classifications represent an improvement on previous classifications and lend themselves to research in learning disability. However, there has been no systematic study of their applicability in this field.

Clinical Aspects

General Considerations

There is an enormous variation in personality and temperament in adults with learning disability and Reid's comments are still true: 'Some retarded patients may be abnormally shy and withdrawn by nature and this may sometimes be a function of institutionalization; others may be excessively friendly and forward. Some are timid, others are touchy, irritable, liable to lose their temper and quickly provoked to aggression. Some are impatient and cannot brook delays. Some are excessively quarrelsome; others are passive and cannot stand up for themselves. Some may be manipulative, bossy, obstinate and prone to sulks. An occasional patient may show traits of malicious sadism or masochism. Some chatter incessantly, others can be abnormally quiet to the point of selective mutism. Some are invincibly convinced of their superiority, others are all too aware of their educational failings. Many retarded people are charming, considerate and gentle and virtually all are likeable in some respect.'[6]

Reid comments that some of these attributes of personality and temperament are probably organically determined and related to structural brain damage. To date, there has been no systematic study of this, although ICD-10 does provide a possible framework within which to start. Contrary to popular assumptions, however, there is no obvious relationship with epilepsy. No evidence of any statistically significant increase in prevalence of personality disorder among the epileptic population was found in a study of 100 adults with learning disability.[14] There was a trend towards an association between epilepsy and explosiveness, but this trend did not attain statistical significance. These findings were substantially confirmed in a study of psychopathology in people with mental handicap and epilepsy in Aberdeen where the investigators were unable to find 'any significant difference in the prevalence of personality disorders between epileptic and non-epileptic patients'.[20] That said, most clinicians who have significant experience in the field of learning disability have encountered typical cases of 'epileptic personality' characterized by rigidity and egocentricity, moodiness, explosive irritability, pedantry, circumstantiality, argumentativeness and religiosity.[21] The significance of the small number of individual cases such as these tends to be lost in large-scale, statistically based studies.

Issues of personality and temperament frequently play a key role in determining the success or otherwise of community living, management and quality of life, for adults with learning disability. Using Mann's SAP it was shown that 63% of a cohort group with either normal or only minimal personality abnormalities were successfully discharged from hospital within 1 year, compared with only 4.6% of those with definite personality disorder.[22] The Aberdeen group also concluded that 'personality disorder is a major exclusion criteria for the rehabilitation and integration of mentally handicapped people from hospital to community'.[20] As a corollary to these investigations, it has been demonstrated that serious personality disorder is the commonest diagnostic category among adults with learning disability leading to a requirement for care in hospital (Table 5.3).[23]

Antisocial Personality Disorder (Dissocial Personality Disorder; Asocial, Psychopathic, Sociopathic, Personality Disorder)

There is a small but well-recognized group of adults with mild learning disability, predominantly but not exclusively male, who come within this rubric and who pose major problems of management, containment and public safety, in whatever residential milieu they live. Their behaviour is characterized by a callous lack of concern for the feelings of others, gross irresponsibility and disregard for social norms and obligations, inability to maintain enduring relationships, a very low tolerance of frustration and a

Table 5.3. ICD-9 psychiatric diagnosis and long-term hospital care needs of 100 mentally handicapped people.

	Number with main psychiatric diagnosis	Number needing in-patient care
Organic psychosis (290,294)	3	0
Schizophrenia (295)	5	1
Affective psychosis (296)	5	2
Paranoid states (297)	3	0
Psychosis of childhood (299)	12	8
Personality disorder (301)	17	8
Sexual deviation and disorders (302)	4	2
Special symptoms or syndrome (307)	5	0
Non-psychotic mental disorder following brain damage	2	0
Disturbance of conduct (312)	15	0
Hyperkinetic syndrome of childhood (314)	9	7
None	20	2

low threshold for violence and aggression, an inability to experience guilt or to profit from experience or punishment, and a tendency to blame others for their errant behaviour. On interviewing these patients the lack of any sense of right or wrong, and of moral responsibility, can be deep-rooted, obvious and pervasive. This inability to empathize with the feelings of others, and a lack of imagination as to the consequences of their behaviour, can lead to serious considerations of public safety for which treatment efforts are of uncertain efficacy and have to be secondary to considerations of security and containment. Some of these psychopathic adults with learning disability are to be found among the population of persistent fire-raisers and sex offenders (particularly offenders with children).[24] The Reed Report specifically recognizes the need for medium secure services for small but significant numbers of such patients.[25] These issues are more fully considered in Chapter 12.

Phenotypic Personalities

As our knowledge of genetics has developed, there has been increasing interest in phenotypic (genetic) personality attributes and profiles.[26]

Down's Syndrome

People with Down's syndrome are traditionally said to be charming, friendly, affable, given to mimicry and free of personality problems. That may sometimes be so but with the increase in life expectancy it has become clear that this stereotype is only partly true, and people with Down's syndrome are prone to a range of psychiatric disorders including personality problems, affective disorders and Alzheimer's disease.[27]

Fragile-X Syndrome

Fragile-X is predominantly, but not exclusively, a syndrome of males. Sufferers may show certain personality characteristics including sensory defensiveness, social anxiety, speech and language abnormalities including delayed echolalia and repetitive speech, stereotypy and insistence on routine.[28] These characteristics have lain behind the association of fragile-X syndrome with autistic type disorders.

Prader–Willi Syndrome

People with Prader–Willi syndrome show, in addition to the disturbed behaviour related to hyperphagia, impairments in psychosocial adjustments and relationships, perhaps related to sensitivity about physical appearance, and also feelings of worthlessness and inferiority. Other characteristics are said to include skin-picking, belligerence, stubbornness, irritability and impulsiveness.[29]

Other Associations

There are many other associations: self-injury by biting in the Lesch–Nyhan syndrome, 'chatterbox' phenomena in hydrocephalus, and unprovoked laughing in the Angelman (puppet) syndrome. Criminality and tall stature has been linked with the XYY syndrome although the association has now been questioned and appears to be linked more with impulsivity.

Summary

Studies into phenotypic personality are problematic but potentially very informative. They need to be longitudinal, based on large numbers and carefully controlled, otherwise there is the possibility of faulty stereotypes about genetically determined personality and behaviour which can breed therapeutic nihilism.

Treatment and Management

There are no reliably effective treatment techniques for personality disorder, whether it be in people of normal intelligence or with learning disability. This is hardly surprising bearing in mind the deeply ingrained and long-standing nature of the disorder inherent in the definition. In general, as much depends on the temperament and aptitude of the therapist, as on any particular treatment technique. One should never underestimate the potential benefits to be derived from an improved and more normal quality of life for the person with learning disability. What may be labelled as originating in personality disorder may be the consequence of deprived, artificial and unsatisfying lifestyles.

It is important also to identify and treat any associated psychiatric disorder such as a functional psychosis, bereavement or a dementia, for example. The underlying personality structure may modify and influence the presentation, and the response to treatment, but that does not lessen the importance of establishing and diagnosing these associated psychiatric conditions.

Insight-based Psychotherapy

Individual, group and family therapy may all have a potential contribution to make. In recent years there has been increasing interest in the applicability of these treatment techniques to people with learning disability and there has been some progress. The group setting is particularly suitable for patients with associated neurotic difficulties; family therapy is an appropriate forum in which to explore issues such as the loss of the anticipated perfect child, and the family life-cycle.[30, 31]

Behaviour Therapy

People with learning disabilities, whether or not there is an associated personality disorder, may benefit from a range of behavioural treatment techniques including social skills training, assertiveness training, cognitive therapy and anger management. The experience of progress, achievement and success can modify some external manifestations of personality disorder.

Occupational Therapy, Time Structuring and Vocational Training

Learning disabled adults with personality disorder benefit, as does the rest of the population, from the experience of meaningful training, a structured day and gainful activity. Occupational therapists have a particularly important contribution to make in this area.

Drug Treatments

There are no established psychopharmacological treatments for personality disorder but any secondary or associated psychiatric disorders should be identified and treated with appropriate medication. There are some nonspecific indications for treatment with psychoactive drugs, and more are likely to emerge. There are anecdotal reports of the successful treatment of aggression with neuroleptics, and drug trials showing benefit from such preparations as thiothixene, haloperidol and trifluoperazine for brief psychotic episodes and episodes of severe behaviour dyscontrol.[32,33] Investigators have reported some response to the treatment of 'characterological' depression with tricyclic antidepressants and monoamineoxidase inhibitors.[34,35] Lithium has been shown to have a usual effect on some retarded people with problems of hyperactivity, aggression and self-mutilation.[36] In some patients self-injury appears at least partly to be an obsessional phenomenon and there may be some response to treatment with clomipramine. Benzodiazepines are largely contraindicated in the treatment of personality disorders because of their propensity to cause rage reactions.[37] The newer anticonvulsants such as carbamazepine, and β-blockers, have been reported as beneficial in dyscontrol syndromes, rage reactions, impulsive assaultiveness, self-injury and mutilation by cutting.[38] The newer generation of selective serotonin re-uptake inhibitors (SSRIs) may also have a contribution to make in the management of nonspecific aggressiveness, but this has yet to be established in the field of learning disability. The topic has been recently extensively reviewed.[37,41]

Containment and Limit Setting

Most people with learning disability and an associated personality disorder pose management problems for their carers, and diminish the quality of their own lives through their personality disorder, but do not pose any great hazard to the public. A few with antisocial personality disorder may, however, pose some hazard and for them the treatment and management approach has to be set against a background of issues such as limit setting, containment and, if necessary, detention under the Mental Health Act. The priority then becomes the most acceptable quality of life for the individual concerned, which is consonant with public safety. Management of these people requires qualities of consistency, goal setting and rewards which are earned in response to the establishment of sustained socially acceptable behaviour patterns. This can be a time-consuming and painfully slow process.

References

1. Freeman CPL (1993) Personality disorders. In Kendell RE & Zealley AK (eds) *Companion to Psychiatric Studies*, 5th edn, pp. 587–615. Edinburgh: Churchill Livingstone.
2. Cattell PB & Butcher HJ (1968) *The Prediction of Achievement and Creativity*. London: Bobbs-Merrill.
3. Tyrer P (1988) *Personality Disorders: Diagnosis, Management and Course*. London: Butterworth/Wright.
4. Earl CJC (1961) *Subnormal Personalities: Their Clinical Investigation and Assessment*. London: Baillière, Tindall and Cox.
5. Corbett JA (1979) Psychiatric morbidity and mental retardation. In James FE & Snaith RP (eds) *Psychiatric Illness and Mental Handicap*, pp. 11–25. London: Gaskell Press.
6. Reid AH (1982) *Psychiatry and Mental Handicap*, pp. 111–4. Oxford: Blackwell Scientific Publications.
7. Gostason R (1985) Psychiatric illness among the mentally retarded: a Swedish population study. *Acta Psychiatrica Scandinavica Supplement* No. 318.
8. Day K (1985) Psychiatric disorder in the middle-aged and elderly mentally handicapped. *British Journal of Psychiatry* **147**, 660–7.
9. Eaton LF & Menolascino FJ (1982) Psychiatric disorders in the mentally retarded: types, problems and challenges. *American Journal of Psychiatry* **139**, 1297–303.
10. Zigler E & Burack JA (1989) Personality development and the dually diagnosed. *Research in Developmental Disabilities* **10**, 225–40.
11. Mann AH, Jenkins R, Cutting JC & Cowan PJ (1981) The development and use of a standardised assessment of abnormal personality. *Psychological Medicine* **11**, 829–47.
12. World Health Organization (1978) Mental disorders: glossary and guide to their classification in accordance with the ninth revision of the international classification of disease. Geneva: WHO.
13. Ballinger BR & Reid AH (1987) A standardized assessment of personality disorder in mental handicap. *British Journal of Psychiatry* **152**, 577.
14. Reid AH & Ballinger BR (1987) Personality disorder in mental handicap. *Psychological Medicine* **17**, 983–7.
15. Dana L (1993) Personality disorder in persons with mental retardation: assessment and diagnosis. In Fletcher RJ & Dosen A (eds) *Mental Health Aspects of Mental Retardation*, pp. 130–40. New York: Lexington Books.
16. Pilgrim J & Mann A (1990) Use of the ICD-10 version of the Standardized Assessment of Personality to determine the prevalence of personality disorder in psychiatric in-patients. *Psychological Medicine* **20**, 986–92.
17. Goldberg B, Gitta MZ & Puddephatt A (1995) Personality and trait disturbances in an adult mental retardation population: significance for psychiatric management. *Journal of Intellectual Disability Research* **39**, 284–94.

18. APA (1994) *Diagnostic Criteria from DSM-IV*. Washington DC: American Psychiatric Association.
19. WHO (1992) *ICD-10. Classification of Mental and Behavioural Disorders*. Geneva: World Health Organisation.
20. Deb S & Hunter D (1991) Psychopathology of people with mental handicap and epilepsy. III: Personality disorder. *British Journal of Psychiatry* **159**, 830–4.
21. Batchelor IRC (1994) *Henderson and Gillespie's Textbook of Psychiatry*, 10th edn, pp. 430–1. London: Oxford University Press.
22. Ballinger BR & Reid AH (1988) Standardized assessment of personality in mental handicap. *British Journal of Psychiatry* **152**, 577.
23. Ballinger BR, Ballinger CB, Reid AH & McQueen E (1991) The psychiatric symptoms, diagnoses and care needs of 100 mentally handicapped patients. *British Journal of Psychiatry* **158**, 251–4.
24. Day K (1984) Male mentally handicapped sex offenders. *British Journal of Psychiatry* **165**, 630–9.
25. Reed J (1994) Report of the Working Group on High Security and Related Psychiatric Provision. London: Department of Health.
26. Einfeld SL & Aman M (1995) Issues in the taxonomy of psychopathology in mental retardation. *Journal of Autism and Developmental Disorders* **25**, 143–67.
27. Holland AJ (1994) Down's syndrome and Alzheimer's disease. In Bouras N (ed) *Mental Health in Mental Retardation: Recent Advances and Practices*, pp. 154–67. Cambridge: Cambridge University Press.
28. Turk J, Hagerman RJ, Barnicoat A & McEvoy J (1994) The fragile X syndrome. In Bouras N (ed) *Mental Health in Mental Retardation: Recent Advances and Practices*, pp. 135–53. Cambridge: Cambridge University Press.
29. Fraser W & Nolan M (1994) Psychiatric disorders in mental retardation. In Bouras N (ed) *Mental Health in Mental Retardation: Recent Advances and Practices*, pp. 79–92. Cambridge: Cambridge University Press.
30. Sinason V (1990) Individual psychoanalytical psychotherapy with severely and profoundly handicapped patients. In Dosen A, Van Gennep A & Zwanniken G (eds) *Treatment of Mental Illness and Behavioural Disorder in the Mentally Retarded*, pp. 71–80. The Netherlands: Logon.
31. Hollins S, Sinason V & Thompson S (1994) Individual, group and family psychotherapy. In Bouras N (ed) *Mental Health in Mental Retardation: Recent Advances and Practices*, pp. 233–43. Cambridge: Cambridge University Press.
32. Goldberg SC, Schulz SC & Schulz PM *et al.* (1986) Borderline and schizotypal personality disorders treated with low dose thiothixene vs placebo. *Archives of General Psychiatry* **43**, 680–6.
33. Soloff PH (1981) Pharmacotherapy of borderline disorders. *Comprehensive Psychiatry* **22**, 535–43.
34. Akiskal HS, Rosenthal TL & Haykal RF (1980) Clinical and sleep EEG findings separating 'subaffective dysthymias' from 'character spectrum disorders'. *Archives of General Psychiatry* **37**, 777–93.
35. Cowdry R & Gardner DL (1988) Pharmacotherapy of borderline personality disorder. *Archives of General Psychiatry* **45**, 111–9.
36. Wickham EA & Reed JV (1987) Lithium in the control of aggression and self mutilating behaviour. *International Clinical Psychopharmacology* **2**, 181–90.
37. Stein G (1993) Drug treatment of the personality disorders. In Tyrer P & Stein G (eds) *Personality Disorder Reviewed*, pp. 262–304. London: Gaskell/Royal College of Psychiatrists.
38. Ratey JJ, Mikkelsen EJ & Smith GB *et al.* (1986) Beta-blockers in the severely and profoundly retarded. *Journal of Clinical Psychopharmacology* **6**, 103–7.
39. Reid AH, Naylor GJ & Kay DSG (1981) A double-blind, placebo controlled, crossover trial of carbamazepine in overactive, severely mentally handicapped patients. *Psychological Medicine* **11**, 109–13.
40. Gardner DL & Cowdry RW (1986) Positive effects of carbamazepine on behavioural dyscontrol in borderline personality disorder. *American Journal of Psychiatry* **143**, 519–22.
41. Crabbe HF (1994) Pharmacotherapy in mental retardation. In Bouras N (ed) *Mental Health in Mental Retardation: Recent Advances and Practices*, pp. 187–204. Cambridge: Cambridge University Press.

6

Organic Behaviour Disorder

Stephen G. Read

The nosological disorders of general psychiatry are useful for the diagnosis of learning disabled people down to an IQ of about 50. It is about 50 because the transformation between severely learning disabled and mildly learning disabled people is made over a broader range of IQ than is indicated by the expression of a single number such as IQ 50. Nevertheless, it is at about IQ 50 that the transition occurs and this is because at that stage there is a serious loss of speech and communication ability. Mildly learning disabled people can therefore also be said to suffer from schizophrenia, from personality disorders and from bipolar disorders and autism. All of these conditions can give rise to aggressive and self-injurious behaviour. The corollary of this is that when we are confronted by aggressive behaviour in mildly learning disabled people, we should seek to explain this by using the diagnostic categories of general psychiatry which include the above nosological disorders. It may be difficult to reach a diagnosis because of difficulties with communication in this group but, nevertheless, theoretically and in practice a diagnosis is usually possible, given patience and the use of simple vocabulary.

However, the situation changes below around IQ 50 because of the distinct and calamitous loss of language and communication abilities. It is generally accepted that it is not possible to diagnose schizophrenia below an IQ of about 50 (although this border is being pushed back) or at any rate in a situation where a person is incapable of describing their own mental events as a series of self-reports. Likewise, it is thought inappropriate to refer to people below IQ 50 who have considerably diminished capacity to form a full personality, the term 'personality disorder' and this is usually avoided. However, there are three diagnostic groups which appear to be applicable to those people below IQ 50 who show extremely severely disordered, or loosely termed 'psychotic', behaviour; these are manic depressive psychosis, autism and organic behaviour disorder.

Manic depressive psychosis is diagnosed mainly on the likelihood of a possible mania being the explanatory factor in a person's severe aggressive behaviour by the concomitant or previous existence of a depressive disorder, which is diagnosable even in people down to and including profound learning disability. There is, of course, an almost total preoccupation in diagnosis with biological symptoms but, nevertheless, it is quite possible to make a diagnosis of depression and hence there is a possibility of bipolar disorder in somebody who is displaying overactivity and aggression. It is very difficult in itself to differentiate a manic disorder from an organic behaviour disorder in the absence of any suggestion from past history that depression has been present. However, there may be indicators, in the presence of euphoria, that a manic state persists, as a euphoric attitude is seemingly uncommon in those people who suffer from organic behaviour disorder yet produce very similar destructive and aggressive behaviour.

Autism should be more readily definable as a separate entity because of the personal characteristics and the communication deficits, but in the severely handicapped many have made the mistake of diagnosing an autistic person who also has explosively violent behaviour as suffering from organic behaviour disorder. Autism and manic depressive disorder are a part of general psychiatric nosology which continues with validity into the group of learning disabled people with low IQs. However, organic behaviour disorder is a diagnosis which is limited to people with IQ below 50. Organic behaviour disorder is understood to be a biological psychiatric condition which produces a characteristic clinical picture of violence and self-injury through a final common pathway imposed upon a number of different possible aetiologies.

It is a moot point as to whether this condition conforms to the requirements of the term 'psychosis', although often in the past and sometimes still today it is referred to as 'organic psychosis'. It is certainly a disorder, but not perhaps in itself what is understood to be a mental illness. It may be unfortunate that it has a psychological terminology including the words 'behaviour disorder', but at least the term 'organic' suggests that it is produced by brain damage. The former might suggest that the behaviour is a result of aberrant learning but the latter suggests that cerebral impairment is the cause.

Epidemiology

There is no distinct category within either Diagnostic and Statistical Manual, 4th Edn (DSM-IV), or International Classification of Diseases, 10th Edn (ICD-10), for this peculiar condition. Although many practitioners may find that this is the most common condition with which they are concerned when severely learning disabled people are encountered, formal recognition has yet to be given to its existence. ICD-10 does have a category which could possibly be used and this is FO9, 'Unspecified Organic or Symptomatic Mental Disorder'. This is said to include organic psychosis not otherwise specified. It may not be seen as much of an advance to have gained such a small toe-hold within the ICD-10 compared with no recognition whatsoever, but it is likely that this is the start of the recognition of this syndrome. Conversely, DSM-IV does not appear to provide any diagnostic category which could be used for this purpose.

It is partly for this reason that diagnosis of behavioural disorders within a learning disabled population has been such an imprecise process. A large study was carried out in New York of learning disabled patients in institutions, in sheltered accommodation of all sorts and living at home.[1]

Jacobson examined 35 007 prescription returns relating to learning disabled people. Of this population 3341 representing 9.5% were classified as psychiatric. Of these psychiatric disorders 52.7% were unspecified. That is, 52.7% of 3341 learning disabled people were suffering from unspecified psychiatric disorder. The percentage of the psychiatric group who were taking medication was 62.3%. However, this formed only 25% of the total number of learning disabled people who were receiving psychotropic medication. That is, 75% of the subjects receiving psychotropic medication had received no psychiatric classification and of those who had received psychiatric classification 50% were unspecified. If this study is at all representative of practice in the field then it strongly suggests that the behaviour of learning disabled people, while considered sufficiently disordered to merit psychotropic drug treatment, is not receiving an accompanying diagnosis.

How then is it possible to assess the prevalence of this disorder among learning disabled people? It is necessary to look at specific studies on defined populations of learning disabled people to see what the incidence of disordered behaviour is amongst them. Sigafoos *et al.*[2] produced a survey of aggressive behaviour among a population of persons with intellectual disability in Queensland, Australia, in 1994. A total of 2412 individuals with intellectual disability were studied, of which 261 were identified who engaged in at least one form of aggressive behaviour. This yielded an overall prevalence of 11%. Most of these persons were described as functioning in the severe/profound (54%) or moderate (31%) range of intellectual disability; 34% displayed self-injury. There was a distinct difference between the relative prevalence of aggressive behaviour in institutionalized individuals (35%) when compared with those living in group homes (17%) or other community facilities (3%).

These results compare favourably with those of Harris,[3] who published a paper on the nature and extent of aggressive behaviour amongst people with learning difficulties in a single health district in 1993. The study group was 1362 people within the health district who were known to have a learning difficulty. Here, the overall prevalence of aggressive behaviour was 17.6% with, again, a markedly different rate being identified between hospitals in the district (38.2%) and day facilities (9.7%). Whereas Sigafoos *et al.*[2] found that the aggressive behaviour sample included a higher percentage of males (64%), Harris[3] found there was no significant evidence of an association between a person's gender and the presence of aggressive behaviour within schools or hospitals, but did identify a disproportionate number of men within day facilities.

A different approach was taken by Gillberg[4] and others who studied in a more detailed fashion a smaller number, this time of children, aged between 13 and 17 years. They examined 164 Swedish urban children with IQs of less than 70, born between 1966 and 1970. Gillberg *et al*[4] described seven main psychiatric conditions with which he classified this group: (1) psychotic behaviour, (2) depressive syndrome, (3) conduct disorder, (4) emotional disorder, (5) psychosomatic disorder, (6) hyperkinetic disorder, and (7) other psychiatric disorder. Tables 6.1 and 6.2 show the prevalence of the various psychiatric classifications, first for the severely learning disabled group and second for the mildly learning disabled group. The designation 'psychotic behaviour' was given to half of the severely learning disabled group. Only 26% of this group were thought not to suffer from a psychiatric disorder. A psychiatric prevalence rate of 64% is one of the highest for any group ever encountered. The frequency of psychotic disorder is three times higher in the severely learning disabled group than it is in the mildly learning disabled group. Conversely, the prevalence of neurotic disorders is considerably higher in the mildly learning disabled group than it is in the severely learning disabled group. Thus, what started out as a practical difference between the two groups based on language and IQ is shown upon further study to reflect a different distribution of psychiatric disorders between the two groups, severely and mildly learning disabled. Clearly, the two descriptions of 'psychotic behaviour' and 'aggression' are not the same. But the conclusion to be drawn from these studies would seem to be that there exists a highly significant proportion of severely mentally handicapped people who show such disordered behaviour as to be described as 'psychotic' and that some of this group show behaviour which is undoubtedly aggressive or violent and may include self-injury.

Table 6.1. Rates of psychiatric disorder in severe mental retardation.

	n	% Epilepsy	% Down's syndrome
Too severe to rate	7 (11%)	57	29
No psychiatric disorder	71 (26%)	0	53
Psychotic behaviour[a]	33 (50%)	39	12
Depressive disorder	1 (1.5%)	100	0
Emotional disorder	3 (4.5%)	0	67
Total psychiatric disorder (autism 5)	42 (64%)	33	17

[a]Calculated frequency for severe mental retardation (SMR) + psychotic disorder in general population = 0.15% in 13–17-year age range.

Table 6.2. Rates of psychiatric disorder in mild mental retardation.

	n	% Epilepsy	% Down's syndrome
No psychiatric disorder	36 (43%)	8	6
Psychotic behaviour[a]	12 (14%)	17	0
Depressive disorder	3 (4%)	0	0
Emotional disorder	8 (10%)	13	0
Conduct disorder	10 (12%)	0	0
Total psychiatric disorder	47 (57%)	11	0

[a]Calculated frequency for psychotic disorder + mild mental retardation (MMR) in general population = 0.05% in 13–17-year-olds.

Natural History

Although referral to a psychiatrist may not take place until some years later, history-taking from the parents of aggressive severely learning disabled children usually shows that this type of behaviour pattern began between the ages of 2 and 4 years. This is reflected in the work of Dosen,[5] who examined a population of mentally retarded children that underwent clinical observation because of serious aggressive, destructive, negativistic and hyperactive behaviour. The pattern is of the development of temper tantrums that are more prolonged, more intense and more frequent than is normal. Indeed, the aggressive behaviour during these temper tantrums may be so severe that other siblings are threatened. Parents may not only be worried about younger siblings that have been born in the meantime, but may also worry about older siblings, so ferocious can the behaviour be while the index child is in a tantrum. The child is also very liable to self-injury during one of these tantrums and the usual response provoked in parents is that of brief physical restraint. This the parent is able to carry out because of the large discrepancy in weight and strength between the child and the parent. The procedure usually safely aborts what might otherwise be a dangerous situation in which the child might injure itself or other people. It is usually apparent at this stage that the child is learning disabled, but even if it is not it is certainly apparent by the time the child goes to nursery school or to infant school. Such children in the UK always receive special education from an early age. Teachers and educational psychologists are skilled in tackling these particular behavioural problems and the high staff ratios and sympathetic surroundings go to making a behavioural approach in these early years successful. The child is often affectionate or even over-affectionate, being somewhat promiscuous in the way they behave, showing that they are disinhibited in emotions as well as in behaviour. Some children are too aggressive and/or self-injurious and an early referral to a child psychiatrist or a psychiatrist specializing in learning disabilities is made. Sometimes the parents have unwittingly been told that it is a problem that the child will grow out of and they look forward to the day which they expect some time in the child's teens when they will be free of this worrying and irksome problem.

However, it is in the teens that this disorder is really exaggerated. What was before a turbulent and troublesome young child often in need of restraint, now becomes a burly, aggressive and dangerous teenager. The result of this transformation, caused by puberty, is often a referral to the psychiatrist. It is often as a last resort that such a referral would have been made and the social and personal situation of the patient is often very precarious. The patient is likely to be on the verge of being expelled from school or training centre and the family is likely to be in disarray as the relationship between the parents crumbles under the ferocious assault of the child's behaviour. Siblings may be despairing at their inability to have a normal home life to do their homework from school or to have friends into the house. The very substance of the house will have deteriorated because of the repeated impact of the destructive behaviour of the patient.

The aggressive and destructive behaviour need not be absolutely profligate as regards all surroundings in which the patient finds himself. Predilection may be found for acting out such behaviour in a particular place such as a school or at home. It is not unusual to find out that either one 'escapes' relative to the other. Because there is an element of environmental determination one must be wary of jumping to the conclusion that the disorder is psychosocial.

Kobe et al.[6] in their study of non-ambulatory persons with profound mental retardation point out that they have a high prevalence of physical and medical problems along with high rates of self-injurious, stereotypic and aggressive behaviour. It is wise to recall that such aggressive behaviours can occur not only in the fully mobile, severely handicapped person but also in the non-ambulatory, profoundly learning disabled person who has even greater medical and physical problems.

Sometimes, during late childhood and early teens, and often during the teenage years but usually during early adult life, the question of drug therapy for this condition is raised. The purpose of such therapy is to reduce aggression and self-injury and as such it may help to keep the family together and permit them to endure life in a more acceptable fashion. Often the situation has reached such a pitch by the time referral has been made that a decision has already been entered into regarding the child's future care in an institution. Such a decision may also be made during treatment. In previous years the patient would be likely to be consigned to a mental handicap hospital or other such institution and remain there for the rest of his days. The back wards of such institutions were full of these patients where uncontrolled aggression was the order of the day. Now, at least in the UK, many such patients continue to live productive lives in the community and still enjoy reasonable relationships with their parents and their siblings. Modern methods of treatment may be more effective but the course of the disorder remains and it will continue to afflict the individual until the fifth or sixth decade. In these later decades there is a slow dissipation of the disorder and aggression and self-injury tend to reduce leaving an individual who is devoid of much motivation.

Diagnosis of Violent and Self-injurious Behaviour

Of the various behavioural checklists and scales available in the literature few have been found to be suitable for the task of diagnosis of violence and self-injury in the severely learning disabled. During the 1980s a small number of scales were developed with the intention of assessing aggressive behaviour or behaviour with social skill deficits in learning disabled adults.

The Social Performance Survey Schedule (SPSS) was a scale consisting of 100 items which measured positive and negative social behaviours and was developed by Lowe and Cautela in 1978.[7] Matson attempted to adapt this scale in producing a 57-item scale of a roughly equivalent number of positive and negative items for use with mildly learning disabled people.[8]

As regards violence and self-injury in severely learning disabled people this scale has two faults. First, it is designed to deal with the behaviour that they present and is far more socially oriented, and second it is appropriate only to mildly learning disabled people who understand language.

The Aberrant Behaviour Checklist was produced in 1985 by Aman *et al.*[9] The scale is made up of five subscales: (1) irritability, agitation, crying (15 items); (2) lethargy, social withdrawal (16 items); (3) stereotypic behaviour (seven items); (4) hyperactivity, non-compliance (16 items); and (5) inappropriate speech (four items). There was a total of 58 items. The rating scale was scored simply by summing the obtained ratings (0–3) for the relevant items to obtain totals for each subscale. There was no attempt to weight the various items according to seriousness. For diagnostic assessment of violent and self-injurious behaviour in the severely learning disabled, this scale also fell somewhat short. There is no pertinent assessment of aggression and violence either to the self or to others as it may be performed by a patient.

In 1987 Brizer *et al.*[10] produced a rating scale for reporting violence on psychiatric wards. The Scale for the Assessment of Aggressive and Agitated Behaviours (SAAB) was produced as an instrument capable of quantifying the nature and frequency of violent behaviours and in particular the interactive nature of these behaviours. The SAAB is a 17-item scale that records aggression in just five items. The scale is completed after direct observation of violent events and is not suitable for diagnostic purposes.

The Overt Aggression Scale, or OAS, for the objective rating of verbal and physical aggression was published in 1986 by Yudofsky *et al.*[11] There are five subscales within this rating scale and all have four levels of severity except for that relating to intervention. The first is verbal aggression, the second is physical aggression against objects, the third is physical aggression against self, and the fourth is physical aggression against other people. The final subscale relates to the intervention that is taken with regard to the aggressive event. With regard to the diagnostic assessment of violence and self-injury in severely learning disabled patients, this scale has a somewhat redundant subscale in verbal aggression. There are only four levels of severity for physical aggression against self. The sums of weighted behaviour and intervention scores do provide a composite rating which suggests a level of severity for an aggressive episode. However, there is no detail as to how this weighting is made. The rating scale is completed following an episode of aggression and it might well be that the diagnostic validity of such information lies as much in the number of ratings made as in their content.

The author has drawn up a Hostility Checklist of the symptoms that in his experience are characteristic of organic behaviour disorder. It is noteworthy that organic behaviour disorder is not the same as challenging behaviour. Anyone can produce challenging behaviour and it is often produced in conditions such as schizophrenia and bipolar disorder. Certainly, it is also produced in personality disorders. The core symptoms of organic behaviour disorder are aggression or violence and self-injury. Aggression is defined as 'the offensive action or procedure directed toward another individual or object with the intent to

Table 6.3.   Hostility checklist.

	Negative	Moderate	Severe
1 Invasion of personal space (stands too close, approaches from behind)	0	0	1
2 Loud use of voice (shouts, swears, screams, etc)	0	0	1
3 Fast gesticulation (rapid movement of limbs, etc)	0	1	2
4 Fast locomotion (runs, jumps, etc)	0	1	2
5 Forceful throwing (throws objects, tips tables)	0	1	2
6 Smashes objects (windows, crockery, etc)	0	1	3
7 Hits people (punches, slaps, etc)	0	2	3
8 Scratches people (wheals, or draws blood with nails)	0	2	4
9 Kicks people (anywhere on body)	0	2	4
10 Bites people (indents skin or draws blood)	0	3	5
11 Throttling attempts (forcefully holds around the neck)	0	4	7
12 Serious combined assaults (attacks without weapon)	0	4	8
13 Uses 'non-dangerous' weapons (picks up household objects and hits)	0	4	8
14 Uses dangerous weapons (picks up knife, scissors, etc and uses)	0	5	10
TOTAL			
15 Bites hand repetitively (scars as a result)	0	1	3
16 Hits head with hands repeatedly (bruises and swellings to head)	0	2	4
17 Hits head against objects repeatedly (bruises, cuts and swellings to head)	0	2	4
18 Picks at cavities of head repetitively (including eyes)	0	2	5
19 Scratches or nips limbs or body repeatedly (wheals or blood drawn)	0	2	5
20 Produces ulcers anywhere (by whatever means)	0	4	7
21 Swallows inorganic objects (causing concern in caregiver)	0	4	7
22 Falls heavily due to excitement (rushes around oblivious to furniture)	0	4	7
23 Attacks self with 'non-dangerous' weapons (hits self with household objects)	0	4	8
24 Attacks self with dangerous weapons (razor blades, glass, knives, scissors, etc)	0	5	10
TOTAL			

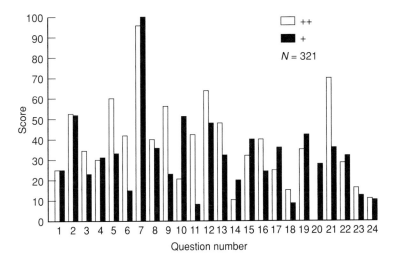

Figure 6.1 Cumulative scores (moderate and severe) for each hostility checklist item in 321 learning disabled patients.

control, threaten or do harm'. Violence is defined as 'the forceful infliction of abuse or damage to another individual or object'.[12] From this it would seem to follow that 'self-injury is the forceful infliction of abuse or damage to the self'. Consequently, there are two sections to this Hostility Checklist (Table 6.3), the first being that related to aggression and violence and the second being that related to self-injury. The checklist was administered to

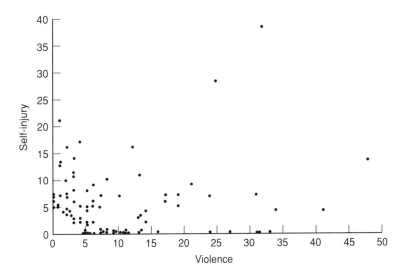

Figure 6.2 Correlation of violence with self-injury in the 88 learning disabled patients who scored 4 or more on the hostility checklist. Spearman's rank correlation coefficient = 0.264; 95% confidence interval for the correlation coefficient = 0.058 to 0.449; $n = 88$.

321 mentally handicapped patients in a mental handicap hospital. The cumulative scores of moderate and severe recordings for each hostility checklist item in these 321 mentally handicapped patients is shown in Figure 6.1. It is clear that there is a broad overall spread of relevance for each of the items in the questionnaire. Cronbach's α is 0.8690 for this checklist, indicating a high degree of internal consistency. On test re-test comparison, Spearman's rank correlation coefficient was 0.830 indicating that this is a robust instrument.[13]

If the symptoms are as displayed above, what then is their mode of delivery? The unit of diagnosis is the temper tantrum. Temper tantrums occur as relatively short-lived outbursts of disordered behaviour, producing the symptoms outlined above. It is useful to know what a person does during a temper tantrum, how long it lasts and how often they occur; together these will produce a summary of the severity of the disorder. The disorder itself is episodic and episodes may occur frequently or infrequently, sometimes with many months between episodes and at other times a few days. Violence is usually associated with some degree of self-injury, although either may be free of the other. As can be seen from Figure 6.2 there is a positive correlation between violence and self-injury with some significant numbers of hospitalized patients showing purely violence. A small number of patients show purely self-injury. However, the majority of patients show a mixture of violence and self-injury. In a further study of 907 learning disabled people in the community the correlation was 0.5 Pearson *P*<0.001, showing a significant and strong correlation between violence and self-injury. Violence and self-injury were also shown to be correlated with degree of handicap as 0.3 Pearson *P*<0.001.

Differential Diagnosis

Epilepsy

Many severely learning disabled people suffer epilepsy, that is, they have seizures. 'A seizure is a sudden, involuntary, time-limited alteration in behaviour including change in motor activity or autonomic function, consciousness or sensation, accompanied by an abnormal electrical discharge in the brain'.[12] Fundamental to the concept of a seizure is that stereotyped behaviour is produced by stereotyped discharge. The behaviour is usually primitive, non-goal directed, non-organized and physiologically consistent with a hypersynchronous cortical discharge. A fundamental question then is whether severely learning disabled people who are subject to episodic rages are suffering from a form of epilepsy. That means that there must not merely be an association between fits and violent behaviour but there must be evidence that the aggression and violence so produced are ictal in nature. In fact, there are no documented cases of ictal aggression in which an organized directed attack of individual or object occurred as the initial or sole manifestation of an epileptic seizure. It would seem that the more organized, directed and modifiable by the environment a behaviour is, the less likely it is to be epilepsy.

Mendez *et al.*[14] go even further in questioning whether interictal violence among epileptic patients could result from factors other than epileptiform activity. They examined 44 patients who presented for psychiatric evaluation because of violent behaviour. When compared with 88 age- and sex-matched epileptic patients without prior violent behaviour they found a considerable excess of mental illness and mental retardation in the former group. However, violent and non-violent patients did not differ on seizure variables such as type and frequency of seizures or as electroencephalographic changes, age of onset of epilepsy or anticonvulsant therapy. They suggested that interictal violence is associated more with psychopathology and mental retardation than with epileptiform activity or other seizure variables.

The association between violence and epilepsy may not rest entirely with the underlying brain damage. It has been shown that the social interaction of patients who have frequent seizures is subject to the additional incursion of behaviour problems and that these behaviour problems are associated with polypharmacy in pursuit of seizure reduction.[15]

Personality Disorder

Personality disorder as a concept is useful when applied to mildly and moderately learning disabled people.[16] A number of learning disabled people were formally rated as to the presence or absence of a personality disorder in the descriptive terms of ICD-9 Section 301. The predominant personality disorders were affective, explosive and hysterical. The authors commented that most of the medication was aimed either against quiescent affective disorders or against personality disorders. Importantly, they commented that they did not think that the concept of personality disorder, as published in current literature, was applicable to learning disabled people who were severely rather than mildly or moderately affected.

Bipolar Disorder

Differential diagnosis of bipolar disorder in severely learning disabled people from the diagnosis of organic behaviour disorder can be very difficult. Organic behaviour disorder by its nature is episodic and in a true cyclical bipolar disorder it may not be difficult to distinguish between them. Emphasis may have to be made on the truly cyclical nature of bipolar disorder compared with the more varied episodic nature of organic behaviour disorder. However, bipolar disorder may not be truly cyclical and even in the literature what may be described as chronic bipolar disorder can be virtually indistinguishable from organic behaviour disorder.[17] Reliance for a diagnosis of bipolar disorder must often be made upon the previous or concomitant existence of a diagnosis of depression. Wieseler et al.[18] suggested the use of a rating scale to assess the presence or absence of bipolar affective disorder in learning disabled people. In 1983, Kazdin et al.[19] evaluated several scales and inventories. All the scales looked at were found to correlate well with the diagnosis of depression and in particular the Beck Scale and the Zeung Scale were found useful for mildly learning disabled people, while the Hamilton Rating Scale was found particularly suitable for severely learning disabled people. In 1986, Sireling[20] continued this work by further emphasis on the Hamilton Rating Scale. He eliminated low-scoring symptoms and symptoms heavily dependent on verbal report and produced a 10-item scale of strict relevance to severe learning disability. Examination of the mental state of a patient currently in the active phase of an organic behaviour disorder or in a manic phase of a bipolar disorder can give some hints as to which of the diagnoses is the true one. Bipolar disorder is suggested by the presence of marked euphoria and pressure of vocal production, whereas in organic behaviour disorder the high levels of arousal may not be so sustained nor may there be such high levels of euphoria.

Schizophrenia

In 1972 Reid[21] came to the firm conclusion that it was not possible to diagnose schizophrenia in the severely learning disabled. He found that schizophrenia and paranoid psychosis could be diagnosed on the usual clinical grounds in mildly and moderately learning disabled people but not in severely learning disabled people who could not communicate verbally. It might be thought that hallucinatory behaviour when occurring in the severely learning disabled could indicate the presence of a schizophrenic illness. Certainly, this symptom, when coupled with other indicators, is very suggestive of a schizophrenic illness in a person who has little or no language. As diagnostic acumen increases it may be possible to diagnose more and more aggressive and self-injurious learning disabled individuals as suffering from schizophrenia when their language is very poor or virtually absent. It is difficult to concur with the conclusion that severely learning disabled people cannot suffer from schizophrenia because it is impossible to diagnose it, but that tends to be the situation that one meets in clinical practice.

Autism

Autism is a syndrome of multiple aetiologies, and several disease entities – genetic, metabolic and structural – are associated with it. Examples include infantile hydrocephalus, tuberous sclerosis and fragile-X syndrome. In 1991 Fernell et al.[22] examined a population-based series of children with infantile hydrocephalus with respect to the occurrence of autistic symptoms. Autistic symptomatology was evaluated according to a modified short version of the so-called Autism Behaviour Checklist. This comprised 17 short statements, each indicating a symptom consistent with autism. The 17 symptoms chosen were those with the highest loadings on the original Autism Behaviour Checklist. It can be seen from the symptoms on this checklist that none of them are characteristic of organic behaviour disorder. Indeed, the central 'aloneness' of autism is characteristically absent in organic behaviour disorders as patients with the latter are as disinhibited in their promiscuity of affection as they are disinhibited in their temper tantrums. Differentiation between organic behaviour disorder and autism should not be difficult unless one is persuaded by the intensity and frequency of violent behaviour to forget that autistic patients can produce this picture also.

Self-Injurious Behaviour

It is uncertain whether purely self-injurious people with a learning disability form a separate group from those with organic behaviour disorder. They certainly form a more severely and profoundly handicapped group as a whole than those who exhibit a predominance of aggression. In 1986, Griffin et al.[23] examined a state-wide prevalence of self-injurious behaviour in learning disabled individuals in residential institutions in Texas, USA. They found that 90% of the patients were severely and profoundly learning disabled. Of these patients 55% were also aggressive towards others. It seems that where it occurs, self-injury is usually accompanied by aggression, but there is a subgroup where there is almost only self-injury. Consequently, self-injurious behaviour has been treated as if it were almost a separate entity and, to some extent, this is supported by the different treatment modalities used for it. In children, at least, there appears to be a sex bias towards males: a study by Griffin et al.[24] suggested that 59% were males and only 41% were females and most of them exhibited self-injurious behaviour at least daily.

Gualtieri and Schroeder[25] consider that self-injurious behaviour is no more than the occasion for a neuropsychiatric differential diagnosis. They consider that first of all there should be enquiry as to environmental, medical and psychiatric circumstances and then consideration of specific syndromes and neurochemical hypotheses.

Psychopharmacological Treatment

Synopsis

Since the development of psychoactive medication, many drugs have been employed in an attempt to reduce the intensity and severity of violence and self-injury exhibited by some learning disabled people. Prior to their introduction, paraldehyde, a hypnotic and sedative with anticonvulsant effects, and a range of opiates were tried with limited success. The use of minor tranquillizers and antidepressants to lessen the frequency of incidents of self-injurious behaviour initially met with some success.[26] Biederman and Jellinek,[27] in reviewing the effects of anti-anxiety agents, considered that because these agents tended to produce disinhibition, resulting in increased restlessness and more disturbed behaviour, they were of limited value.

The place of lithium in the management of aggression in learning disabled patients prone to aggression and self-mutilation has been noted by several authors.[28–33] The multiple references to lithium therapy for aggressive disorders in learning disabled people is some indication of the extent to which its usage has become established.

In nonepileptic learning disabled patients, there are reports of anticonvulsant therapy producing beneficial effects in reducing the level of overactivity and self-injury, initially with sulthiame[34] and later with carbamazepine.[17,35]

The use of the γ-aminobutyric acid derivative, baclofen, has been reported by Primrose[36] in the management of self-injury in learning disabled patients.

A small number of favourable results have also been reported using the β-adrenergic blocking drug, propranolol.[37]

More recently, reports have appeared in the literature of the use of opiate antagonists in the treatment of purely self-injurious syndromes.[38] However, it has been noted that only some patients respond.

Antipsychotic medications have probably been the most widely prescribed psychoactive agents in the management of aggressive behaviour and in particular the phenothiazine neuroleptics, chlorpromazine and thioridazine, and the butyrophenone, haloperidol. Early reports on chlorpromazine described it as effective and predictable[39] and Schiller[40] considered it to be more effective than reserpine in reducing aggressiveness, self-injury and uncooperativeness. In a controlled trial, Hunter and Stephenson[41] found both chlorpromazine and trifluoperazine to be significantly effective in the control of hyperactivity and behavioural abnormalities in severely learning disabled children. In a double-blind study comparing haloperidol with thioridazine published in 1969, Ucer and Kreger[42] observed that haloperidol significantly reduced hyperactivity, anxiety, aggressiveness and impulsiveness in emotionally disturbed learning disabled children. However, in a placebo-controlled comparison between haloperidol and thioridazine in adult patients,[43] few differences in clinical response or side-effect profile were found. Since the first UK report by Jancar in 1965,[44] haloperidol has been shown to be effective in the treatment of both psychotic and nonpsychotic behavioural disorders in the learning disabled.[45]

Since depot neuroleptics became available, several workers have noted their beneficial effects in controlling disturbed and aggressive behaviour and these findings were confirmed by Kinnell (1977)[46] in an essentially learning disabled population. A large multicentre study[47] reported on patients treated with depot phenothiazine and although other writers have commented on the methodological imperfections in the study design, the results appear to show the beneficial effects of depot medication. In a more recent double-blind study using piperazine, a phenothiazine derivative, Lynch et al.[48] demonstrated the marked superiority of depot medication over placebo in the management of aggressive symptoms. This was soon followed by a report of the efficacy of clopenthixol decanoate in the management of aggressive learning disabled patients[49] and a report of the efficacy of haldol decanoate in the management of severe violence and self-injury.[50]

Trends

Lithium – Alone and Combined

The use of lithium in the treatment of serious behaviour disorders in the learning disabled has made steady progress since early reports suggested that it was most effective when it was accompanied by polydipsia.[51] In their review of the literature and description of two case studies, Sovner and Hurley[32] suggested that blood levels of 1.0 millimole (mmol) per litre were needed. In a retrospective study over a 10-year period of 38 subjects, Spreat et al.[52] showed over 63% of patients proved to have more than 30% reduction in the frequency of their aggression. They noted that higher serum levels were associated with a favourable response as was the presence of hyperactivity and violent and destructive behaviour. They went on to review the literature of other trials of lithium in this disorder and suggested that serum levels of 0.7–1.3 mmol l^{-1} were necessary for adequate treatment.

Lithium therapy has been used in combination with carbamazepine for treatment of particularly severe cases of violent and self-injurious behaviour.[53] In this case report a patient was prescribed carbamazepine in a dose sufficient to keep the serum level at 10 µg ml^{-1} when she became friendly and interactive. The authors reported that they thought lithium and carbamazepine had a synergistic effect but that it was necessary to keep the serum levels of carbamazepine high to achieve benefit. In a further report[54] lithium was prescribed for 2 months followed by lithium and carb-amazepine. The results of this trial show that two patients out of the original 10 recovered on a combination of lithium and carbamazepine, while three patients were improved on this same combination.

Sodium Valproate

In 1989, Sovner[55] described five cases treated with sodium valproate. He reported that four had a marked response to the medication and one had a moderate response. Kastner et al.[17] described three cases treated successfully with sodium valproate.

Propranolol

The first reports of the efficacy of an adrenergic β-blocker, propranolol, in the treatment of aggressive and violent behaviour of learning disabled patients came from Yudofsky et al. in 1981.[37] They described four cases which had been treated with propranolol. There has been a small series of single case studies and open trials of propranolol since these initial observations were made and these studies are adequately reviewed by Ruedrich et al.[56] Apart from the usual reservations regarding diagnostic specificity and the use of objective rating scales, these authors make the valid point that in all the reports concerning the use of propranolol in the treatment of aggression, violence and self-injury in learning disabled people, there is always the co-prescription of other agents, usually antipsychotic drugs. Side-effects may be aggravated by the concomitant administration of antipsychotics. It is wise to point out that the side-effects of bradycardia, hypotension and bronchospasm are potentially serious.

Naltrexone

The suggestion that morphine and other opioids may induce self-mutilation in animals and that in humans higher concentrations of β-endorphin were found in the cerebrospinal fluid (CSF) of children who had self-injurious behaviour led to the first clinical trials of opiate antagonists for the treatment of that condition.[57] Naloxone has a very short half-life and it was not until the longer-acting naltrexone became available that treatment with opiate antagonists became a practical proposition. A number of case studies were reported in the years prior to a more definitive double-blind crossover trial reported in 1990 by Kars et al.[38] There was a significant response in one-third of the patients in this small trial. In 1990, Sandman et al.[58] performed a double-blind trial of four fixed doses of naltrexone on four patients with self-injurious behaviour. All the patients had decreased self-injurious behaviour when treated with naltrexone and three patients decreased their self-injurious behaviour as the dose of naltrexone increased. Interestingly, there were no consistent effects of naltrexone on stereotypy. However, it may be that it will prove possible clinically to separate those subjects who show a peculiar form of self-injurious behaviour and are likely to produce a positive response to opiate antagonists.

Clozapine

The use of the atypical antipsychotic clozapine in a learning disabled population with aggression and self-injurious behaviour was examined in 1994 by Cohen and Underwood.[59] It led to a significant reduction in both aggression and self-injurious behaviour. Side-effects were minimal, but the incidence of white cell disorder is high (2%) and the prospect of nursing such patients in a bone marrow unit is daunting.

Depot Antipsychotics

Young[60] produced the first substantial investigation of the effect of depot antipsychotics on aggression in learning disabled people. His patients were mixed mentally ill and learning disabled. Some of his learning disabled subjects showed improvement with fluphenazine enanthate. In 1980, Craft and Schiff[47] published a report on the use of depot antipsychotics in more than 100 patients who were learning disabled. Their stated intention was to clarify the indications for depot antipsychotics and to assess their effects – both primary effects and side-effects. For this, their sole criterion for entry was that all neuroleptics had been ineffective in alleviating a patient's condition, which might be a behaviour disorder and might also be a psychosis. The problem of assessment and diagnosis dogged this clinical trial for the treatment of aggression and self-injury in learning disabled people. Nevertheless, one clinical observation that may well be of worth was that the widely held assumption that patients with manifest organic brain damage were more susceptible to drug-induced extrapyramidal disturbance was not supported by the results of this trial. The first double-blind placebo-controlled crossover trial of a depot antipsychotic with placebo in the management of aggressive learning disabled patients took place in 1985.[48] The overall impression is of a tight convincing trial demonstrating the effectiveness of pipothiazine palmitate compared with placebos. In 1986, Read and Batchelor[50] produced the first report of success with haloperidol decanoate and in that same year Miele and Wiley[49] gave a report of the successful use of zuclopenthixol decanoate. One reason why better responses may be obtained by giving a drug by the parenteral route rather than the oral route may be that higher concentrations are achieved at receptor level because of the avoidance of first pass metabolism and the provision of relatively steady serum levels, effectively increasing the side-effects threshold.

Prescribing Practice

A number of studies[1,61-63] have shown that antipsychotic prescription for learning disabled individuals may have been carried out in a profligate and irresponsible manner for a number of years. Antipsychotics may have been used widely for so-called 'behaviour disorder' without regard to side-effects – short and long-term – and with little consideration for the indications for their prescription.

The wide range of psychoactive drugs now available can produce a series of side-effects which may present behaviour disorder itself.[64] These include Parkinsonism, dystonia, akathisia and tardive dyskinesia, all produced by dopamine blockers, mania which may be produced by tricyclics, aggressiveness which may be produced by benzodiazepines, and incontinence which may be produced by lithium. A further area of concern regards litigation, in particular with regard to the production of tardive dyskinesia by prolonged use of dopamine blocking agents.[65] It is suggested here that what is most concerning about prescribing trends to the learning disabled is the lack of specificity of psychiatric diagnosis, from which it follows that there will be disordered prescribing.

Behaviour Therapy

If these patients are indeed chronically over-aroused as suggested by Read and Batchelor[50] and one effect at least of antipsychotic medication is to reduce this level of arousal, then this indeed is of great benefit for the use of alternative therapies. Behaviour therapy is extremely difficult, if not impossible, to carry out effectively in someone with very high arousal levels and it certainly benefits from the reduction of these levels. Early and less severe forms of organic behaviour disorder can indeed be dealt with by behaviour therapy alone. Behaviour therapy and pharmacotherapy can therefore work together in a synergistic fashion. Behaviour therapy programmes should form an integral part of management regimens for this disorder. The techniques of behaviour therapy are dealt with in Chapter 13.

Games

There are other forms of social treatment and mention must be made of the effects of socialization games on proximity and social behaviour of aggressive learning disabled people. Edmonson and Han[66] examined the effect of socialization games to find that the rate of friendly behaviour was significantly greater after the games.

Exercise

Baumeister and MacLean[67] implemented a jogging exercise programme for two severely learning disabled adults who showed high rates of self-injurious behaviours. Daily response rates were lower after the exercise compared with before. When the programme was terminated self-injurious behaviour again increased.

Conclusion

The existence of organic behaviour disorder may not yet be recognized by the major diagnostic classifications, but to those in clinical practice its existence is a matter of fact. It presents as a recognizable syndrome in the severely and even profoundly learning disabled and although it may not be defined as a mental illness as such it is certainly a psychiatric disorder which merits diagnosis and treatment. The patient is usually so aroused or arousable that behaviour therapy is insufficient on its own, but needs to be employed in a harmonious and synergistic fashion with psychoactive medication. The use of that psychoactive medication needs to be eclectic, informed and careful. There needs to be a positive diagnosis of this syndrome and an astute use of the agents that are available. Only then can redundant polypharmacy and the overuse and misuse of drugs be avoided. However, those that need these medications must have them for otherwise not only are their own lives in abject misery, but also the lives of those around them.

References

1. Jacobson J (1988) Problem behaviour and psychiatric impairment within a developmentally disabled population 3: Psychotropic medication. *Research in Developmental Disabilities* **9**, 23–38.
2. Sigafoos J, Elkins J, Kerr M & Attwood T (1994) A survey of aggressive behaviour among a population of persons with intellectual disability in Queensland. *Journal of Intellectual Disability Research* **38(4)**, 369–81.
3. Harris P (1993) The nature and extent of aggressive behaviour amongst people with learning difficulties (mental handicap) in a single health district. *Journal of Intellectual Disability Research* **37(3)**,: 221–42.
4. Gillberg C, Persson E, Grufman M & Themner U (1986) Psychiatric disorders in mildly and severely retarded urban children and adolescents: epidemiological aspects. *British Journal of Psychiatry* **149**, 68–74.
5. Dosen A (1983) Negative destructive behaviour in young retarded children (Dutch). *Tijdschrift voor Kindergeneeskunde* **51(1)**, 13–8.
6. Kobe FH, Mulick JA, Rash TA & Martin J (1994) Nonambulatory persons with profound mental retardation: physical, developmental and behavioural characteristics. *Research in Developmental Disabilities* **15(6)**, 413–23.
7. Lowe M & Cautela J (1978) A self-report measure of social skills. *Behaviour Therapy* **9**, 535–7.
8. Matson JL, Helsel WJ, Bellack AS & Senatore V (1983) Development of a rating scale to assess social skill deficit in mentally retarded adults. *Applied Research in Mental Retardation* **4**, 399–407.
9. Aman M, Singh N, Steward A & Field C (1985) Aberrant Behaviour Checklist – A behaviour rating scale for the assessment of treatment effects. *American Journal of Mental Deficiency* **89(5)**, 485–91.
10. Brizer D, Convit A, Krakowski M & Volavka J (1987) A rating scale for reporting violence on psychiatric wards. *Hospital and Community Psychiatry* **38(7)**, 769–70.
11. Yudofsky S, Silva J, Jackson W, Endicott J & Williams D (1986) The Overt Aggression Scale for the objective rating of verbal and physical aggression. *American Journal of Psychiatry* **143**, 1, 35–9.
12. Treiman D (1991) Psychobiology of ictal aggression. *Advances in Neurology* **55**, 341–56.
13. Read S (1996) MD thesis. Leeds University.
14. Mendez MF, Doss RC & Taylor JC (1993) Interictal violence in epilepsy. Relationship to behaviour and seizure variables. *Journal of Nervous and Mental Disease* **181(9)**, 566–9.
15. Esbe C, Gillies J & Montgomery J (1990) Anti-epileptic polypharmacy, psychosocial behaviour and locus of control orientation among mentally handicapped adults living in the community. *Journal of Mental Deficiency Research* **34**, 351–60.
16. Reid A & Ballinger B (1987) Personality disorder in mental handicap. *Psychological Medicine* **17**, 983–7.
17. Kastner T, Friedman D, Palmer A, Ruiz M & Henning D (1990) Valproic acid for the treatment of children with mental retardation and mood symptomatology. *Paediatrics* **86(3)**, 467–72.
18. Wieseler NA, Campbell GJ & Soniss W (1988) Ongoing use of an affective rating scale in the treatment of a mentally retarded individual with a rapid cycling bipolar affective disorder. *Research in Developmental Disabilities* **9(1)**, 47–53.

19. Kazdin A, Matson J & Senatore V (1983) Assessment of depression in mentally retarded adults. *American Journal of Psychiatry* **140(8)**, 1040–3.
20. Sireling L (1986) Depression in mentally handicapped patients: diagnostic and neuro-endocrine evaluation. *British Journal of Psychiatry* **149**, 274–8.
21. Reid A (1972) Psychoses in adult mental defectives II. Schizophrenic and paranoid psychoses. *British Journal of Psychiatry* **120**, 213–8.
22. Fernell E, Gillberg C & van Wendt L (1991) Autistic symptoms in children with infantile hydrocephalus. *Acta Paediatrica Scandinavica* **80(4)**, 451–7.
23. Griffin JC, Williams DE, Stark MT, Altmeyer BK & Mason M (1986) Self injurious behaviour: a state-wide prevalence survey of the extent and circumstances. *Applied Research in Mental Retardation* **7(1)**, 105–16.
24. Griffin JC, Ricketts RW, Williams DE, Locke BJ, Altmeyer BK & Stark MT (1987) A community survey of self-injurious behaviour among developmentally disabled children and adolescents. *Hospital and Community Psychiatry* **38(9)**, 959–63.
25. Gualtieri C & Schroeder S (1989) Pharmacotherapy for self-injurious behaviour: Preliminary tests of the D1 Hypothesis. *Psychopharmacology Bulletin* **25(3)**, 364–71.
26. Galamboss M (1965) Long-term clinical trial with diazepam on adult mentally retarded persons. *Diseases of the Nervous System* **26**, 305–9.
27. Biederman J & Jellinek M (1984) Psychopharmacology in children. *New England Journal of Medicine* **310(15)**, 968–72.
28. Campbell M, Fish B, Korein J, Shapiro T, Collins P & Coh C (1972) Lithium and chlorpromazine: A controlled cross-over study of hyperactive severely disturbed young children. *Journal of Autism and Childhood Schizophrenia II* 234–263.
29. Cooper A & Fowlie H (1973) Control of gross self-mutilation with lithium carbonate. *British Journal of Psychiatry* **1222**, 370–1.
30. Worrell E, Moody J & Naylor G (1975) Lithium in non-manic depressives: anti-aggressive effect and red blood cell lithium values. *British Journal of Psychiatry* **126**, 464–8.
31. Dale P (1980) Lithium therapy in aggressive mentally subnormal patients. *British Journal of Psychiatry* **137**, 469–74.
32. Sovner R & Hurley A (1981) The management of chronic behaviour disorders in mentally retarded adults with lithium carbonate. *Journal of Nervous and Mental Disease* **169(3)**, 191–5.
33. Tyrer SP, Walsh A, Edwards DE, Berney TP & Stephens DA (1984) Factors associated with a good response to lithium in aggressive mentally handicapped subjects. *Progress in Neuro-psychopharmacology and Biological Psychiatry* **8**, 751–5.
34. Al-Kaisi A & McGuire R (1974) The effect of sulthiame on disturbed behaviour in mentally subnormal patients. *British Journal of Psychiatry* **124**, 45–9.
35. Reid A, Naylor G & Kay D (1981) A double blind placebo controlled cross-over trial of carbamazepine in over-active severely mentally handicapped patients. *Psychological Medicine II* 109–13.
36. Primrose D (1979) Treatment of self-injurious behaviour with a GABA (gamma-aminobutyric acid) analogue. *Journal of Mental Deficiency Research* **23**, 163–74.
37. Yudofsky S, Williams D & Gorman J (1981) Propranolol in the treatment of rage and violent behaviour in patients with chronic brain syndromes. *American Journal of Psychiatry* **138**, 218–20.
38. Kars H, Broekema W, Glauderman-vans Gelderen I, Verhoeven W & van Ree J (1990) Naltrexone alleviates self-injurious behaviour in mentally retarded subjects. *Biological Psychiatry* **27**, 747–56.
39. Adamson W, Nellis B, Runge G, Cleland C & Killian E (1958) Use of tranquillisers for mentally deficient patients. *American Medical Association Journal of Diseases of Children* **96**, 159–64.
40. Schiller H (1959) Reserpine, chlorpromazine and the mentally retarded. *Psychiatric Quarterly* **33(10)**, 684–99.
41. Hunter H & Stephenson G (1963) Chlorpromazine and triflluoperazine in the treatment of behavioural abnormalities in the severely subnormal child. *British Journal of Psychiatry* **109**, 411–7.
42. Ucer E & Kreger K (1969) A double blind study comparing haloperidol with thioridazine in emotionally disturbed, mentally retarded children. *Current Therapeutic Research* **11**, 278–83.
43. Vaisenen K, Viukari M, Rimon R & Raisanen P (1981) Haloperidol, thioridazine and placebo in mentally subnormal patients – serum levels and clinical effects. *Acta Psychiatrica Scandinavica* **63**, 262–71.

44. Jancar J (1965) The use of haloperidol in the treatment of severe behaviour disorders in mental deficiency. *Clinical Trials Journal* **2(2)**, 153–5.
45. Grabowski S (1973) Safety and effectiveness of haloperidol for mentally retarded, behaviourally disordered and hyperkinetic patients. *Current Therapeutic Research* **15(11)**, 856–61.
46. Kinnell H (1977) Depot tranquillisers for disturbed behaviour. *British Medical Journal II* 578.
47. Craft M & Schiff A (1980) Psychiatric disturbance in mentally handicapped patients. *British Journal of Psychiatry* **137**, 250–5.
48. Lynch D, Eliatamby C & Anderson A (1985) Pipothiazine palmitate in the management of aggressive mentally handicapped patients. *British Journal of Psychiatry* **146**, 525–9.
49. Miele T & Wiley Y (1986) Clopenthixol decanoate in the management of aggressive mentally handicapped patients. *British Journal of Psychiatry* 373–6.
50. Read S & Batchelor D (1986) Violence and self-injurious behaviour in mentally handicapped patients: Psychopharmacological control. *International Clinical Psychopharmacology Supplement I* **1(1)**, 63–74.
51. Dostal T (1972) Anti-aggressive effect of lithium salts in mentally retarded adolescents. In Annell A (ed) *Depressive States in Childhood and Adolescence*, pp. 491–8. Stockholm: Almquist and Wiksell.
52. Spreat S, Behar D, Renesk B & Niazzo P (1989) Lithium carbonate for aggression in mentally retarded persons. *Comprehensive Psychiatry III* **6**, 505–11.
53. Buck O & Havey P (1986) Combined carbamazepine and lithium therapy for violent behaviour. *American Journal of Psychiatry* **143(11)**, 1487.
54. Glue P (1989) Rapid cycling affective disorders in the mentally retarded. *Biological Psychiatry* **26**, 250–6.
55. Sovner R (1989) The use of valproate in the treatment of mentally retarded persons with typical and atypical bipolar disorders. *Journal of Clinical Psychiatry* **50(3, Suppl.)**, 40–3.
56. Ruedrich S, Grush L & Wilson J (1990) Beta adrenergic blocking medications for aggressive or self-injurious mentally retarded persons. *American Journal of Mental Retardation* **95(1)**, 110–9.
57. Richardson J & Zaleski W (1983) Naloxone and self-mutilation. *Biological Psychiatry* **18**, 99–101.
58. Sandman CA, Barron JL & Colman H (1990) An orally administered opiate blocker, naltrexone, attenuates self-injurious behaviour. *American Journal of Mental Retardation* **95(1)**, 93–102.
59. Cohen SA & Underwood MT (1994) The use of clozapine in a mentally retarded and aggressive population. *Journal of Clinical Psychiatry* **55(10)**, 440–4.
60. Young E (1970) Hospital experience with fluphenazine enanthate. *Diseases of the Nervous System* **31(10)**, 705–9.
61. Altmeyer B, Locke B, Griffin J, Rickets R, Willliams D, Mason M & Stark M (1987) Treatment strategies for self-injurious behaviour in a large service delivery network. *American Journal of Mental Deficiency* **91(4)**, 333–40.
62. Stone R, Alvarez W & Ellman G (1989) Prevalence and prediction of psychotropic drug use in California Developmental Centres. *American Journal of Mental Retardation* **93(6)**, 627–32.
63. Wressell S, Tyrer S & Berney T (1990) Reduction in antipsychotic drug dosage in mentally handicapped patients. *British Journal of Psychiatry* **157**, 101–6.
64. Sovner R (1982) Psychotropic drug side-effects presenting as behaviour disorders. *Psychiatric Aspects of Mental Retardation I* **12**, 45–48.
65. Cohen S, Khan A, Zheng Y & Chiles J (1991) Tardive dyskinesia in the mentally retarded: Comparison of prevalence, risk factors and topography with a schizophrenic population. *Acta Psychiatrica Scandinavica* **83**, 234–7.
66. Edmonson B & Han SS (1983) Effects of socialization games on proximity and prosocial behaviour of aggressive mentally retarded institutionalized women. *American Journal of Mental Deficiency* **87(4)**, 435–40.
67. Baumeister AA & MacLean WE Jr (1984) Deceleration of self-injurious and stereotypic responding by exercise. *Applied Research in Mental Retardation* **5(3)**, 385–93.

7

Autism and Asperger's Syndrome

Thomas P. Berney

Introduction

Public awareness of autism is increasing. Here is a diagnosis which explains what was previously inexplicable, which justifies a demand for appropriate and intensive teaching and which brings social and emotional support. Improvements in diagnostic technique and a growing awareness of behavioural phenotypes have encouraged a more careful dissection of symptomatology in people with learning disability. In the media, the diagnosis previously limited to *Rain Man* and the occasional documentary, is being used more widely. Not all publicity is positive: like schizophrenia, autism is being linked to tragedy, violence and crime. However, even this notoriety brings a wider awareness of the prevalence, not just of the core condition, but also of its more subtle variants.

What is autism? Initially, it was identified as a syndromal collection of observed, behavioural symptoms which emphasized the relative impairments of social relationships and language. It is 50 years since Kanner[1] identified autism in America and Asperger[2] wrote about his eponymous syndrome in Vienna. Itard had probably identified it even earlier, distinguishing children with mutism from those with simple retardation. He left us a detailed clinical account which emphasizes the language deficit, and then went further to explore the management of the disorder.[3] However, despite the clarity of these descriptions autism was perceived as a childhood form of schizophrenia. In 1971 Kolvin and his colleagues demonstrated that these were separate disorders,[4] but the belief in a unitary psychosis persisted for a further decade outside Britain. The subsequent description of Schizoid Personality in Childhood and its identification both with Asperger's syndrome and with the schizophrenia spectrum blurred the relationship further, particularly as it was considered a potential precursor to schizophrenia.[5]

It has become clear that both autism and schizophrenia represent disorders that include a spectrum of syndromes.[6] Although some overlap has been suggested, usually on the basis of cross-sectional phenomenology,[7,8] the two disorders have their own characteristic and distinct courses and probably do not coincide more than might be expected on the basis of chance.[9]

A greater awareness of autism, together with the identification of more subtle, subjective symptoms, psychological deficits and associated neuro-biological anomalies, has led to a broader definition. At the same time, a separate initiative, the identification of a (potentially unifying) genetic basis, is moving from a behavioural syndrome towards a discrete disorder with the possibility of a laboratory diagnosis.

Initially disparate, there has been a convergence of diagnostic criteria. The publication of ICD-10[10] and DSM-IV[11] heralds this international agreement on definition although, with some controversy, the Autistic Disorders have been renamed as Pervasive Developmental Disorders and grouped together with Rett syndrome.

Clinical Characteristics

Autism is a disorder identified early in development. Furthermore, it usually coexists with significant learning disability. Any deficits must be measured against this background. It must be stressed that symptoms are never simply present or absent. This gradation of intensity of symptomatology results in a continuum of disorder which shades into normality. Furthermore, as each individual symptom can manifest to a different degree, their varying proportions result in the protean presentations of the spectrum of autism.[6]

Wing[12] has described a characteristic triad of impairments – of social relationships, language and of imagination – as well as sensory and motor abnormalities. These form the basis of the latest diagnostic criteria (ICD-10 and DSM-IV) although the check-list of symptoms places greater weight on the restricted and repetitive quality of the person's activity that substitute for the varied activities that require imagination.

Social Impairment

The lack of social relationships, expressed in attachments and friendships, varies in degree and nature. *Difficulty with social cues* affects reciprocal social interaction, joint interactive play and joint attention behaviour and there is an unconcern for the interests/activities of others or, for that matter, in sharing pleasure or achievement. They go their own egocentric way, not pointing out objects that give them interest or pleasure. The *failure to recognize emotional cues* results in an inappropriate response to distress in others which may reflect a wider lack of empathy.

This gives us the basis for three clinical subtypes:[13]

(a) *the aloof*, whose aversion to social interaction corresponds most closely to the autistic withdrawal described by Kanner[1]
(b) *the passive*, who can be drawn into interaction but only for as long as they are prompted
(c) *the active but odd*, who spontaneously engage with people but, lacking the ability to develop more than a superficial relationship,

talk at rather than to them. This is the group which might be identified with Asperger's syndrome or Schizoid Disorder of Childhood.[14]

Language Abnormality

The whole sphere of language is affected, both verbal and nonverbal, although expressive may be more afflicted than receptive language. Overall, there is less language, ranging from a difficulty in building conversation to complete mutism. Where speech is present, there is usually abnormal prosody, the lack of variation in pitch, rate, rhythm and emphasis giving it a mechanical quality. Semantic shortcomings spoil the person's ability to respond automatically to their name or to understand jokes or colloquial speech. A pragmatic deficit may pass unrecognized but impedes social communication with diminished synchronicity and reciprocity. The result is a computer-like, unmodulated, impassivity with less use of social gaze, posture and gesture. Another consequence is an anxiety-generating incomprehension of the messiness of the everyday life that surrounds us all.

Language is deviant and delayed, emerging in abnormal syntax. Echolalia (and echopraxia) can be immediate or delayed, the latter resulting in the tape-recorder-like replay of whole scenes observed on television or in real life. The resulting quotes may have all the life and emotional expression that the person's speech normally lacks and can dominate their communication to the extent that they mask the real severity of the condition. Pronominal reversal and the use of the third person cause confusion, and jargon or idiosyncratic and unusual terms can make the person incomprehensible to those who do not know them well.

Limited Imagination

Imagination is expressed in an individual's play, fantasy, interests and activities. In the autistic disorders this is restricted to a few and circumscribed themes and there is a lack of spontaneity, imaginativeness and creativity. Left to themselves the individual's activities are typically repetitive and stereotyped; they may rock or tap, post objects, sort them or order them by their size, colour or some other characteristic, and have more interest in some part of the object than in its function as a whole. Compulsive routines can involve others in a set of questions and answers, a catechism which has to be completed before anything else can happen. Unusual attachments, for example to balls or a magpie series of objects, result in large collections and storage problems. This imposition of rigidity and routine on the whole daily life is a consequence, as well as a cause, of an individual's inability to cope with the complexity, novelty and messiness of everyday life. Faced with anything unexpected the result may be an excess of distress in the form of a catastrophic rage.

Sensory Characteristics

Although only touched on by the diagnostic criteria, a distortion of sensory perception may underlie the selective response to stimuli in various modalities but particularly of hearing and vision. Thus, there is often an excessive interest in shiny, spinning or swinging objects, in unusual textures, smells and tastes and a preference for peripheral gaze. Thresholds are altered and the result can be stimulus overload in which everyday noises have an effect akin to that of chalk screeching on a blackboard, or a stun grenade. Alternatively there may be an inability to make sense of a perception because of the distracting effects of the surround – to distinguish signal from noise. However, the reverse may also be true so that the individual ignores strong stimuli (such as a loud noise or their name being called) or be able to select some detail, such as a thread, from the complex background of a patterned carpet. The awareness of pain (as distinct from the threshold) is frequently diminished, particularly in early childhood. The result is a pattern of perception, specific to that individual at that time, which sets them at odds with those around.

More subtle is the lack of internal structure gained from an appreciation of time and space. This leaves the person with autism struggling to comprehend the passage of time, both in its extent and in how to relate it to events in an abstract, sequential framework. Although puzzling to those for whom such an understanding has always been a part of their natural world, it can lead to a preoccupation with routines and predictability as well as an intolerance of delay. A similar difficulty in perceiving the spatial relationships of objects leaves the individual unable to understand the size and shape of their environment or how objects relate geographically within it.[15]

Motor Characteristics

Motor dysfunction ranges from the graceful and agile to the clumsy child who cannot run or climb. Abnormal tone reveals itself in unusual postures, toe-walking (which may sometimes be so sustained and severe as to require eventual surgical tendon release) and dysphagia. Mannerisms and repetitive and stereotypic movements are common, notably hand-flapping while bouncing up and down, and gyration. These are most marked when aroused whether by excitement, anxiety or distress.

Underlying this symptomatology there is a much broader movement disorder apparently rooted in subjective experience rather than simply being a motor phenomenon. At the centre is the individual's level of motivation, with unthinking, involuntary actions often being attainable where more deliberate actions are impossible – the *kinesia paradoxica*, well recognized in Parkinson's disease, or the ability to ride a bicycle or type fluently as long as the person does not concentrate on their actions. In autism this separation of automatic from deliberate applies to communication so that, on an isolated occasion, the very relaxed or very anxious mute may briefly speak, using complex language, leaving the bystanders wondering what they had really heard.[16]

Tics may occur in autism and, with the development of a verbal tic, evolve into Tourette's syndrome. Taken with the obsessive–compulsive qualities accompanying autism, it is suggested that the association is more than coincidence[17] and that there may be a fundamental link, perhaps in abnormal serotonin metabolism.

Pattern of Development

In most children the features of autism can be discerned from birth, although it may require the hindsight that goes with diagnosis to recognize very early symptoms such as the failures to use gaze for signalling, to imitate gesture or facial expression, to engage in joint attention with pointing, or to anticipate being picked up. However, there are children who appear to develop normally and acquire some speech, only later to lose it and withdraw. Where this happens it is usually at about 18–24 months but, by definition, should be before 36 months. Delayed recognition appears to be linked to higher ability. Where there is clearly a delayed onset and this occurs after 24 months, the child may be the victim of the separate pathogenetic subgroup of disintegrative disorders.[18]

Thereafter the features of autism tend to peak at 2–5 years and subsequently soften and evaporate with age so that often, by adulthood, many of the positive features have been lost. Where the developmental history has been omitted the result can be confused with chronic schizophrenia[7] or personality disorder.[19]

Diagnosis

Criteria

As concepts have changed so they have been reflected in the revised criteria and terminology of successive editions of ICD and DSM. The consequence has been some adjustment to the boundaries of the population identified.

The latest addition has been the identification and provisional separation of Asperger's Autistic Psychopathy. Asperger considered this to be a personality disorder in contrast to the psychotic process of autism, the children being identified relatively late (not before their third year), and their speech developing normally in contrast to their motor skills – they talk before they walk. Although he did not exclude learning disability, his description was of someone with an innovative and original cognitive approach.[20] This definition subsequently broadened to include anyone with good, spontaneous, syntactical speech[21,22] even if there had been early speech delay. ICD-10 and DSM-IV have since redefined Asperger's syndrome by the absence of significant delays in both speech and cognition. Needless to say, the differing criteria have led to some confusion and many studies fall foul of circularity, simply demonstrating the presence of the symptoms used to identify the disorder in the first place. Given the criteria, it is not surprising that recognition of Asperger's syndrome should occur later and it remains unclear whether its onset is delayed. Comparative studies with autism have found differences in social isolation, fluency[23] and neuropsychological characteristics.[24] It has been suggested that whereas autism is primarily a disorder of language function and the dominant hemisphere, Asperger's syndrome affects visuomotor, nondominant hemispheric function.[25] Although clumsiness has been suggested to be a distinctive feature[26] closer scrutiny has not confirmed this in those identified on ICD-10 criteria.[27]

Instruments

Whatever the criteria, most diagnostic inconsistency results from variance in the way they are applied. A number of schedules and questionnaires have been promoted. The most thorough is probably the Autism Diagnostic Schedule (ADI), a 111-item structured interview schedule which is used to take a detailed account from the person's carers.[28,29] This is complemented by the Autism Diagnostic Observation Schedule (ADOS)[30] which uses a structured interview with the individual to derive a systematic set of observations relevant to autism. The interview, graded to suit the developmental level, leads the person through a series of tasks and presses which elicit the symptomatology of autism. This has subsequently been refined and provides modules for the assessment of the pre-linguistic person (the PLADOS).[31]

The Medical Research Council's Handicaps, Behaviour and Skills (HBS) Schedule is the main alternative instrument. This assesses not only those areas concerned with autism but also the developmental level (a Vineland Quotient can be derived) and quantifies the wide range of behavioural disturbance associated with learning disability.[32] An extensively revised version is about to be released.

The Childhood Autism Rating Scale (CARS)[33] is a semistructured schedule for rating children on 15 items which derive from various diagnostic scales including DSM-III-R. As a framework it is designed to be widely used by a variety of professionals in different settings including carer interview, classroom observation and case history review. It has been extensively tested and compared with other systems.[34,35]

The Autism Behaviour Checklist (ABC)[36] has been criticized for a variety of reasons, particularly for its yes/no approach to symptoms. Based on a statistical selection of relevant items, it remains an effective screening instrument which has not yet been supplanted,[37,38] particularly if the parents fill it in for the child as he/she was at 3–5 years.[39]

Can autism be detected in the routine health surveillance done by health visitors and general practitioners? A retrospective survey of their records showed that the autistic children were more likely to show 'problems' in the social category but otherwise there was little to distinguish them, particularly from those children with a mild learning disability. Indeed, the latter were more likely to show 'problems' in the hearing category than any other group. This may reflect either an absence of symptomatology before about 18 months or the insensitivity of routine screening.[40] The latter might be improved by the Checklist for Autism in Toddlers (CHAT),[41] a screening instrument, designed to be used by primary health care professionals at 18 months. Nine questions addressed to the carer are supplemented by five observations by the professional covering points such as pretend play and joint attention. This will select children with early autism from those whose development is normal; a trial is in progress to test its ability to distinguish them from those with other forms of developmental disability.

Differential Diagnosis

The presence of learning disability in about 80% of people with an autistic disorder obscures the clarity of the diagnosis. The more severe the degree of disability, the more frequent the coexistent autism and the more the diagnosis is dependent on the symptoms of deficit and delay (as against the positive, deviant symptoms). This is complicated by the need to define the symptomatology in the context of the normal developmental process. Many will be categorized as Atypical Autism, a group identified by its failure to meet the full criteria for autism in all three areas (or by an onset after 3 years). However, some will fall into the grey area of Overactive Disorder associated with Learning Disability and Stereotyped Movements, a category created by ICD-10. The title provides a fairly comprehensive description of a disorder which is of uncertain validity. In DSM-IV the residual group of Pervasive Development Disorder Not Otherwise Specified (PDD-NOS) provides a catch-all for both of these categories.

The label of Multiplex Developmental Disorder has been suggested for another diagnostic grouping.[42] This early-onset disorder would include those with a combination of: (1) disturbed social relationships equivalent to Avoidant Disorder (DSM-IV), (2) poor regulation of their anxiety, and (3) disturbances in cognitive processing similar to Schizotypal Personality (DSM-IV).

The boundaries of Asperger's syndrome cause some difficulty. Has it a protean presence, embracing most of the odd personalities associated with the autistic triad, or are there adjacent, more specific disorders? The clinical definition of these alternatives are frequently limited by the lack of early developmental history leaving it unclear how far growth has blurred an earlier, more clear-cut picture of autism. The lack of standardized assessment (sometimes because of an inability to obtain the subject's cooperation) also blurs the distinctions. The thoroughly investigated group of schizoid children appears to include and extend this group.

Over the last decade Newson[43] has been delineating a syndrome named after its principal characteristic – Pathological Demand Avoidance syndrome. This she distinguishes from autism by the presence of a superficial sociability with an awareness of the reactions of others and an ability to be involved in role-play. All of this is dedicated to resisting the tasks and demands of everyday life.

In the absence of impaired sociability, Bishop[44] has identified a specific language disorder, Semantic-Pragmatic Disorder. It is debatable whether such a separate disorder exists or whether it is merely a variation on Asperger's syndrome.[15,45]

Again, starting from the framework of specific learning disability, there has developed the concept of the Nonverbal Learning Disability[46,47] or the Right Hemisphere Disorder.[48] These identify a group who have good verbal intelligence but a cluster of social, motor and cognitive deficits (particularly visuo-spatial and arithmetic) which sound very like the pedagogic perception of Asperger's syndrome.

The Disintegrative Disorders

Rett's syndrome is a condition, probably with a genetic basis, which appears to afflict only girls (although this may mean simply that boys do not survive early pregnancy). There is a loss of hand skills and speech starting at 7–24 months. A progressive motor deterioration follows, producing truncal ataxia, abnormal spinal curvature and eventual spastic paraplegia. Hand-wringing stereotypy (so marked as to form the logotype of the parent association) and phasic hyperventilation are characteristic.

Other childhood disintegrative disorders exist as an ICD-10 category which forms a 'rag-bag' of rare, residual conditions some of which will stem from various encephalopathies. These are defined by a period of normal development, usually taken as 2 years, prior to the onset of a global developmental deterioration which includes the loss of acquired skills (such as continence and self-feeding) and, for some, motor deterioration. Although there may be a degree of recovery, the prognosis is poor compared with late onset autism, with cases becoming and remaining significantly more retarded.[18,49,50]

In acquired aphasia with epilepsy (Landau–Kleffner syndrome) both receptive and expressive language skills are lost while general intelligence is retained. The behavioural picture can be very similar to that of autism. A paroxysmal, epileptiform electroencephalogram (EEG) abnormality may predate the language loss and is most marked in sleep. Clinical seizures take varied forms but occur only in about 75% of cases.[51] The publication of a case study of a child who had neither EEG nor clinical evidence of epilepsy but who improved on steroid treatment, broadens this diagnostic area.[52–56]

Epidemiology

The epidemiology of autism has always been at the mercy of its diagnostic methods and criteria. Such surveys as have been made have been geographically uneven, being largely in Europe (particularly England and

Sweden) and Japan with only one survey in the USA (in Wisconsin).[57] Lotter, in the first and unusually thorough, community study in 1963 found a prevalence of 4.5 per 10 000 of whom 2 per 10 000 had the nuclear features of social aloofness and resistance to change. Support came from a similar study by Wing and Gould[58] in Camberwell, an area of London. Other studies followed from Japan,[59] West Berlin,[60] Göteborg (Sweden)[61] and France.[62] An American survey of Wisconsin was unusual in finding only 0.7 cases per 10 000, possibly by a readier ascription of cases to the category of atypical autism.[63]

As wider criteria are used the stated prevalence increases. Thus, the Camberwell study found Wing's triad of impairment to be present in 22 per 10 000 and a subsequent Swedish study found Asperger's syndrome to be present in 36 per 10 000 although, if all possible cases were included, this doubled to 71 per 10 000.[64] The combination of these figures gives a total prevalence for all autistic disorders of nearly 1% (L. Wing, personal communication). At face value such a level of prevalence would carry hugely different implications for the management of a disorder which otherwise has been seen as sufficiently rare to warrant unusually intensive, individual and specialized resources. This revised perception is supported by Wolff's estimate that schizoid personality of childhood accounts for 2% of the child population, with about 25% eventually developing schizophrenia.[5]

Ability Level

Autism is associated with a wide range of ability but its distribution varies with the survey, again reflecting the breadth of the diagnostic criteria. The English survey[58] found about 70% to have severe learning disability whereas it was only 27% in Sweden.[61] A significant degree of learning disability was present in about 70% of the French subjects[62] but in only 45% of those in Berlin.[60]

Gender

Autism is more frequent in males but the ratio is dependent on ability, falling from a ratio of 15:1 where there is a minimal degree of learning disability to about 2:1 in those with a severe learning disability. The latter is close to the bias found in nonautistic subjects who have an equivalent degree of learning disability. Wing suggests that this may be interpreted in the light of gender differences in cognitive skills.[65] Thus girls, less vulnerable to the loss of language skills, are less frequently affected by autism. However, when afflicted, the disorder affects their cognitive ability more severely because of a lack of compensatory visuo-spatial skills. This would accord with the increased risk of recurrence reported if the autistic child is a girl (7% as against 3.7% for a boy).[66]

Social Class

Kanner's original observation of an upward bias in the parents of his children was thought to be the result of selection pressures; these being the parents who would seek further opinions and were likely to obtain a definitive diagnosis. Although the bias was confirmed by Lotter's study, it was not found in the other English or in the Swedish surveys. If present it may reflect innate parental characteristics which, bringing success in their wake, give an upward social drift. This would give the suggested autistic genotype a survival value thereby ensuring its maintenance in the population. The wider recognition of the broader phenotype may allow this hypothesis to be tested.

Affective Disorder

Increasingly, affective disorder is being reported in the relatives of those with autistic disorder.[67] This includes both depressive and anxiety disorders, which often predate the birth of the child with autism, and can occur outside the immediate family and may be limited to those with hyperserotonaemia.[68]

One study tightly relates a high prevalence of bipolar affective disorder in relatives to those cases of autism without evidence of associated neurological disorder.[69,70] Where it occurs in the autistic person there may be two overlapping mechanisms. First, the genetic predisposition to autism may also predispose to affective disorder. Second, bipolar affective disorder may be both caused and coloured by cerebral disorder in general and learning disability in particular, resulting in an early onset, rapid cycling and an atypical presentation.[71]

Neurobiology

Neuropsychology

Cognitive deficits abound in autism and may be broadly divided into those which are narrow and highly specific, primarily affecting social-cognitive functioning, and those which are rather broader, such as poorly developed executive function.[72] Their relationship raises two crucial questions: first, are they specific to autism and, second, do they occur in every case. Only then is it worth asking how far any deficit goes towards providing a comprehensive explanation of the features of autism which include not only the basic triad of impairment but other elements such as the extreme variation in ability.

Learning Disability

Autism is associated with learning disability. Despite the hopes for realizable potential, IQ scores have been shown to be as stable over time as they are for the general population. They are good predictors of educational

attainment, and remain unchanged in the face of improved social functioning or any form of teaching or training.[73]

In autism, the disparity in the subtest scores often makes a nonsense of
any overall figure. This leaves many studies open to challenge about the
way in which their subjects were matched, whether by verbal or nonverbal
ability. Verbal ability is usually the more impaired in autism. The reverse
may apply in Asperger's syndrome but confusion about its definition and
the uneven spikiness of the subtest profiles combine to impede any clear
conclusion.

Learning disability is no longer a sufficient explanation either for the
presence of the symptomatology or for the exclusion of the diagnosis – the
label of 'learning disability with autistic traits' is not helpful. This view is
reinforced by the finding that the lower the IQ, particularly verbal, the
higher the subject's familial loading for autism, indicating an intrinsic
genetic link between the two diagnoses.[74]

Conversely, individuals with autism sometimes have a special skill in
which they excel, sometimes even when compared with the normal population. An unusual rote memory is most frequent but other skills are the
ability to calculate, work out dates, read fluently (although not necessarily
with comprehension), to perceive, remember or play music and to draw.
Such skills, rather over-promoted by the film *Rain Man*, although not
exclusive to autism, are particularly frequent occurring in 10–25% of the
population.

Delayed Development of a Theory of Mind

In 80% of people with autism there is a delay in the development of a
Theory of Mind. This is the ability to appreciate that, because others think
in a similar way, you can 'mentalize'; that is, by putting yourself in their
shoes you can understand their thoughts and feelings and, consequently,
explain and predict their actions. It is a complex ability that can be broken
down into various components and orders of difficulty – the Sally–Anne
test is an example of one means to identify deficits at first-order level.
Using dolls, the subject is given a short vignette in which Sally leaves her
marble in a box before leaving the room. Her friend, Anne, then moves it
to another box. Sally returns and the subject has to say where Sally will
look for the ball ('she thinks that. . . .'). A more complex vignette is used
to identify problems at the second-order level, in which the subject has to
work out how one character will behave, taking into account the view of
a second character ('she thinks that he thinks. . . .').[75]

Theory of Mind is a property that is acquired over time and in the same
predictable sequence as in normal children. Failure to pass the tests therefore might be explained partly by the general developmental delay associated with autism, particularly in language. Furthermore there is evidence
that, given sufficient verbal ability or a simplified test, autism itself is not
a barrier even at the level of second-order reasoning.[76,77] Nor does it prevent
a person from telling whether someone is joking or lying provided,

however, that it is in a test: real life situations are a different matter.[78] Similarly, although the test may distinguish people with Asperger's syndrome from people with High Functioning Autism,[24] it is not a clear indicator of social impairment.[79]

The absence of Theory of Mind – 'mind-blindness' – is a very specific disability which might relate to early developmental deprivation. This is supported by the discovery of similar deficits in children of normal ability who, because of prelingual deafness, developed without the benefit of everyday conversation. The implication is that there might be a more fundamental communicative deficit in autism which deprives the child of early conversational tuition in their own mental state and that of others.[80] An example of the complexity of this area is the critical importance of the way in which the question is put to a subject whose understanding may differ from the experimenter. Asking the child 'where will Sally look first for her marble' rather than simply 'where will Sally look for her marble' dramatically improves the success rate.[77] This brings out the importance in these tests of taking into account both verbal and performance ability.

Weak Central Coherence

Stimuli and events are interpreted in a global context. In autism the failure to take this context into account and to perceive an overall meaning or pattern, has been identified as deriving from a weak drive for 'central coherence'.[81] The result is a person able to perform well on those tasks (such as Block Design in the Wechsler Intelligence Scale or the Embedded Figures Test) where most are hampered by their tendency to look for a gestalt. Conversely it also results in a semantic–pragmatic deficit which undermines their ability to communicate.

Impaired Executive Function

Executive Function is the ability to identify a goal, to work out how to accomplish it, to pursue it flexibly while coping with set-backs and, ignoring distractions, to stay focused on it until the task is completed. It includes the ability to shift from one concept to another, to change behaviour, to use acquired knowledge and to manage multiple sources of information. It encompasses abilities necessary for central coherence, such as perceiving the relationship between isolated details and their integration into a coherent whole. Defects occur in autism[82] but these are not specific and, indeed, occur in any condition that affects frontal-lobe function, be it a post-traumatic encephalopathy, schizophrenia, attention deficit hyperactive disorder or developmental immaturity. This may simply indicate the imprecision of the tests used to define the deficits that occur in different conditions, the need to make allowance for the developmental status of the subject and the lack of population norms, especially in childhood.[83]

These approaches to the underlying psychology of autism are not mutually exclusive and, indeed, it seems unlikely that any single theory can provide a comprehensive explanation of autism. The difficulty that children with autism have in recognizing facial emotional expression, led Hobson[84] to suggest that the prime deficit might be a failure to develop a social and emotional relationship with people. The process would require the perception of the signals of emotional expression, its affective recognition and its reciprocal expression. From this early disruption follows a failure to develop a 'concept of persons', the equivalent (viewed in an emotional rather than in a cognitive framework) of the failure to develop Theory of Mind. The end-result would be an inability to relate to people and the characteristic autistic isolation. Weak central coherence would complement this in explaining other aspects of autism, particularly the problems in perception and the uneven abilities.[85] It is unclear how central a part impaired executive function might play. These relationships are discussed in more depth by Happé[86] and by Bailey and his colleagues.[72]

Neuroanatomy

There are several reports of an increase in brain size, in both volume and weight. This is probably the result of cortical thickening and is in marked contrast to the reduced size usually associated with learning disability syndromes.[72,87,88]

Post-mortem studies have given us tantalizing hints and their scarcity has lent them a disproportionate weight. Reports of Purkinje cell loss[89–91] have been complicated by the high prevalance of epilepsy (which is associated with cell loss in its own right) but they have served to focus attention on the cerebellum. Unfortunately, neuroimaging, with its access to a larger number of subjects, has not yet given its hoped-for, unequivocal answer. Courchesne has reported folia VI–VII of the cerebellar vermis to be hypoplastic and, subsequently, that vermal hyperplasia occurs in a smaller group of subjects, giving an overall bimodal distribution of abnormal vermal size.[92] Other studies, using stringently selected control subjects, have not confirmed this.[93–97] Courchesne's rebuttals claim the confirmatory support of a Japanese study[98,99] which, although it does indicate cerebellar abnormality, is of a substantially different nature.[100] If there is cerebellar abnormality, the absence of gross brainstem pathology suggests it to be primary rather than as the result of changes elsewhere.[101] At the heart of this debate is the potentially central role for the cerebellum in a wide range of mental activity, but, in particular, in controlling the attention-shifting aspect of executive function.[102] This might furnish a neurophysiological explanation for most of the abnormalities of autism.

Reports of late-onset autism secondary to acquired lesions of the temporal lobe[103,104] have intensified the interest in that area. They coincide with reports of increased neuronal density in the hippocampus and in other limbic areas.[105] As with many other findings this awaits replication by other centres. Reports of ventricular dilation, indicating medial temporal atrophy, remain unconfirmed.[106]

The parietal lobe has also come under scrutiny. Courchesne and his colleagues found evidence of localized cortical thickening[107] and also a reduction in the callosal fibres serving that area.[108] Single Positron Emission Computer Tomography (SPECT) scanning shows reduced perfusion in the temporal and parietal areas.[109]

Taken together the mass of unconfirmed reports, implicating the temporo-parietal, limbic lobe and cerebellar areas of the brain, provide fertile ground for speculation and further research but, as yet, no clear dominant pattern for autistic neurology.

Neurophysiology

Varied studies have produced inconsistent and conflicting results which simply indicate the variety of populations examined and, in particular, differences in their age and ability. Thus, SPECT identified reduced frontal cerebral perfusion, suggesting maturational delay, at the age of 3–4 years but such differences had disappeared within three years.[110] Nearly all the studies make no allowance for the selection pressures which give varied mixes of primary and secondary autism which, in turn, are reflected in the very differing rates of medical disorders such as epilepsy or tuberose sclerosis.

Epilepsy occurs in 20–30% of people with autism[111–113] and is unusual in that about one-half of the cases have their onset in adolescence or early adulthood, a contrast with the early age of onset more usual in learning disability.[114] Inconsistencies of diagnosis limit the conclusions that might be drawn from the comparison of studies of different populations. Generally, other than in those with profound learning disability, the prevalence of epilepsy is not associated with the severity of disability.[72] However, the *early-onset seizures*, predominantly generalized tonic–clonic in form,[112] may relate not only to the degree of disability, both mental and physical,[115] but also to the presence of verbal auditory agnosia rather than to the autistic deficit in sociability,[116] although this was not confirmed by a subsequent study.[113] It is the *later-onset seizures* which might differ, occurring in the more able person and being predominantly of complex partial type.[112] The frequency of EEG abnormality will depend on how it is defined and on the intensity of the investigation. However, 30–60% of subjects show abnormalities which tend to be epileptiform, bilateral and not usually localized. In some, improved seizure control will improve the autism to the extent that it begs the question as to whether the epilepsy or the autism was the primary condition.[104]

The results of auditory-evoked brainstem potentials have been mixed although one study found a delayed response in young children.[117] Auditory and visual novelties result in a lack of autonomic arousal[118,119] with a corresponding lack of electrophysiological responsiveness in the cortical association areas.[120,121]

Neurochemistry

Raised whole-blood serotonin occurs in about 30% of people with autism and is constant over time.[122] Its presence may indicate an increased genetic predisposition to autism[123,124] as it appears to segregate within families. It has more than one cause, in some being the result of increased uptake and, in others, the result of decreased binding.[125] However, it is not specific to autism, occurring in about 50% of people with severe learning disability.[126] Its significance is unclear as it is difficult to relate the abnormal peripheral levels of a compound to its more central function: for example, a low level may reflect either deficient synthesis or increased utilization.

Abnormal dopaminergic transmission is central to hypotheses about schizophrenia. Together with autism's motor abnormalities (which have some similarity to those of Parkinson's disease) this has led to attention being directed to dopamine. However, the core symptoms of autism do not show the same response to dopaminergic-blocking drugs (the neuroleptics). Furthermore, assay results are inconsistent and nonspecific. Raised levels of homovanillic acid (dopamine's principal metabolite) in the cerebrospinal fluid (CSF) suggest an increased central turnover.[127]

There is little evidence that the noradrenergic systems have a central role in autism.

The similarity between autistic behaviour and that induced by injecting young animals with exogenous opioids led Panksepp to propose that autism might result from excessive striatal opioid activity. There is some support in the discovery of abnormal endorphin levels in the CSF,[128] and in the therapeutic effectiveness of naltrexone, a long-acting receptor blocker.[129] Although the relevance of opioids to autism has yet to be confirmed, it has been proposed that peptide derivatives might cause individuals with autism to have a characteristic urinary chromatographic profile,[130] although this was not confirmed in the one carefully controlled, blind study.[131]

Aetiology

There is now general acceptance that autism is a neurodevelopmental disorder with an organic basis. The association with epilepsy, the presence of neurobiological abnormality, the lack of gross environmental pathology, and the associations with a genetic basis and with various medical causes of learning disability all combine to indicate both a primary, inherited disorder and a secondary, symptomatic one. The subject of debate is the relative proportions of these two aetiological groups.

The evidence that the majority of cases of autism have a genetic basis is now overwhelming. There is markedly increased familial risk of autism and a 3% probability that a further sibling will be affected. A series of twin studies have shown a marked disparity between the 60% concordance of monozygotic (MZ) pairs and the 3% concordance of dizygotic (DZ) pairs.[132] Their concordance increased to 92% and 10% when, rather than autism, a wider range of cognitive and social deficits were identified. This is in agreement with the results of family studies which show a high prevalence of the lesser variants of autism in first-degree relatives.[74,133] The pattern of inheritance is characteristic of several genes and further calculation suggests that the broader phenotype may be based on three or four interacting genes.[134] Further complicating matters are the hints of genetic heterogeneity – that there may be several genic subtypes of autism such as those demarcated by hyperserotonaemia (and even within that group)[123,125] and differences in familial loading between verbal and nonverbal probands.[74]

Obstetric complications are a symptom of the autistic state rather than the cause. However, in about 10% of cases autism is secondary to other medical causes, that usually act early in embryogenesis.[135] An autistic phenotype has been associated with most of the genetic causes of learning disability including Down's syndrome although, in the last, it is present in only 3–10% of the population.[136,137] A more specific link with fragile-X syndrome has turned out to be founded on clinical confusion (particularly because of the shyness associated with fragile-X syndrome) and laboratory overdiagnosis. In tuberose sclerosis autism occurs in up to 50% of cases.[138,139] Here, it is unclear whether the association is with the tuberose sclerosis genotype or with the infantile spasms that often accompany it.

The case for an infectious agent started with the association with congenital rubella[140] and was furthered by the suspicion of a post-immunization onset. Adult-onset autistic disorder was described following herpes encephalitis.[141] However, a meticulous search has failed to find any evidence of the seasonality which might have supported an infective component either as cause or as activating trigger.[142]

The debate about the relative frequencies of primary, genetic autism and autism secondary to medical disorders is still unresolved and, in part, is a debate about the narrowness of diagnosis and the population under study. Medical disorder appears to be more frequent where the autism is atypical or associated with severe learning disability.[135]

Pathogenesis

A wide variety of hypotheses have been proposed as to how an innate abnormality might lead to the phenotype of autism. Each is promoted by an enthusiastic prophet convinced that the cause is well-founded. The diversity of findings suggests that there are several possible pathways from aetiology to the final common outcome. It is also likely that many of the disparate findings are the result rather than the cause of the process producing autism. In embryonic development an early anomaly can cause a subsequent cascade of pathology: the trick is to distinguish the early anomaly from both the ensuing distortion of the system and its more direct effects. One suggestion is that, rather than being a unitary disorder, autism might be a compilation of deficits on at least two main dimensions: mechanical language skills (arising from the left hemisphere) and sociability, play and nonverbal communication (arising from the right hemisphere).[143] Courchesne proposes a syndrome arising from a cerebellar fault and the resultant deficits in the parietal and temporal cortex and the corresponding callosal white matter.[102]

The twin and family studies carried out by Rutter and his colleagues have led to a better appreciation of the extent of the autistic spectrum which includes a broader phenotype that is associated with neither learning disability nor epilepsy.[72] However, this leaves us with no clear diagnostic boundary. In the twin study, the diversity within monozygotic pairs parallels that between pairs, indicating that the variation is not simply the result of a genetic heterogeneity. Reviewing this, they[72] point out that any explanation must take into account the characteristic triad of impairment, the association with learning disability, the specific psychological deficits together with the occurrence of unusual skills, and the great diversity in presentation ranging from the aloof child with severe retardation to Asperger's syndrome. The extent to which any model, no matter how intellectually appealing, gets beyond speculation will depend on its degree of empirical support.

The psychological approaches largely emphasize the social and linguistic deficits that would arise from the lack of a particular skill. Although explaining some of the special talents they ignore the relationship with learning disability except as a coincident complication.

An ethological analysis of autistic behaviour led to the suggestion that autism results in a child whose social behaviour is dominated by avoidance. The effect is to retard the acquisition of language as well as other communication and cooperation skills[144] resulting in a form of deprivation. This is a theme which, although robustly challenged,[145] has been pursued by the Tinbergens.[146,147] There are certainly abnormalities in attachment behaviour which might arise from conflict between approach and avoidant behaviours. However, a systematic study suggests that their nature is consistent with this.[148] The ethological approach explains features such as stereotypies which might represent a form of displacement activity and decrease arousal,[149] an avenue encouraged by impaired executive function.

Reichelt has taken the opioid theory further, suggesting that the opioids might be exogenous, deriving from incompletely digested gluten and casein proteins.[150,151] It is now clear that biologically active peptides are produced in the bowel and can be absorbed intact.[150,151] This opens the possibility that autism might result from a variable environmental challenge in the form of exposure to the foods with which the body is innately unable to cope. Autism might also be the result of a number of possible breaches of a series of protective barriers. Of these, the first is the bowel where it has been suggested that mucosal sulphation defects might increase permeability.[152] Next is the potential for circulating peptidases, both in plasma and in red cells, to effect a functional barrier although this has been little-recognized or researched. Finally there is the blood–brain barrier. In addition to a genetic defect, the barriers might be affected by a variety of other agents, including viral infections, allowing exogenous opioids access to the central nervous system. In the end, much of this is based on evidence which has yet to be systematically and independently replicated.

Management of Autism

Assessment

Diagnosis must be the starting point for any programme. It gives the individual and his carers an identifiable and blame-free reason for their difficulties, membership of a group with similar afflictions, a range of potential remedies and a better idea of the outcome.

Misdiagnosis carries such far-reaching consequences that a clinically efficient, systematic assessment is essential. The failure to recognize autism, especially in its more subtle presentations, can be disastrous for a child who is blamed for his shortcomings and expected to cope with unsympathetic peers, with bullying and teasing being frequent presentational complaints. It is equally disastrous for the family who alternately blame themselves and their child for his behaviour. In the present climate, with its emphasis on family psychopathology, it seems inevitable that the professional's thought should turn towards child abuse and inappropriate investigation amounting to a form of therapeutic abuse.[153]

The initial assessment also provides a baseline against which progress is measured and requires a combination of:

- a full account from the carers / teachers which should include global judgements as well as specific items
- direct observation, preferably in several situations including one of everyday familiarity such as at school or in the home
- psychometric testing which should include both ability and communication.

Performance will depend on motivation. In autism this carries its own peculiar difficulties taking it beyond the individual's enthusiasm. It depends on the balance between voluntary and involuntary intent and all too frequent is the question 'is it that he can't do it, or that he won't do it?'. Consequently, it is essential for any assessment to get as wide-ranging a picture as possible of the individual's function in different circumstances.

General Education/Training

There are a large number of treatment programmes on the market, many of which are very expensive both in terms of money and in the amount of time a family needs to dedicate to the afflicted child. Coming from different theoretical standpoints and addressing different aspects of autism, they all claim global improvement with little comparative or objective evaluation. Any assessment of a programme's effectiveness should take into account:

- the innate change that the programme has brought about
- the superficial change that results from a change of environment: for example, the imposed structure that accompanies a behavioural programme

- the background change that would have occurred anyway as a consequence of natural development
- transient change due to spontaneous fluctuation.

as well as any other factors that might be happening outside the programme itself. No therapy is pure and it is important to recognize the extent to which a programme's effectiveness depends on the charisma of its enthusiastic advocate.

The essential elements of a teaching programme have been well described[154,155] and can be summarized as:

(1) Systematic and well structured: the programme should be presented in a series of clearly defined steps, each addressing a specific target. Only the essential cues should be given to help the student for whom it will be difficult to distinguish the key signal from the surrounding noise. The process should be enjoyable and failure-free and with active participation so that they learn by doing. It should strike a balance between under-stimulation and excessive demand.

(2) An appreciation of the fundamental handicaps: difficulty with the motivation to carry out a task, problems with executive function, difficulty in generalizing what is learned to other settings as well as other difficulties, such as in perception. Rewards should be tailored to the student, harnessing the person's own special interests, with intermittent reinforcement being more effective than continuous. Punishers are dangerous, opening the door to a punitive philosophy and they may not be received in the spirit the carer intended;[156] thus, pain may be perceived as pleasurable and an angry outburst as excitement.[157] Engagement should not depend on the student's initiative but, at the same time, the emphasis should be on self-direction, self-monitoring, and the independent use of skills. Once something is learned it is difficult to apply it to other circumstances. Teaching should take place in multiple and varied settings to avoid getting into routines which are stimulus or situation specific. Experiences should be natural, meaningful and directly relevant to everyday life, emphasizing the utility of a task rather than on rote-learning and routine.

(3) Any work must be family oriented as long-term gains depend on the long-term carer (whether parent or residential worker) being the primary therapist. This means the programme must include a home-based approach with the carers as co-therapists. The changing presentation of autism requires that they are constantly adapting and modifying their skills and strategies so that sustained follow-up is required if gains are not to be lost. There is the risk that this may increase the burden of caring if not approached carefully. The relationship with the carers must be supportive and adapt to a number of roles.[158]

(4) There is general agreement that intervention should be early[159] and intense.[160] However, although poorly quantified, there must

be the suspicion that some part of its success might lie in the recruitment of children who would have made a spontaneous recovery in any event. Any claims should be based on comparative studies.

Social Interaction

This is best taught by involvement and example, in short, in the person's own home with the help of his carers. Thus, activities need to be organized to be reciprocal and social, rather than solitary, making the carers essential to their completion. Social signals and social skills need to be taught both with real-life coaching and with more formal rehearsal such as in role-play, perhaps using video-recording to increase self-awareness. For those individuals integrated into the main-stream education, the use of a buddy system can increase supervision and support and complements the use of adults.[161] Throughout, it is essential to keep the outcome in mind. Anything taught should be useful and normal as, for example, it is not helpful to convert an aversive gaze to a fixed glare.[162]

Holding therapy has developed over the last 40 years as a means of improving attachment and social relationships in a number of forms of childhood disturbance. The Tinbergens saw in this a means to overcome the social avoidance central to autism and suggested the use of 'taming', a form of desensitization.[147] In practice the more confrontational 'holding' was employed with the child being held firmly for periods of up to 1 h, until there was a form of resolution. It is arguable whether the results from this technique, which has much in common with flooding and catharsis, warrant the distress and whether there might be more humane ways of achieving the same end.[163–166]

Communication

Central to any programme is the aim of developing better communication whether by speech, sign or gesture. Therapy must also target comprehension, although this is frequently better than expression. Much will depend on where the person is starting from. Thus, someone who is mute may first need to learn to point and to touch the appropriate sign cards to indicate their basic needs such as for food or the toilet. Expressive speech might be shaped from simple sounds or be built on echolalic speech. Although echolalic and jargon speech have a place in the development of language, they carry the risk of becoming entrenched and habitual, particularly if maintained by the responses of those around; it is too easy for carers to fall into a habitual style of response. Common failings are for carers either not to use speech or else to use too complex a form, flooding the individual with an incomprehensible mass of words which submerges the key phrases that carry the message.

At a different level, there are the people with semantic–pragmatic deficits. They can be taught formally such aspects as the additional meanings of colloquial speech, the recognition of nonverbal signals, and the use of gesture. As importantly, they can learn the scope there is for unintentional misunderstandings and the etiquette of who to talk to, for how long and about what topics.

Augmented communication has long been used, including sign language. Although some may be helped by its introduction, others may find it a distracting hindrance. It is so unpredictable as to who will benefit from it that it is a matter of experiment to discover its usefulness to an individual.

Facilitated communication is one form that is being vigorously explored. The claims being made by and through it, together with a lack of evidence for its effectiveness, make it controversial. It requires the physical assistance of a facilitator to introduce the process to the person with autism and it may be some years, if ever, before the facilitator can withdraw. The assumption is that there is an inherent motor/volitional block which can be overcome by working against the physical resistance of a restraining hand coupled with the confidence engendered by the relationship with the facilitator.[16] Unsurprisingly, for a method that is dealing with motivation, it has not been easy to assess the effectiveness of the method. There are repeated studies showing that, for many, the technique has more in common with the ouija board, expressing the facilitator's thoughts rather than those of the client.[167] Yet, the matter is not straightforward: first, there is occasional evidence of a subject's authorship, and next there is some unease about the validity of the test procedures. Overcoming motivational block is not a straightforward matter, even with a normal subject, and 'stage-fright' is a more complicated matter with someone who has autism. What is clear is that we cannot be certain at any given time or with any given subject, of the authorship of a communication. However, once more trivial messages have been accepted, it is difficult to ignore a claim, no matter how unreliable, that (for example) the subject has been abused. The result must be an understandable unease about the implications of embarking on a programme.[168,169] Of equal importance, although passing without comment, is the effect of a programme on a person's longer-term functioning, development and overall welfare.

Restricted, Repetitive Behaviour

Stereotyped and ritualistic activities interfere with learning and are also disruptive. It is difficult to tell to what extent they are a source of comfort and pleasure to the person but the aim should be their reduction rather than their elimination and gradual change rather than head-on confrontation. Success results from the enrichment of a boring environment and diversion with other activities as well as restricting the extent of the undesired activities.

The need for predictability encourages the development of fixed routines which can be very situational, for example, only occurring at home. There they can dominate the life of the whole family. The solution lies in arranging the person's life to give it order and pattern. This provides a background against which it is possible to ensure that there are sufficient small changes to accustom him to variation. This becomes the basis of eventual compromise allowing the individual to maintain some activities without limiting the family's functioning.

Behavioural Problems

Medical disorders are frequent in autism, the more so the greater the degree of disability. Limited communication and an altered perception, particularly of pain, means that the first concern must be for the health of the individual. Epilepsy is common, may present in an atypical way, and the prodromal build-up may be more of a problem than the seizure. Affective disorders are not uncommon and their treatment may transform the autism.[170]

Aggression is frequent and may represent a means of communication, of gaining attention, of relieving boredom, or be the response to a perceived threat. It is essential to appreciate the perspective of the person with autism whose interpretation of threat may be very unusual. Thus, standard responses, such as time-out, may provide a paradoxical reward for someone who wishes nothing other than to withdraw. Any strategy adopted should be based on a sympathetic functional analysis of the underlying problem, made with the help of carers who know the person well. The standard response to a standard symptom taken from a behavioural cook-book, is particularly likely to misfire.

Phobias can be more bizarre and intense than those usually seen in normal development. This may be the result of unusual perception: for example, an aversion to the head being touched is so frequent that it may reflect an atavistic hypersensitivity. Desensitization can be effective, particularly if the feared circumstance is mixed with something desired – for example, eating or watching a favourite video while having their hair or nails cut.

Sleep problems may simply indicate a disturbed biological rhythm, although this may sometimes be due to an affective disorder. The former may be corrected by confidence, routine and training possibly assisted by melatonin.[171]

Medical Treatment

Views differ about the extent of routine, baseline investigation. In the more able group, with no physical stigmata it is difficult to justify many tests unless medication is contemplated. This would warrant the collection of baseline values for those functions which might be affected: full blood count, liver and renal function tests, as well as electrocardiography (ECG) and EEG. The prevalence of epilepsy might justify the last, provided that it is clear what the clinical response is going to be to an abnormal record (not easy if there is no clinical sign of a seizure). Another consideration is that, should the routine, waking record be negative, a sleep-activated EEG should follow, along with more specialized recordings depending on the results; it therefore becomes a decision to engage in a potential chain of EEG investigations rather than in a single investigation. There is a greater likelihood of a medical disorder in the less able group or where there is organic symptomatology. Here, a variety of clinical investigations, including genetic and biochemical screens, are necessary. Otherwise, it is doubtful whether there is any justification for routine neuro-imaging or CSF investigations except for research. This carries its own requirements for consent, including ethical clearance.[135]

Drug treatment is usually long-term and raises the issue of adequate consent. Attitudes to medication often become polarized about whether the eventual cost to health, often hypothetical, warrants the benefit and, less often, about whose benefit. Recommended dosages are often irrelevant in a population who often are unusually sensitive or insensitive to the drug. Thus, a dosage schedule can be very specific to the individual who may have a very small window between the minimum effective dosage and the onset of toxicity. A therapeutic U-curve can result whereby a paradoxical response occurs at a higher dosage – the Goldilocks phenomenon in which too much of the drug is as ineffective as too little. Compliance is a problem, especially in autism, with the patient who is stronger willed (or simply stronger) than their carer. Finally, even where drugs are effective, the response may be partial or fleeting, lasting a few weeks or months before leaving the therapist with the problems of weaning the patient off the drug.

The neuroleptics have been the most potent drugs advocated. Chlorpromazine was too sedative, impairing learning and social interaction as well as the undesirable behaviour for which it was often a blanket prescription. Thioridazine is probably the most popular drug in the field[172] because of its reputation as less likely to cause tardive or withdrawal dyskinesias. However, except for one study which showed it to be effective for stereotyped behaviours,[173] little of the evidence for its value is derived directly from autism. The butyrophenones, and haloperidol in particular, have been more systematically researched by Campbell and her colleagues; they have found long-term haloperidol, given with intermittent dosage, to be effective with aggression[174] although associated with facial stereotypies which are very frequent in autism.[175] Under trial are newer neuroleptics, such as risperidone, which claim effectiveness with less risk.

Fenfluramine, selected because it depleted serotonin, had its moment of glory when a large multicentre trial confirmed earlier reports of its effectiveness.[176] However, this was followed by a flurry of null reports. A re-examination of the methodology of the original trial[177] failed to rehabilitate a drug whose positive effects were too subtle to merit its prescription.[178] Fenfluramine probably owes any effectiveness it does have to dopaminergic blockade (a property of the laevorotatory form and one which is achieved more effectively by the neuroleptics) or to its action as a stimulant.

Naltrexone is a long-acting opioid antagonist with a characteristic taste which limits compliance. Its effectiveness in autism was confirmed in a double-blind trial using very low dosage (0.5 mg kg^{-1} 48 h^{-1})[179] and in self-injury at higher doses.[180,181] Further trials have not confirmed the former but this may have reflected the position of a higher dosage on a therapeutic U-curve.[182,183]

On the same theoretical basis the incompletely digested peptides from dietary gluten and casein have been postulated to be a source of exogenous opioids which cause or exacerbate autism. Success has been claimed for dietary restriction[184] but the results await independent replication.

Analogue adrenocorticotrophic hormone (ORG 2766) is a drug which appears to have considerable potential but is still at the experimental level. Rather than directly altering a subject's behaviour, it alters their response to the environment, a property which is often under-rated in other drugs.[185]

Effectiveness has been claimed for a large number of other compounds, particularly vitamins. Vitamin B$_6$ (pyridoxine) (with a magnesium supplement) is reported to produce a global improvement in a minority of children.[186] Folate has been recommended[187] but may simply be acting as a mild stimulant. Tetrahydrobiopterin is being tried in autism as in a large number of other conditions.[188]

Other drugs are used in treating the symptomatology associated with autism. Adequate seizural control can produce an associated improvement in the autism.[189] Where anxiety is prominent, especially with panic states, anxiolytics in general, and β-adrenergic blockers in particular, are effective.[190,191]

Support

Family Work

The parents require all the help needed by the parents of any child with learning disability.[192] However, over and above this, their child is disconcertingly different to those of the others, being less responsive and rewarding, often more disruptive, and much more perplexing and frustrating.[193] There may be difficulty in distinguishing the problems arising from autism from the usual problems inherent in any person of the same age. Therefore, the care of a child with autism is difficult and puts unusual stress on a family and marriage. This, in turn, may be either offset or exacerbated by parental genetic traits, although these do not appear to bring any consistent trend towards a greater or lesser hardiness or resilience.[194] In addition, the advent of the disorder may have been after a period of apparently normal development, matters may have been further inflamed by delayed diagnosis and, in the longer term, by a failure to respond to a particular programme or strategy of management.

It is natural for parents to become over-protective and to be guilty about not spending sufficient time with their child, let alone for them to remain objective. Most helpful are an outside view, reassurance and practical ideas and advice. Joining a local parent support group and the National Autistic Society helps to remove the sense of isolation as well as furnishing practical ideas about specific forms of help and how to obtain these. Books are useful and two that have been written with carers and teachers in mind are those by Wing[15] and Attwood.[195] Close liaison between staff and parents is essential to minimize the confusing inconsistencies in policy and attitude. As with other parents of children with a disability, help is required with the morass that is the system of benefits and services. The greater difficulty in finding suitable placements, particularly residential, means that parents have to confront many of these issues much earlier, with adjustment being driven by an administrative rather than a clinical timetable.

Most cases of autism have a genetic basis, allowing some estimate of the probability of further children being affected. Investigation and counselling are important as for any other form of disability.

Services

Integration into mainstream education implies that the child is able to make use of a normal school environment. In autism the need for structure and predictability, the inability to take the initiative and the difficulty in coping with other people, combine to make the mainstream school unsuitable without considerable modification and support. Conversely, specialized schools for children with autism have difficulty in providing a full range of curricular activities and, for the more sociable child, a peer group to practise on.

Later should come a combination of resources which might include further education or employment. Any placement has to be sufficiently structured and supported for it to continue long enough to discover whether it is suitable. Occupational/vocational services are essential as are the support and enthusiasm of a variety of people: inter-agency disagreements usually result in the person with autism remaining at home with his parents.

Outcome

There is a well-recognized developmental spurt at about the age of 4–5 years, frequently credited to the initiation of some coincident educational/treatment programme. Thereafter, progress is slower. As in the nonautistic population, adolescence brings increasing social and educational demands and the issues of autonomy and self-awareness. For about one-third, it represents a set-back, with the development of depression, anxiety, or behavioural disturbance and epilepsy may make a belated appearance.[196,197] Catatonia may represent an insidious and malignant worsening of the motor indecision but may also represent a comorbid depression, responding to treatment.[198] Early adulthood often brings another developmental surge.[197]

There are two useful predictors of long-term attainment and social functioning. The first is the child's adaptive or nonverbal ability which remains as constant as it would for any group. Second is the development of useful language or symbolic play which, if they are not present by the age of 5 years, are unlikely to develop later.[197,199] The degree of improvement is the greater the more able the person and the milder their initial autism.[200]

Very few adults with autism achieve complete independence – about one-half of those of normal ability and who had developed useful language by the age of 5 years (about 10–15% of those with clear autism).[111] However, this does not take into account the much larger, and largely unrecognized, population of those with Asperger's syndrome, autistic variants or the broader phenotype.

There have been two notable controlled treatment studies. The first, in London, compared 16 children aged 3–11 years with groups of matched controls over a period of 18 months. A home-based intervention programme, using the parents as the primary therapists, produced marked improvement in the nonspecific emotional and behavioural problems. However, the programme effected little change in the core, autistic elements of sociability, language and rigid behaviour. In these areas much of the change was the result of maturation and also occurred in the untreated controls. Treatment improved the use of existing language, amplifying such communication as had already started and bilaterally developed usage in both child and mother.[199]

The second, in California, reports the progress of 19 children who had a mean age of 32 months and IQ of 53 (range 30–80) at the start of their intensive programme. Again the parents were co-therapists but the focus was on discrete trial learning carried out in the home for a 40-h week by students over a minimum of 2 years. The long term follow-up claims an average gain of 20 IQ points in the experimental group above the controls.[160] There has been substantial criticism of the methodology of the study. This focused especially on whether the subjects were randomly allocated, the diagnosis of these very young autistic children, the duration of the treatment, the demands on the family and the actual mechanism of change.[201] The study assumes that all children will respond to the same type of programme and makes no allowance for the effect of altered family attitudes or for the charisma of the therapist. However, in the end, the results are startling with complete integration of seven of the subjects into the normal educational system. Replication is awaited.

Conclusion

It is 50 years since autism was generally acknowledged and it is only in the last decade that the extent of the genetic basis has been recognized. The increasing expertise identifies the inconsistencies as much as the larger pattern. Are we are dealing with a continuum of disorder, shading gradually into normality, or a range of separate but overlapping diagnostic categories? The latter may form a spectrum, ranging from Asperger's syndrome to aloof autism analogous to the light spectrum in which a range of colours can be identified on the background continuity. The range of form and severity is so great that some clinical subgrouping, whether by category or by symptom dimension, is necessary to account for the varying outcomes and the apparently idiosyncratic responses to a wide battery of treatment.

Autism will continue to provide many scientists with a series of Rorschach images on which they can project their pet theories. It will also give the charismatic therapist some of his most lucrative successes. Despite this, a central core of evidence is slowly building up which is defining the model developmental disorder. Meanwhile individuals with autism have to navigate their way between a number of agencies, including health, social services, education and the charities; some competing and others reluctant. The effect is to encourage parental polarization which either drives towards residential placement or else produces an irrational resistance to the child ever leaving home.

All too often treatment is aimed at the removal of undesirable behaviours. Of more importance is the fostering of normal development, the ability to integrate specific skills to engage in normal, intuitive social relationships and, that grail of treatment, to enjoy the experience of everyday life.

References

1. Kanner L (1943) Autistic disturbances of affective contact. *Nervous Child* **2**, 217–50.
2. Asperger H (1944) Die autistischen Psychopathen im Kindesalter. *Archiv für Psychiatrie und Nervkrankheiten* **117**, 76–137.
3. Carrey NJ (1995) Itard's mémoire on 'mutism caused by a lesion of the intellectual functions': A historical analysis. *Journal of the American Academy of Child and Adolescent Psychiatry* **34(12)**, 1655–61.
4. Kolvin I, Ounsted C, Humphrey M & McNay A (1971) Studies in childhood psychoses. II. The phenomenology of childhood psychoses. *British Journal of Psychiatry* **118**, 385–95.
5. Wolff S (1995) *Loners: The Life Path of Unusual Children*. London: Routledge.
6. Wing L (1982) The autistic continuum. In Wing L (ed) *Aspects of Autism: Biological Research*, 3rd edn, pp. v–viii. London: Gaskell/Royal College of Psychiatrists, Gaskell Psychiatry series.
7. Petty LK, Ornitz EM, Michelman JD & Zimmerman EG (1984) Autistic children who become schizophrenic. *Archives of General Psychiatry* **41**, 129–35.
8. Tantam D (1988) Lifelong eccentricity and social isolation: II. Asperger's syndrome or schizoid personality disorder? *British Journal of Psychiatry* **153**, 783–91.
9. Volkmar FR & Cohen DJ (1991) Comorbid association of autism and schizophrenia. *American Journal of Psychiatry* **148(12)**, 1705–7.
10. World Health Organisation (1992) *The ICD-10 Classification of Mental and Behavioural Disorders: Clinical Descriptions and Diagnostic Guidelines*. Geneva: World Health Organisation.
11. American Psychiatric Association (1994) *Diagnostic and Statistical Manual of Mental Disorders (DSM-IV)*, 4th edn. Washington DC: American Psychiatric Association.
12. Wing L (1979) Differentiation of retardation and autism from specific communication disorders. *Child Care, Health and Development* **5(1)**, 57–68.
13. Attwood A & Wing L (1987) Syndromes of autism and atypical development. In Cohen DJ & Donellan AM (eds) *Handbook of Autism and Pervasive Developmental Disorders*, vol. 25, pp. 3–19. New York: Wiley.
14. Wolff S & McGuire RJ (1995) Schizoid personality in girls: a follow-up study – what are the links with Asperger's syndrome. *Journal of Child Psychology and Psychiatry* **36(5)**, 793–818.

15. Wing L (1996) *The Autistic Spectrum*. London: Constable.
16. Attwood T (1992) Movement disorders and autism: a rationale for the use of facilitated communication. *Communication* **26(3)**, 27–9.
17. Comings DE & Comings BG (1991) Clinical and genetic relationships between autism-pervasive developmental disorder and Tourette syndrome: A study of 19 cases. *American Journal of Medical Genetics* **39**, 180–91.
18. Volkmar FR & Cohen DJ (1989) Disintegrative disorder or 'late onset' autism. *Journal of Child Psychology and Psychiatry and Allied Disciplines* **30(5)**, 717–24.
19. Tantam D (1988) Lifelong eccentricity and social isolation: I. Psychiatric, social and forensic aspects. *British Journal of Psychiatry* **153**, 777–82.
20. van Krevelen DA (1962) Early infantile autism and autistic psychopathy. *Journal of Childhood Autism and Schizophrenia* **1(1)**, 82–6.
21. Gillberg IC & Gillberg C (1989) Asperger syndrome: Some epidemiological considerations: A research note. *Journal of Child Psychology and Psychiatry and Allied Disciplines* **30(4)**, 631–8.
22. Wing L (1981) Asperger's syndrome: A clinical account. *Psychological Medicine* **11(1)**, 115–29.
23. Szatmari P, Archer L, Fisman S, Streiner DL & Wilson F (1995) Asperger's syndrome and autism: differences in behaviour, cognition, and adaptive functioning. *Journal of the American Academy of Child and Adolescent Psychiatry* **34(12)**, 1662–71.
24. Ozonoff S, Rogers SJ & Pennington BF (1991) Asperger's syndrome: Evidence of an empirical distinction from high-functioning autism. *Journal of Child Psychology and Psychiatry and Allied Disciplines* **32(7)**, 1107–22.
25. Everard MP (1976) Mildly autistic young people and their problems. International Symposium on Childhood Autism. St. Gallen, Switzerland.
26. Gillberg C (1989) Asperger syndrome in 23 Swedish children. *Developmental Medicine and Child Neurology* **31(4)**, 520–31.
27. Ghaziuddin M, Butler E, Tsai L & Ghaziuddin N (1994) Is clumsiness a marker for Asperger syndrome? *Journal of Intellectual Disability Research* **38(5)**, 519–27.
28. le Couteur A, Rutter M & Lord C et al. (1989) Autism Diagnostic Interview: A standardized investigator-based instrument. *Journal of Autism and Developmental Disorders* **19(3)**, 363–87.
29. Lord C, Rutter M & le Couteur A (1994) Autism Diagnostic Interview – Revised: A revised version of a diagnostic interview for caregivers of individuals with possible pervasive developmental disorders. *Journal of Autism and Developmental Disorders* **24(5)**, 659–85.
30. Lord C, Rutter ML & Goode S et al. (1989) Autism Diagnostic Observation Schedule: A standardized observation of communicative and social behaviour. *Journal of Autism and Development Disorders* **19(2)**, 185–212.
31. DiLavore PC, Lord C & Rutter M (1995) Pre-linguistic Autism Diagnostic Observation Schedule. *Journal of Autism and Developmental Disorders* **25(4)**, 355–79.
32. Wing L (1996) Wing Schedule of Handicaps, Behaviour and Skills (HBS). In Rapin I (ed) *Preschool Children with Inadequate Communication*. London: Mac KeithPress.
33. Schopler E, Reichler RJ & Renner BR (1988) The Childhood Autism Rating Scale (CARS). Los Angeles: Western Psychological Services.
34. Sturmey P, Matson JL & Sevin JA (1992) Analysis of the internal consistency of three autism scales. *Journal of Autism and Developmental Disorders* **22(2)**, 321–8.
35. van-Bourgondien ME, Marcus LM & Schopler E (1992) Comparison of DSM-III-R and Childhood Autism Rating Scale diagnoses of autism. Special Issue: Classification and diagnosis. *Journal of Autism and Developmental Disorders* **22(4)**, 493–506.
36. Krug DA, Arick J & Almond P (1980) Behaviour checklist for identifying severely handicapped individuals with high levels of autistic behaviour. *Journal of Child Psychology and Psychiatry and Allied Disciplines* **21(3)**, 221–9.
37. Volkmar FR, Cicchetti DV & Dykens E et al. (1988) An evaluation of the Autism Behaviour Checklist. *Journal of Autism and Developmental Disorders* **18(1)**, 81–97.
38. Wadden NP, Bryson SE & Rodger RS (1991) A closer look at the Autism Behaviour Checklist: Discriminant validity and factor structure. *Journal of Autism and Developmental Disorders* **21(4)**, 529–41.
39. Yirmiya N, Sigman M & Freeman BJ (1994) Comparison between diagnostic instruments for identifying high-functioning children with autism. *Journal of Autism and Developmental Disorders* **24(3)**, 281–91.

40. Johnson MH, Siddons F, Frith U & Morton J (1992) Can autism be predicted on the basis of infant screening tests? *Developmental Medicine and Child Neurology* **34(4)**, 316–20.
41. Baron-Cohen S, Allen J & Gillberg C (1992) Can autism be detected at 18 months? The needle, the haystack, and the CHAT. *British Journal of Psychiatry* **161**, 839–43.
42. Cohen DJ, Paul R & Volkmar FR (1986) Issues in the classification of pervasive and other developmental disorders: Toward DSM-IV. *Journal of the American Academy of Child Psychiatry* **25(2)**, 213–20.
43. Newson E (1996) Pathological Demand Avoidance syndrome: A statistical update. In: Shattock P (ed) *Therapeutic Intervention in Autism: Perspectives from Research and Practice.* University of Durham, UK: National Autistic Society.
44. Bishop DV (1989) Autism, Asperger's syndrome and semantic–pragmatic disorder: Where are the boundaries? Special Issue: Autism. *British Journal of Disorders of Communication* **24(2)**, 107–21.
45. Brook SL & Bowler DM (1992) Autism by another name? Semantic and pragmatic impairments in children. *Journal of Autism and Developmental Disorders* **22(1)**, 61–81.
46. Rourke BP (1988) The syndrome of Nonverbal Learning Disabilities: Developmental manifestations in neurological disease, disorder, and dysfunction. *Clinical Neuropsychologist* **2(4)**, 293–330.
47. Rourke BP (1995) *Syndrome of Nonverbal Learning Disabilities: Neurodevelopmental Manifestations.* New York: Guilford Press.
48. Semrud-Clikeman M & Hynd GW (1990) Right hemisphere dysfunction in nonverbal learning disabilities: social, academic and adaptive functioning in adults and children. *Psychological Bulletin* **107**, 196–209.
49. Hill AE & Rosenbloom L (1986) Disintegrative psychosis of childhood: Teenage follow-up. *Developmental Medicine and Child Neurology* **28(1)**, 34–40.
50. Kurita H, Kita M & Miyake Y (1992) A comparative study of development and symptoms among disintegrative psychosis and infantile autism with and without speech loss. *Journal of Autism and Developmental Disorders* **22(2)**, 175–88.
51. Appleton RE (1995) The Landau–Kleffner syndrome. *Archives of Disease in Childhood* **72(5)**, 386–7.
52. Stefanatos GA, Grover W & Geller E (1995) Case study: Corticosteroid treatment of language regression in pervasive developmental disorder. *Journal of the American Academy of Child and Adolescent Psychiatry* **34(8)**, 1107–11.
53. Volkmar FR, Cooke E & Lord C et al. (1996) Autism and related conditions. *Journal of the American Academy of Child and Adolescent Psychiatry* **35(4)**, 401–2.
54. Stefanatos GA (1996) Autism and related conditions (reply to Volkmar et al.). *Journal of the American Academy of Child and Adolescent Psychiatry* **35(4)**, 404–5.
55. Deonna T (1996) Autism and related conditions. *Journal of the American Academy of Child and Adolescent Psychiatry* **35(4)**, 403–4.
56. Stefanatos GA (1996) Autism and related conditions (reply to Deonna). *Journal of the American Academy of Child and Adolescent Psychiatry* **35(4)**, 402–3.
57. Zahner GEP & Pauls DL (1987) Epidemiological surveys of infantile autism. In: Cohen DJ & Donellan AM (eds) *Handbook of Autism and Pervasive Developmental Disorders,* pp. 199–207. New York: Wiley.
58. Wing L & Gould J (1979) Severe impairments of social interaction and associated abnormalities in children: Epidemiology and classification. *Journal of Autism and Developmental Disorders* **9(1)**, 11–29.
59. Hoshino Y, Kumishiro H, Yashima Y, Tachibana R & Watanabe M (1982) The epidemiological study of autism in Fukushima-ken. *Folia Psychiatirica et Neurologica Japonica* **36**, 115–24.
60. Steinhausen HC, Gobel D, Breinlinger M & Wohlleben B (1986) A community survey of infantile autism. *Journal of the American Academy of Child Psychiatry* **25(2)**, 186–9.
61. Gillberg C (1984) Infantile autism and other childhood psychoses in a Swedish urban region: Epidemiological aspects. *Journal of Child Psychology and Psychiatry and Allied Disciplines* **25(1)**, 35–43.
62. Fombonne E & du-Mazaubrun C (1992) Prevalence of infantile autism in four French regions. *Social Psychiatry and Psychiatric Epidemiology* **27(4)**, 203–10.
63. Treffert DA (1970) Epidemiology of infantile autism. *Archives of General Psychiatry* **22**, 431–8.
64. Ehlers S & Gillberg C (1993) The epidemiology of Asperger syndrome: A total

population study. *Journal of Child Psychology and Psychiatry and Allied Disciplines* **34(8)**, 1327–50.

65. Wing L (1981) Sex ratios in early childhood autism and related conditions. *Psychiatry Research* **5**, 129–37.

66. Jorde LB, Hasstedt SJ & Ritvo ER *et al.* (1991) Complex segregation analysis of autism. *American Journal of Human Genetics* **49**, 932–8.

67. Smalley SL, McCracken J & Tanguay P (1995) Autism, affective disorders, and social phobia. *American Journal of Medical Genetics* **60(1)**, 19–26.

68. Cook EH, Charak DA & Arida J *et al.* (1994) Depressive and obsessive–compulsive symptoms in hyperserotonemic parents of children with autistic disorder. *Psychiatry Research* **52(1)**, 25–33.

69. DeLong R & Nohria C (1994) Psychiatric family history and neurological disease in autistic spectrum disorders. *Developmental Medicine and Child Neurology* **36(5)**, 441–8.

70. DeLong R (1994) Children with autistic spectrum disorder and a family history of affective disorder. *Developmental Medicine and Child Neurology* **36(8)**, 674–87.

71. Berney TP & Jones PM (1988) Manic depressive disorder in mental handicap. *Australia and New Zealand Journal of Developmental Disability* **14**, 219–25.

72. Bailey A, Phillips W & Rutter M (1996) Autism: Towards an integration of clinical, genetic, neuropsychological, and neurobiological perspectives. *Journal of Child Psychology and Psychiatry* **37(1)**, 89–126.

73. Rutter M (1983) Cognitive deficits in the pathogenesis of autism. *Journal of Child Psychology and Psychiatry and Allied Disciplines* **24(4)**, 513–31.

74. Bolton P, Macdonald H & Pickles A *et al.* (1994) A case-control family history study of autism. *Journal of Child Psychology and Psychiatry and Allied Disciplines* **35(5)**, 877–900.

75. Baron-Cohen S (1989) The autistic child's theory of mind: A case of specific developmental delay. *Journal of Child Psychology and Psychiatry and Allied Disciplines* **30(2)**, 285–97.

76. Sparrevohn R & Howie PM (1995) Theory of mind in children with autistic disorder: Evidence of developmental progression and the role of verbal ability. *Journal of Child Psychology and Psychiatry and Allied Disciplines* **36(2)**, 249–63.

77. Tager-Flusberg H & Sullivan K (1994) A second look at second-order belief attribution in autism. *Journal of Autism and Developmental Disorders* **24(5)**, 577–86.

78. Leekham SR & Prior M (1994) Can autistic children distinguish lies from jokes? A second look at second-order belief attribution. *Journal of Child Psychology and Psychiatry and Allied Disciplines* **35(5)**, 901–15.

79. Bowler DM (1992) 'Theory of mind' in Asperger's syndrome. *Journal of Child Psychology and Psychiatry and Allied Disciplines* **33(5)**, 877–93.

80. Peterson CC & Siegal M (1995) Deafness, conversation and theory of mind. *Journal of Child Psychology and Psychiatry and Allied Disciplines* **36(3)**, 459–74.

81. Frith U (1989) *Autism: Explaining the Enigma*. Oxford: Blackwell.

82. Ozonoff S, Strayer DL, McMahon WM & Filloux F (1994) Executive function abilities in autism and Tourette syndrome: An information processing approach. *Journal of Child Psychology and Psychiatry and Allied Disciplines* **35(6)**, 1015–32.

83. Kelly TP, Borrill HS & Maddell DL (1996) Development and assessment of executive function in children. *Child Psychology and Psychiatry Review* **1(2)**, 46–51.

84. Hobson RP (1993) *Autism and the Development of Mind*, Essays in Developmental Psychology. Hove, UK: Lawrence Erlbaum.

85. Frith U & Happé F (1994) Autism: Beyond 'theory of mind'. *Cognition* **50(1–3)**, 115–32.

86. Happé FGE (1994) Annotation: Current psychological theories of autism: The 'Theory of Mind' account and rival theories. *Journal of Child Psychology and Psychiatry and Allied Disciplines* **35(2)**, 215–29.

87. Filipek PA, Richelme C & Kennedy DM *et al.* (1992) Morphometric analysis of the brain in developmental language disorders and autism. *Annals of Neurology* **32**, 475.

88. Piven J, Arndt S, Bailey J, Havercamp S, Andreasen N & Palmer P (1995) An MRI study of brain size in autism. *American Journal of Psychiatry* **152**, 1145–49.

89. Bauman M (1991) Microscopic neuroanatomic abnormalities in autism. *Pediatrics* **87**(Suppl.), 791–6.

90. Ritvo ER, Freeman BJ & Scheibel AB *et al.* (1986) Lower Purkinje cell counts in the cerebella of four autistic subjects: Initial findings of the UCLA-NSAC research report. *American Journal of Psychiatry* **143(7)**, 862–6.

91. Williams RS, Hauser SL, Purpura DP, DeLong GR & Swisher CM (1980) Autism and

mental retardation: neuropathologic studies performed in four retarded persons with autistic behavior. *Archives of Neurology* **37**, 749–53.

92. Courchesne E, Townsend J & Saitoh O (1994) The brain in infantile autism: Posterior fossa structures are abnormal. *Neurology* **44(2)**, 214–23.

93. Garber HJ, Ritvo ER & Chiu LC *et al.* (1989) A magnetic resonance imaging study of autism: Normal fourth ventricle size and absence of pathology. *American Journal of Psychiatry* **146(4)**, 532–4.

94. Garber HJ & Ritvo ER (1992) Magnetic resonance imaging of the posterior fossa in autistic adults. *American Journal of Psychiatry* **149(2)**, 245–7.

95. Kleiman MD, Neff S & Rosman NP (1992) The brain in infantile autism: Are posterior fossa structures abnormal? *Neurology* **42(2)**, 753–60.

96. Piven J, Nehme E & Simon J *et al.* (1992) Magnetic resonance imaging in autism: Measurement of the cerebellum, pons, and fourth ventricle. *Biological Psychiatry* **31(5)**, 491–504.

97. Piven J & Arndt S (1995) The cerebellum and autism. *Neurology* **45(2)**, 398–99.

98. Courchesne E, Townsend J & Saitoh O (1995) 'The cerebellum and autism': Reply. *Neurology* **45(2)**, 399–402.

99. Courchesne E (1995) New evidence of cerebellar and brainstem hypoplasia in autistic infants, children and adolescents: The MR imaging study by Hashimoto and colleagues. *Journal of Autism and Developmental Disorders* **25(1)**, 19–22.

100. Hashimoto T, Tayama M & Murakawa K *et al.* (1995) Development of the brainstem and cerebellum in autistic patients. *Journal of Autism and Developmental Disorders* **25(1)**, 1–18.

101. Hsu M, Yeung-Courchesne R, Courchesne E & Press GA (1991) Absence of magnetic resonance imaging evidence of pontine abnormality in infantile autism. *Archives of Neurology* **48(11)**, 1160–3.

102. Courchesne E, Townsend J & Akshoomoff NA *et al* (1994) Impairment in shifting attention in autistic and cerebellar patients. *Behavioral Neuroscience* **108(5)**, 848–65.

103. Gillberg C (1986) Brief report: Onset at age 14 of a typical autistic syndrome: A case report of a girl with herpes simplex encephalitis. *Journal of Autism and Developmental Disorders* **16(3)**, 369–75.

104. Hoon AH & Reiss AL (1992) The mesial-temporal lobe and autism: Case report and review. *Developmental Medicine and Child Neurology* **34(3)**, 252–9.

105. Bauman ML & Kemper TL (1994) *Neurobiology of Autism.* Baltimore, Maryland: Johns Hopkins University Press.

106. Saitoh O, Courchesne E, Egaas B, Lincoln AJ & Schreibman L (1995) Cross-sectional area of the posterior hippocampus in autistic patients with cerebellar and corpus callosum abnormalities. *Neurology* **45(2)**, 317–24.

107. Courchesne E, Press GA & Yeung-Courchesne R (1993) Parietal lobe abnormalities detected with MR in patients with infantile autism. *American Journal of Roentgenology* **160**, 387–93.

108. Egaas B, Courchesne E & Saitoh O (1995) Reduced size of corpus callosum in autism. *Archives of Neurology* **52(8)**, 794–801.

109. Mountz JM, Tolbert LC, Lill DW, Katholi CR & Liu HG (1995) Functional deficits in autistic disorder: characterization by technetium-99m-HMPAO and SPECT. *Journal of Nuclear Medicine* **36(7)**, 1156–62.

110. Zilbovicius M, Garreau B & Samson Y *et al.* (1995) Delayed maturation of the frontal cortex in childhood autism. *American Journal of Psychiatry* **152(2)**, 248–52.

111. Gillberg C (1991) Outcome in autism and autistic-like conditions. Special Section: Longitudinal research. *Journal of the American Academy of Child and Adolescent Psychiatry* **30(3)**, 375–82.

112. Gillberg C (1991) The treatment of epilepsy in autism. *Journal of Autism and Development Disorders* **21(1)**, 61–77.

113. Wong V (1993) Epilepsy in children with autistic spectrum disorder. *Journal of Child Neurology* **8(4)**, 316–22.

114. Goulden KJ, Shinnar S, Koller H, Katz M & Richardson SA (1991) Epilepsy in children with mental retardation: a cohort study. *Epilepsia* **32**, 690–7.

115. Elia M, Musumeci SA, Ferri R & Bergonzi P (1995) Clinical and neurophysiological aspects of epilepsy in subjects with autism and mental retardation. *American Journal on Mental Retardation* **100(1)**, 6–16.

116. Tuchman RF, Rapin I & Shinnar S (1991) Autistic and dysphasic children: II Epilepsy. *Pediatrics* **88**, 1219–25.

117. Wong V & Wong SN (1991) Brainstem auditory evoked potential study in children with autistic disorder. *Journal of Autism and Developmental Disorders* **21(3)**, 329–40.
118. van Engeland H (1984) The electrodermal orienting response to auditive stimuli in autistic children, normal children, mentally retarded children, and child psychiatric patients. *Journal of Autism and Developmental Disorders* **14(3)**, 261–79.
119. van Engeland H, Roelofs JW, Verbaten MN & Slangen JL (1991) Abnormal electrodermal reactivity to novel visual stimuli in autistic children. *Psychiatry Research* **38(1)**, 27–38.
120. Courchesne E & Yeung-Courchesne R (1988) Event-related brain potentials. In Rutter M, Hassein TM & Lann IS (eds) *Assessment and Diagnosis in Child Psychopathology*, pp. 264–99. New York: The Guilford Press.
121. Verbaten MN, Roelofs JW, van Engeland H, Kenemans JK & Slangen JL (1991) Abnormal visual event-related potentials of autistic children. *Journal of Autism and Developmental Disorders* **21(4)**, 449–70.
122. Minderaa RB, Anderson GM and Volkmar FR *et al.* (1989) Whole blood serotonin and tryptophan in autism: Temporal stability and the effects of medication. *Journal of Autism and Developmental Disorders* **19(1)**, 129–36.
123. Cook EH, Leventhal BL & Heller W *et al.* (1990) Autistic children and their first-degree relatives: Relationships between serotonin and norepinephrine levels and intelligence. *Journal of Neuropsychiatry and Clinical Neurosciences* **2(3)**, 268–74.
124. Piven J, Tsai G & Nehme E *et al.* (1991) Platelet serotonin, a possible marker for familial autism. *Journal of Autism and Developmental Disorders* **21(1)**, 51–9.
125. Cook EH, Jr, Arora RC & Anderson GM *et al.* (1993) Platelet serotonin studies in hyper-serotonemic relatives of children with autistic disorder. *Life Sciences* **52(25)**, 2005–15.
126. Hanley HG, Stahl SM & Freedman DX (1977) Hyperserotonemia and amine metabolites in autistic and retarded children. *Archives of General Psychiatry* **34(5)**, 521–31.
127. Gillberg C, Svennerholm L & Hamilton-Hellberg C (1983) Childhood psychosis and monoamine metabolites in spinal fluid. *Journal of Autism and Developmental Disorders* **13(4)**, 383–96.
128. Gillberg C (1995) Endogenous opioids and opiate antagonists in autism: Brief review of empirical findings and implications for clinicians. *Developmental Medicine and Child Neurology* **37(3)**, 239–45.
129. Panksepp J & Lensing P (1991) A synopsis of an open-trial of naltrexone treatment of autism with four children. *Journal of Autism and Developmental Disorders* **21(2)**, 243–9.
130. Gillberg C, Trygstad O & Foss I (1982) Childhood psychosis and urinary excretion of peptides and protein-associated peptide complexes. *Journal of Autism and Developmental Disorders* **12(3)**, 229–41.
131. le Couteur A, Trygstad O, Evered C, Gillberg C & Rutter M (1988) Infantile autism and urinary excretion of peptides and protein-associated peptide complexes. *Journal of Autism and Developmental Disorders* **18(2)**, 181–90.
132. Bailey A, Le Couteur A, Gottesman I & Bolton P (1995) Autism as a strongly genetic disorder: Evidence from a British twin study. *Psychological Medicine* **25(1)**, 63–77.
133. Wolff S, Narayan S & Moyes B (1988) Personality characteristics of parents of autistic children: A controlled study. *Journal of Child Psychology and Psychiatry and Allied Disciplines* **29(2)**, 143–53.
134. Simonoff E, Bolton P & Rutter M (1996) Mental retardation: genetic findings, clinical implications and research agenda. *Journal of Child Psychology and Psychiatry* **37(3)**, 259–80.
135. Rutter M, Bailey A, Bolton P & Le Couter A (1994) Autism and known medical conditions: Myth and substance. *Journal of Child Psychology and Psychiatry and Allied Disciplines* **35(2)**, 311–22.
136. Ghaziuddin M, Tsai LY & Ghaziuddin N (1992) Autism in Down's syndrome: Presentation and diagnosis. *Journal of Intellectual Disability Research* **36(5)**, 449–56.
137. Cocchi R (1989) Psychosis in Down children: An epidemiological and clinical survey on 413 subjects. *Italian Journal of Intellective Impairment* **2(2)**, 131–6.
138. Smalley SL, Tanguay PE, Smith M & Gutierrez G (1992) Autism and tuberous sclerosis. *Journal of Autism and Developmental Disorders* **22(2)**, 339–55.
139. Hunt A & Shepherd C (1993) A prevalence study of autism in tuberous sclerosis. *Journal of Autism and Developmental Disorders* **23(2)**, 323–39.
140. Chess S (1977) Follow-up report on autism in congenital rubella. *Journal of Autism and Developmental Disorders* **7(1)**, 69–81.
141. Gillberg IC (1991) Autistic syndrome with onset at age 31 years: Herpes encephalitis as

a possible model for childhood autism. *Developmental Medicine and Child Neurology* **33(10)**, 920–4.

142. Bolton P, Pickles A, Harrington R, Macdonald H & Rutter M (1992) Season of birth: Issues, approaches and findings for autism. *Journal of Child Psychology and Psychiatry and Allied Disciplines* **33(2)**, 509–30.

143. Goodman R (1989) Infantile autism: A syndrome of multiple primary deficits? *Journal of Autism and Developmental Disorders* **19(3)** 409–24.

144. Richer J (1976) The social-avoidance behaviour of autistic children. *Animal Behaviour* **24(4)**, 898–906.

145. Wing L & Ricks DM (1976) The aetiology of childhood autism: A criticism of the Tinbergens' ethological theory. *Psychological Medicine* **6(4)**, 533–43.

146. Tinbergen EA & Tinbergen N (1972) Early childhood autism – an ethological approach. *Beihefte zur Zeitshrift für Tierpsychologie* **10**, 1–53.

147. Tinbergen N & Tinbergen EA (1983) *'Autistic' Children: New Hope for a Cure.* London: George Allen & Unwin.

148. Buitelaar JK (1995) Attachment and social withdrawal in autism: Hypotheses and findings. *Behaviour* **132(5–6)**, 319–50.

149. Hutt C & Hutt SJ (1970) Stereotypies and their relation to arousal. A study of autistic children. In Hutt C & Hutt SJ (eds) *Behaviour Studies in Psychiatry.* Oxford: Pergamon.

150. Gardner MLG (1994) Absorption of intact proteins and peptides. In Johnson LR (ed) *Physiology of the Gastrointestinal Tract,* 3rd edn, pp. 1795–820. New York: Raven Press.

151. Gardner MLG, Knivsberg AM & Reichelt KL (1996) Role of diet in cause and treatment of autistic syndromes. Autism: Hope is not a Dream – the 5th Congress of Autism-Europe. Barcelona: Autism Europe.

152. Waring R & Reichelt KL (1996) The biochemistry of autistic syndromes. Autism: Hope is not a Dream – the 5th Congress of Autism-Europe. Barcelona: Autism Europe.

153. Perkins M & Wolkind SN (1991) Asperger's syndrome: Who is being abused? *Archives of Disease in Childhood* **66(6)**, 693–5.

154. Powers MD (1992) Early Intervention for Children and Autism. In Berkell DE (ed) *Autism: Identification, Education, and Treatment,* pp. 225–52. Hillsdale, New Jersey: Lawrence Erlbaum.

155. Rutter M (1985) The treatment of autistic children. *Journal of Child Psychology and Psychiatry and Allied Disciplines* **26(2)**, 193–214.

156. Royal College of Psychiatrists (1995) *Strategies for the Management of Disturbed and Violent Patients in Hospital.* London: Royal College of Psychiatrists. Council Report CR41.

157. Matson JL & Sevin JA (1994) Issues in the use of aversives: Factors associated with behavior modification for autistic and other developmentally disabled people. In Schopler E & Mesibov GC (eds) *Behavioral Issues in Autism,* pp. 211–25. New York: Plenum Press.

158. Schopler E (1994) Behavioral priorities for autism and related developmental disorders. In Schopler E & Mesibov GC (eds) *Behavioral Issues in Autism,* pp. 55–77. New York: Plenum Press.

159. Fenske EC, Zalenski S, Krantz PJ & McClannahan LE (1985) Age at intervention and treatment outcome for autistic children in a comprehensive intervention program. Special Issue: Early intervention. *Analysis and Intervention in Developmental Disabilities* **5(1–2)**, 49–58.

160. McEachin JJ, Smith T & Lovaas OI (1993) Long-term outcome for children with autism who received early intensive behavioral treatment. *American Journal on Mental Retardation* **97(4)**, 359–72.

161. Simpson RL (1992) Tips for practitioners: Peer tutoring and students with autism. *Focus on Autistic Behavior* **7(4)**, 16–8.

162. Mirenda PL, Donnellan AM & Yoder DE (1983) Gaze behavior: A new look at an old problem. *Journal of Autism and Developmental Disorders* **13(4)**, 397–409.

163. Fell R (1988) The Efficacy of Holding Therapy in the Treatment of Autism. Master of Science (Clinical Psychology). Hull, UK.

164. Richer J & Zappella M (1989) Changing social behaviour: the place of holding. *Communication* **23(2)**, 35–9.

165. Howlin P (1989) Holding Therapy: A reply to Richer and Zapella. *Communication* **23(2)**, 40.

166. Richer J (1989) Changing social behaviour – the place of holding: a reply to Howlin. *Communication* **23(2)**, 40–1.

167. Gould J (1993) Facilitated communication: an overview. *Communication* **27(2)**, 9–15.
168. Prior M & Cummins R (1992) Questions about facilitated communication and autism. *Journal of Autism and Developmental Disorders* **22(3)**, 331–8.
169. Levine K, Shane HC & Wharton RH (1994) 'What if . . .' A plea to professionals to consider the risk–benefit ratio of facilitated communication. *Mental Retardation* **32**, 300–4.
170. DeLong RG & Aldershof AL (1987) Long-term experience with lithium treatment in childhood: Correlation with clinical diagnosis. *Journal of the American Academy of Child and Adolescent Psychiatry* **26(3)**, 389–94.
171. Jan JE & Espezel H (1995) Melatonin treatment of chronic sleep disorders. *Developmental Medicine and Child Neurology* **37(3)**, 279–80.
172. Rimland B (1988) Controversies in the treatment of autistic children: vitamin and drug therapy. *Journal of Child Neurology* 3(Suppl), 68–72.
173. Davis K, Sprague R & Werry J (1969) Stereotyped behaviour and activity level in severe retardates: the effect of drugs. *American Journal of Mental Deficiency* **73**, 721–7.
174. Perry R, Campbell M & Adams P *et al.* (1989) Long-term efficacy of haloperidol in autistic children: Continuous versus discontinuous drug administration. *Journal of the American Academy of Child and Adolescent Psychiatry* **28(1)**, 87–92.
175. Campbell M, Locascio JJ, Choroco MC & Spencer EK *et al.* (1990) Stereotypies and tardive dyskinesia: Abnormal movements in autistic children. *Psychopharmacology Bulletin* **26(2)**, 260–6.
176. Ritvo ER, Freeman BJ & Yuwiler A *et al.* (1987) Fenfluramine treatment of autism: UCLA collaborative study of 81 patients at nine medical centers. *Psychopharmacology Bulletin* **22**, 133–40.
177. du-Verglas G, Banks SR & Guyer KE (1988) Clinical effects of fenfluramine on children with autism: A review of the research. *Journal of Autism and Developmental Disorders* **18(2)**, 297–308.
178. Campbell M (1988) Fenfluramine treatment of autism. *Journal of Child Psychology and Psychiatry and Allied Disciplines* **29(1)**, 1–10.
179. Scifo R, Batticane N, Quattropani MC, Spoto G & Marchetti B (1991) A double-blind trial with naltrexone in autism. *Brain Dysfunction* **4(6)**, 301–7.
180. Barrett RP, Feinstein C & Hole WT (1989) Effects of naloxone and naltrexone on self-injury: A double-blind, placebo-controlled analysis. Special Issue: Drug treatment. *American Journal on Mental Retardation* **93(6)**, 644–51.
181. Benjamin S, Seek A, Tresise L, Price E & Gagnon M. (1995) Case study: Paradoxical response to naltrexone treatment of self-injurious behavior. *Journal of the American Academy of Child and Adolescent Psychiatry* **34(2)**, 238–42.
182. Campbell M, Anderson LT, Small AM, Adams P, Gonzalez NM & Ernst M (1993) Naltrexone in autistic children: Behavioral symptoms and attentional learning. *Journal of the American Academy of Child and Adolescent Psychiatry* **32(6)**, 1283–91.
183. Zingarelli G, Ellman G, Hom A, Wymore M, Heidorn S & Chicz-DeMet A (1992) Clinical effects of naltrexone on autistic behavior. *American Journal of Mental Retardation* **97(1)**, 57–63.
184. Reichelt KL, Knivsberg AM, Lind G & Nodland M (1991) Probable etiology and possible treatment of childhood autism. *Brain Dysfunction* **4(6)**, 308–19.
185. Buitelaar JK, van-Engeland H & de-Kogel KH *et al.* (1992) The use of adrenocorticotrophic hormone (4–9) analog ORG 2766 in autistic children: Effects on the organization of behavior. *Biological Psychiatry* **31(11)**, 1119–29.
186. Martineau J, Barthelemy C, Cheliakine C & Lelord G (1988) Brief report: An open middle-term study of combined vitamin B$_6$–magnesium in a subgroup of autistic children selected on their sensitivity to this treatment. *Journal of Autism and Developmental Disorders* **18(3)**, 435–47.
187. Aman M & Kern RA (1991) Mental retardation: the efficacy of folic acid in fragile X syndrome and other developmental disabilities. *Journal of Child and Adolescent Psychopharmacology* **1**, 285–99.
188. Naruse H, Hayahi T & Takesada M *et al.* (1987) Therapeutic effect of tetrahydrobiotin in infantile autism. *Proceedings of the Japanese Academy* **63(B)**, 231–3.
189. Deonna T, Ziegler AL, Moura-Serra J & Innocenti G (1993) Autistic regression in relation to limbic pathology and epilepsy: Report of two cases. *Developmental Medicine and Child Neurology* **35(2)**, 166–76.
190. Ratey JJ, Bemporad JR & Sorgi P *et al.* (1987) Open trial effects of beta-blockers on speech

and social behaviors in 8 autistic adults. *Journal of Autism and Developmental Disorders* **17(3)**, 439–46.

191. Ratey JJ, Mikkelsen E & Sorgi P (1987) Autism: the treatment of aggressive behaviors. *Journal of Clinical Psychopharmacology* **7**, 35–41.

192. Bicknell J (1983) The psychopathology of handicap. *British Journal of Medical Psychology* **56**, 167–78.

193. Holroyd J & McArthur D (1976) Mental retardation and stress on the parents: A contrast between Down's syndrome and childhood autism. *American Journal of Mental Deficiency* **80(4)**, 431–6.

194. Lyons DM (1995) A survey into the burden of care among parents of children with autism and other learning disabilities: comparing their perceived needs, stress and hardiness. MSc University of Wales.

195. Attwood A (1992) *Why Does Chris Do That.* London: National Autistic Society.

196. Gillberg C (1984) Autistic children growing up: Problems during puberty and adolescence. *Developmental Medicine and Child Neurology* **26(1)**, 125–9.

197. Kobayashi R, Murata T & Yoshinaga K (1992) A follow-up study of 201 children with autism in Kyushu and Yamaguchi areas, Japan. *Journal of Autism and Developmental Disorders* **22(3)**, 395–411.

198. Realmuto GM & August GJ (1991) Catatonia in autistic disorder: A sign of comorbidity or variable expression? *Journal of Autism and Developmental Disorders* **21(4)**, 517–28.

199. Howlin P, Rutter M, Berger M, Hemsley R, Hersov L & Yule W (1987) Treatment of Autistic Children. In Rutter M (ed) Wiley Series on Studies in Child Psychiatry. Chichester: John Wiley.

200. Szatmari P, Bartolucci G, Bremner R, Bond S & Rich S (1989) A follow-up study of high-functioning autistic children. *Journal of Autism and Development Disorders* **19(2)**, 213–25.

201. Schopler E, Short A & Mesibov G (1989) Relation of behavioral treatment to 'normal functioning': comment on Lovaas. *Journal of Consulting and Clinical Psychology* **57**, 162–4.

8

Schizophrenia

Stephen P. Tyrer and Judith A. Dunstan

Schizophrenia in Those with Learning Disability

History

Phillipe Pinel was the first writer to distinguish clearly those who had learning disability from those with mental illness or insanity. However, it was not until later in the nineteenth century that the co-occurrence of schizophrenia and learning disability was recognized. Hurd made the point that if there was a heritable tendency to psychosis, features of mental illness could occur in 'imbeciles of a milder degree' although not in 'the lowest grades of amentia'.[1] Tredgold reported that considerably more than half of patients admitted to hospitals with learning disability had, at one time or another, been insane.[2] Kraepelin adopted a more deterministic line. He believed that some 7% of cases of dementia praecox, the term he used for schizophrenia, arose on the basis of 'idiocy' and stated that an early onset form of psychosis, which he termed 'pfropfschizophrenie', was the cause of certain forms of idiocy with developed mannerisms and stereotypies.[3] Kraepelin's view was based largely on the similarity between the clinical presentation of the more frequent disorganized and catatonic schizophrenics that were found in the institutions of his day and the manneristic behaviour of those with learning disability. However, he was careful to distinguish between those who had learning disability alone and dementia praecox without intellectual impairment.

Greater clarification of the relationship between schizophrenia and learning disability gradually accumulated through more precise epidemiological surveys and from genetic approaches.

Eliot Slater made the point that the prevalence of schizophrenia was the same in the families of those with normal intelligence and 'defectives' and his conjectures were supported by evidence from Kallman *et al.*,[4] which showed an increased rate of schizophrenia in families with schizophrenics but no increase in the rate of learning disability. In their twin studies they found that there was 'not a single case in this material in which the second twin of a mentally defective proband has been schizophrenic or even psychotic at all'.[4] This carefully carried out research effectively buried the concept of 'pfropfschizophrenie'.

Epidemiology

The early assessments of the prevalence of schizophrenia in those with learning disability were carried out in hospital populations for the good reason that these were easy to study and those individuals with learning disability who had behavioural impairments were, at that time, largely housed in large institutions. An early study by Payne in 1968 found a prevalence rate of 10% for schizophrenia[5] but no criterion for the definition of schizophrenia was given in his study.[5] Later studies by Reid[6] and Heaton-Ward[7] in large hospitals for those with learning disability found 3.2% and 3.4% respectively of individuals had schizophrenia (see Table 8.2, later).

A survey by Wright in 1982 showed a prevalence of 1.8% for schizophrenia.[8] This lower figure may be a reflection of the high proportion of those with severe learning disability which made up almost three-quarters of the population that she described. It should be noted that the diagnosis of schizophrenia requires a level of communication that is not normally associated with more severe degrees of learning disability. A number of patients were also excluded in her survey because of what she described as 'a major impairment of social interaction'. Although from her description many of these patients were clearly autistic, some of these may have been described as schizophrenic in early surveys.

Surveys of patients living in the community are more likely to give truer figures of the prevalence of schizophrenia in learning disability. Corbett, who analysed his data by examining patients on the Camberwell Register, also found that 3% of patients that he surveyed either had a current schizophrenic illness or had had a history of a previous schizophrenic episode.[9] Gostason found four patients with schizophrenia in 131 people who had severe or mild mental retardation,[10] which is very similar to the figures above. A more precise investigation by Lund showed an overall prevalence of 1.3% for schizophrenia, despite the fact that the rate of schizophrenia for individuals in the IQ range 62–85 was 3.3%, 2.6% for those in the IQ range 52–67, with only 1.2% for those in the IQ range 36–50. No cases were found in those with an IQ of less than 35.[11] Again, the difficulty of the diagnosis of schizophrenia in those with poor communication skills may have contributed to the lower figure in this study. In the United States Menolascino *et al.* found that in a community-based learning disability programme in Nebraska 25% had a diagnosis of schizophrenia.[12] Some scepticism is needed in interpreting these results as diagnostic instruments were not described and selection factors were clearly apparent.

The findings overall indicate that schizophrenia is certainly commoner in people with learning disability than in those of normal intelligence. Although the incidence of 3% in most studies has most recently been challenged by the investigation of Lund,[11] who has probably carried out the most precise survey to date, the problem of effectively diagnosing schizophrenia in a population of those with learning disability may have contributed to the reduced under-reporting in this area. This issue is discussed later in this chapter.

Aetiology

The factors leading to schizophrenia in people with learning disability have not been investigated to the extent that the incidence of this condition warrants. Although it seems likely that the organic cerebral disorders that lead to learning disability may also be associated with the development of schizophrenia, a seminal review of schizophrenic syndromes associated with organic disorders by Davison and Bagley did not refer to schizophrenia in learning disability at all.[13] Although Hurd reported over 100 years ago that 'heredity undoubtedly plays an important part'[1] no precise study has been carried out examining the genetic links between schizophrenia and those with learning disability and their first-degree relatives.

In the general population the most compelling evidence that schizophrenia is separate from other mental illnesses is borne out by genetic studies. Odegaard examined the rates of psychotic illness in first-degree relatives of consecutive admissions with a diagnosis of schizophrenia and found that the proportion of relatives that received a similar diagnosis was greatest in patients with no affective symptoms and a large number of negative symptoms.[14] Kraepelin observed nearly a 100 years ago that the course of manic-depressive insanity and dementia praecox (schizophrenia) was different,[3] with patients who had an affective psychotic episode tending to return to their former level of functioning rather than following the deteriorating course of schizophrenia.[15]

Studies in the general population have shown that where a child has one parent with schizophrenia the likelihood of the child being similarly affected is around 12%. Where two parents are affected this figure rises to around 46%.[16] When there is a family history of schizophrenia there is little evidence of cerebral damage, whereas in cases where this is no family history of schizophrenia there is often a history of injury at birth or perinatal complications associated with increased ventricular size and some degree of gyral atrophy.[17]

In the general population there is an increased number of babies born with schizophrenia in the second quarter of the year. A similar pattern has been found in those with learning disability with an excess of 20% of births in the spring.[18] Although this number is not statistically significant, partly because of low numbers, the close correlation between the figures for those born with schizophrenia and those with learning disability is noteworthy. It may be that babies born at this time of the year in the northern hemisphere (the study concerned was carried out in Germany) are more prone to have infections or environmental problems. Alternatively, the parents of individuals suffering from learning disability may be inclined only to take sexual partners in the summer months.

Individuals with schizophrenia in the general population show progressive enlargement of the cerebral ventricles over the course of their illness,[19] have brains at post mortem weighing less than average [20] and their illness is associated with a progressive intellectual decline.[21] This evidence makes the paucity of data regarding cerebral function in those with learning disability and schizophrenia all the more frustrating.

In schizophrenia in those with normal intelligence it has been shown that there is an anomaly or developmental arrest of normal cerebral hemispheric asymmetry[22] and it is possible that the consequence of this abnormal development is a failure to establish dominance of one hemisphere over the other. Schizophrenics exhibit an increased incidence of non-right handedness that is associated with a lesser degree of left cerebral dominance for language.[23] In individuals without schizophrenia the left hemisphere is normally involved in processing language (in right-handers) whereas the right hemisphere is more involved in the analysis and processing of spatial stimuli. If there was a failure of hemispheric specialization the relative dominance of one hemisphere over the other for these tasks would not be so marked.

It has been found that schizophrenics lack the normal hemispheric processing differences that are found in normal subjects in tests of linguistic analysis and facial discrimination.[24] Information must be conveyed from one cerebral hemisphere to the other in order to accurately process afferent input and in the rare condition of agenesis of the corpus callosum this process can be investigated in more detail. Anomalies of corpus callosum structure in schizophrenia have been reported. In the Andermann syndrome, a familial syndrome combining congenital corpus callosum agenesis, learning disability, psychotic episodes, peripheral neuropathy and some dysmorphic features, an opportunity arises to examine the relationship between psychotic symptoms and corpus callosum abnormalities. In a study by Filteau et al.[25] no significant relationship was found between corpus callosum agenesis and psychosis. However, there was a relationship between atrophy of the structures in the posterior fossa, including the cerebellum, and psychosis in this syndrome, suggesting that such defects may be associated with psychotic behaviour.

Certain inborn errors of metabolism that are associated with learning disability provide an opportunity to examine the relationship between such syndromes and psychosis. Homocystinuria, an autosomal recessive disorder, involves abnormal methylation of methionine because of cystathionine β-synthase deficiency. It has been proposed that schizophrenia results from abnormal methylation of methionine. If this is so there should be an increased rate of schizophrenia in individuals suffering from homocystinuria. The incidence of psychiatric disturbance, intelligence, behavioural problems and their responsiveness to vitamin B_6 was investigated in 63 people with homocystinuria.[26] Chronic behaviour disorders, personality disorders, depression and obsessive-compulsive disorder were found in around 50% of subjects, with aggressive behaviour and conduct disorders being particularly common. No mention was made of schizophrenia being diagnosed in those subjects but as most were suffering from severe learning disability, the diagnosis would have been difficult to make.

Isolated reports have appeared of female fragile-X carriers having a greater frequency of schizophrenia spectrum diagnoses[27] and of an association between a high uroporphyrinogen-1-synthetase activity and a strong family history of schizophrenia in a geographically isolated population in northern Sweden.[28]

It has been postulated that there is abnormal immunoreactivity in individuals with schizophrenia and learning disability. There is some relationship between delayed hypersensitivity to neural tissue antigens in both schizophrenia and learning disability;[29] one group found increased immunoglobulin G immunoreactive banding in both schizophrenia and learning disability.[30] However, no firm relationship has been found between the presence of increased immunoreactivity and either schizophrenia or learning disability. In one study the diagnosis of schizophrenia correlated with the presence of antinuclear antibodies much more than the ageing process would predict,[31] and in a study in Northern Ireland antibody titres to herpes simplex virus and cytomegalovirus antibody titres were significantly lower in individuals with learning disability, suggesting an impaired immune response.[32]

Klinefelter's Syndrome

An association has also been reported between schizophrenia and Klinefelter's syndrome, a condition where there is an extra X chromosome in a phenotypic male, and where there is also an increased likelihood of learning disability.[33]

Presentation of Schizophrenia in Those with Learning Disability

The detection and diagnosis of schizophrenia is not difficult in those with a mild degree of disability provided that allowances are made for the reduced vocabulary of the sufferer. When the diagnosis is missed it is in most cases because insufficient weight has been given to the symptoms described or because the behavioural manifestations of the psychotic state may have been mistaken for 'behavioural disorder' perhaps precipitated by environmental stress. This leads to a consistent finding that in the presence of a developmental disability there is a greater likelihood of the diagnosis of schizophrenia being missed.[34] These authors have shown that even experienced professionals working in the field of mental illness were more likely to miss the diagnosis if there was a priori evidence of a developmental disability.

Those working in the learning disability field have stressed consistently that the diagnosis of schizophrenia is not possible in those with limited language.[6] Indeed, it is evident from examining the criteria used for the diagnosis of schizophrenia according to well-established operational schedules (see Tables 8.1 and 8.2) that considerable verbal understanding and facility is required in order to be able to communicate effectively the distressing symptoms and disintegration that characterize the presentation of schizophrenia.

Sovner has also referred to what he describes as 'intellectual distortion'[35] affecting diagnosis in this population. It is not only the impaired

Table 8.1   Diagnostic criteria for schizophrenia.

A. Characteristic symptoms	Two (or more) of the following, each present for a significant portion of time during a 1-month period (or less if successfully treated): (1) Delusions (2) Hallucinations (3) Disorganized speech (e.g. frequent derailment or incoherence) (4) Grossly disorganized or catatonic behaviour (5) Negative symptoms (i.e. affective flattening, alogia, or avolition) Note: only one Criterion A symptom is required if delusions are bizarre or hallucinations consist of a voice keeping up a running commentary on the person's behaviour or thoughts, or two or more conversing with each other
B. Social/occupational dysfunction	For a significant portion of the time since the onset of the disturbance, one or more major areas of functioning such as work, interpersonal relations, or self-care are markedly below the level achieved prior to the onset (or when the onset is in childhood or adolescence, failure to achieve expected level of interpersonal, academic, or occupational achievement)
C. Duration	Continuous signs of the disturbance persist for at least 6 months. This 6-month period must include at least 1 month of symptoms (or less if successfully treated) that meet Criterion A (i.e. active-phase symptoms) and may include periods of prodromal or residual symptoms. During these prodromal or residual periods, the signs of the disturbance may be manifested by only negative symptoms or two or more symptoms listed in Criterion A present in an attenuated form (e.g. odd beliefs, unusual perceptual experiences)
D. Schizoaffective and mood disorder exclusion	Schizoaffective disorder and mood disorder with psychotic features have been ruled out because either: (1) no major depressive, manic, or mixed episodes have occurred concurrently with the active-phase symptoms; or (2) if mood episodes have occurred during active-phase symptoms, their total duration has been brief relative to the duration of the active and residual periods
E. Substance/general medical condition exclusion	The disturbance is not due to the direct physiological effects of a substance (e.g. a drug of abuse, a medication) or a general medical condition
F. Relationship to a pervasive development disorder	If there is a history of autistic disorder or another pervasive developmental disorder, the additional diagnosis of schizophrenia is made only if prominent delusions or hallucinations are also present for at least a month (or less if successfully treated)

Table 8.2 Incidence of schizophrenia in learning disability populations. (Modified from Taylor (1989) *Psychological Medicine* **19**, 301–14.)

	Population (age range)	Size	Percentage schizophrenic
Reid (1972)[6]	0–74 years	>500	3.2
Heaton-Ward (1977)[7]	All adults	1251	3.4
Corbett (1979)[9]	All in community over 15 years	402	3.0 (past) 3.5 (current)
Russell & Tanguay (1981)[85]	Adolescent unit	93	7.0
Wright (1982)[8]	Over 16 years	1507	1.8
Gostason (1985)[10]	20–60 years	131	3.0

communication skills that contribute to the problem but also the inability of those with learning disability to employ abstract reasoning. Heaton-Ward makes the point that some severely handicapped patients 'who have no intelligible speech, in whom emotional lability, noisy outbursts, continuous or periodic disorganized, purposeless activity, including aggression, destructiveness and self-mutilation ... could be considered psychotic'.[7] However, he concludes that in order to diagnose psychosis there needs to be a lack of insight and a reduction in the sense of reality. Unless the patient has some form of intelligible communication it is not possible to determine if this is the case.

The context of symptomatology in schizophrenia is also a factor which influences those assessing psychosis in those with learning disability. Because of their reduced opportunity to engage in normal life experiences and social opportunities their delusions, when they occur, may be bland and unremarkable. This concept has been termed 'psychosocial masking'.[35]

Not all authors believe that it is impossible to diagnose schizophrenia in those with severe learning disability. Eaton and Menaloscino state that they have been able to diagnose paranoid schizophrenia in both verbal and nonverbal patients and cite three adults who drew pictures of their 'attackers', describing them with gestures.[36] These authors state that 'the altered affective responses, bizarre rituals, and use of interpersonal distancing devices clearly marks the observed behaviors as schizophrenic'.[36]

Nevertheless, the majority of the workers in this area, particularly those who have used formal diagnostic schedules, believe that in those people with an IQ below 50, no meaningful diagnosis of schizophrenia can be made.[37] The authors who believe it is possible to diagnose schizophrenia in this population have used diagnostic criteria for schizophrenia which have not been firmly established to be valid in follow-up studies.[38]

In those with a mild degree of learning disability the symptoms exhibited by those with a handicap are not dissimilar to the presentation of schizophrenia in those with normal intelligence. Auditory hallucinations are the most frequent symptom and were reported by over 90% of intellectually impaired schizophrenic individuals in one study which compared the presentation of schizophrenia in learning disability with those of normal intelligence.[39] There was a tendency for patients with intellectual impairment to show less psychopathology, particularly persecutory delusions and formal thought disorder. Conversely, bizarre behaviour was increased in those with disability compared with those of normal intelligence, although this difference was not of statistical significance. Discriminant analysis was unable to show any significant difference between the presentation of schizophrenia in those with learning disability compared with those without.

The unsophisticated examiner may at times diagnose someone with learning disability who is behaving in an unusual fashion as schizophrenic. There are at least two factors that lead to errors in this direction. One is the tendency of those with learning disability to become disorganized under emotional stress and the other is because of the limited ability of the subjects to express their symptoms adequately. Sovner has referred to these two phenomena in the learning disabled population as 'cognitive disintegration' and 'baseline exaggeration'.[35] Sovner also claims that 'stress may overload the patients' cognitive functioning resulting in a breakdown in reality'. Patients can present with the signs and symptoms of psychosis which can mistakenly be labelled as schizophrenia. The psychotic symptoms, apparently precipitated by seemingly minimal stress, are perhaps better conceptualized as 'brief reactive psychosis'. Patients may withdraw and talk to themselves, creating or resurrecting an imaginary friend. This is normal in a young child but when found in an adult who also has learning disability may be mistaken for 'psychosis'.

Differential Diagnosis

The differential diagnosis of schizophrenia in those with learning disability depends upon the age of onset and the degree of intellectual impairment. The mean age of onset of schizophrenic illnesses is in the mid-20s and is earlier in males than in females by some 3 years.[40]

Childhood Schizophrenia and Learning Disability

There has been considerable debate about the existence of childhood schizophrenia in those with learning disability since the turn of the century. As previously noted, Kraepelin's concept of 'pfropfschizophrenie' initially persuaded psychiatrists that children with severe learning disability who developed mannerisms, stereotypies and negativistic features, including 'prominent repellent inaccessibility to all attempts at approach' suffered from this type of schizophrenia.[3]

It is of interest that the concept of very early schizophrenia 'demenza precocissima' was described by de Sanctis in 1906[41] and by Heller who believed that schizophrenia affected very young children, a condition he termed 'dementia infantilis'.[42] It is likely that the primitive behaviour of children with severe learning disability showed resemblance to the behaviours of individuals with the more florid schizophrenic syndromes that were manifest earlier this century[43] and which were, of course, more prevalent before the advent of the neuroleptic group of drugs. However, there appears little doubt that many of these children displayed autistic features and that the aloof behaviour of these children, coupled with their stereotypic behaviour which resembled the catatonic posturing of many schizophrenics of this time, was responsible for the belief that these children had a form of schizophrenia.

Infantile autism is categorized by deterioration in language development after the age of 2 years, a restricted repertoire of activities accompanied by an obsessional desire for sameness. In addition, these individuals are aloof and indulge in stereotypic routines. In most profoundly intellectually disabled children there is no deterioration in language because this is never acquired, but these children object to expressions of affection from their parents or others, although sometimes seek close contact with those most familiar to them, on their own terms. Gillberg has shown that autistic features are most prevalent in those with the most severe forms of learning disability and there is a decreased prevalence in the more intellectually able children.[44] There are many children with learning disability who show a pronounced degree of social withdrawal and stereotypic behaviour but who never acquire useful speech or language because of their degree of handicap. While these children present with 'autistic' features the formal diagnosis of autism cannot be made because they cannot fulfil standard operational criteria as a result of their language deficit.

Other pervasive developmental disorders show some resemblance to schizophrenia. In Asperger's syndrome children show a lack of desire to join in with others but engage in solitary activities with little imaginative play, and these symptoms may be confused with those of schizophrenia. Girls with Rett syndrome, in which there may be apparent normal early development followed by deterioration around the age of 2 years with characteristic hand-wringing movements, reduced mobility and hypotonia, are normally readily distinguished by the characteristic neurological features.

The diagnosis of childhood schizophrenia should be reserved for those who exhibit persistent withdrawal, bizarre behaviour, blunted affect and echolalia and who have clearly regressed from an earlier higher level of functioning.[36] The deterioration in these patients occurs later than is found in autism, usually around the age of 4–6 years. If improvement is shown with neuroleptic drugs, which do not have any major effect on the core symptoms in infantile autism, the diagnosis of schizophrenia is more likely to be present. Considerable doubt must remain about the diagnosis of schizophrenia in the absence of positive symptoms.

In patients where there is a strong family history of schizophrenia, together with a deterioration from a previously better level of functioning, the diagnosis may be more tenable if neuroleptics have, to some extent, restored the previous level of functioning. However, until consistent biochemical evidence of schizophrenia is obtained the jury must remain out on this diagnosis in children with learning disability, particularly in those with more severe handicap.

Schizophrenia in Adults with Learning Disability

The diagnosis of schizophrenia in those with learning disability can only be made confidently in patients with good verbal ability. As most authors in the field have stated, unless patients are able to describe their personal experiences adequately, it cannot be ascertained whether they are experiencing true psychotic perceptions or false beliefs. Their intellectual deficit precludes an adequate description of delusional ideas or unusual perceptions, although hallucinations may be easier to identify if the patient is observed responding to apparent hallucinatory experiences. Reid has stated that it is not possible to diagnose schizophrenia in a person who has an IQ of less than 45.[6] It is not clear why the figure of 45 should have been chosen, rather than (say) 40 or 50, but it is evident in clinical practice that only those with a mild degree of learning disability are able to convey accurately the extremely bizarre and frightening symptoms of a schizophrenic illness.

Differential Diagnosis

The differential diagnosis of schizophrenia in adults with mild learning disability depends both on symptomatology and on the course of the illness. Patients with bipolar affective disorder, particularly when they are in a manic phase, can have delusions and, occasionally, hallucinations, which may lead to diagnostic confusion. The delusions in mania are usually of grandiose type but this distinction may not be possible in severe illness where exploration of abnormal beliefs is difficult. Hallucinations in mania are characteristically self-referential and are in keeping with the patient's belief of their special abilities and powers. Above all, the course of bipolar illness is different from that of schizophrenia. Mania rarely lasts more than a few weeks at most and there is often a history of previous affective spells, either hypomanic or depressive, with intervening periods of normal mood. There is some evidence that there is a greater frequency of rapid-cycling bipolar disorder in those with learning disability[45] but even in these cases there is not the same degree of deteriorating course that is found in schizophrenia, and the episodes of depression and mania can be distinguished from each other and from periods of normal mood.

A problem arises in the diagnosis of schizo-affective disorder. By definition this diagnosis includes those individuals who display symptoms of schizophrenia and affective disorder at the same time. No major investigation has been carried out into those with learning disability within this group but the paucity of reports about its presence in this population group suggests that it is only very rarely exhibited.

It is not uncommon for adults with mild degrees of learning disability to describe unusual ideas or experiences, although these individuals are not truly psychotic. Often these symptoms may arise in response to leading questions. Many people with learning disability want to please those in authority and wish to prolong contact with anyone who shows keen interest in them. It often happens that the increased interest of the examiner in identifying a further 'positive' symptom leads the patient to provide increasingly unusual symptoms. The evidence of staff or relatives working with these patients may be more reliable in these cases. Unless there is behavioural evidence of the apparent psychotic symptom, such as responding to apparently hallucinatory experiences, the diagnosis must be considered suspect.

In other patients wish-fulfilment can lead to the development of apparently 'abnormal beliefs'. A young man with learning disability under our care said convincingly that he was married to the daughter of a prominent TV star and that together they had four children. When he was questioned in more detail about the relationship it was clear that his great desire for such a relationship had persuaded him that his wishes had been fulfilled. This ability of the intellectually disabled person to suspend judgement is not true psychosis and it is often easy to sway their beliefs by appropriate argument. Even when this is not possible these ideas are often ephemeral and are not held with any intensity over a long period of time. These individuals confabulate readily, particularly if they are stimulated by others discussing their symptoms with them. Another young man told his carers that he had seen 'powerful men with green and red clothing' fighting in his presence. He believed that 'these powerful men' would rescue him from his carers whom he did not like. Closer enquiry revealed that he used to play a video game of boxers who wore green and red shorts.

There is usually no difficulty in distinguishing people with autistic disorder from schizophrenia in this population. Those with autism do not exhibit or describe hallucinations or delusions. Neurotic disorder is fundamentally different in presentation from schizophrenia and is not normally a source of confusion. Autistic tendencies are also apparent at a very early age and there is not the characteristic onset of schizophrenia in the late teens or early twenties.

Adults with a Severe Learning Disability

The difficulties of making a diagnosis in this population group has been referred to earlier in this chapter. However, it is important to note that there is progressive intellectual deterioration in schizophrenia in those of normal intelligence[21] and a number of patients who function within the severe range of learning disability and who have symptoms suggestive of schizophrenia may have previously had a higher IQ. Heaton-Ward reported a patient whom he diagnosed as suffering from hebephrenic schizophrenia although she had an IQ of 23.[7] He makes the point that this patient and others were able to express concepts which suggested that they previously had a much higher level of intellectual functioning. In these cases the diagnosis of schizophrenia may depend upon past medical records to illustrate definite evidence of positive schizophrenic features and a history from carers of a higher level of premorbid functioning.

In some patients with an apparent paranoid schizophrenic illness, particularly in the late middle-aged and elderly, there may be evidence of cognitive decline. In these patients an organic paranoid psychosis or dementia may be the diagnosis rather than schizophrenia. Furthermore, it is well established that patients with paranoid delusional disorder have evidence of visual and/or hearing impairment. Heaton-Ward describes one XO–XX chromosome mosaic patient who was deaf and blind and had what he described as a paranoid psychosis.[7]

In other patients who appear to have a paranoid schizophrenic illness the 'paranoid' ideas may be a misinterpretation of reality. A 34-year-old man under our care refused to go into his bedroom and seemed apprehensive about a darkened corner of the room. It was later found that mice were living under the skirting-board and he had been disturbed by their chattering during the night. Similarly, a patient who is convinced that another may be out to harm them may have good reason to believe that they are in danger from this individual. It is not unknown for patients with learning disability to suffer attacks from others, whether physical, verbal or sexual and it is important to be aware of these possibilities. Where patients have suffered sexual or physical abuse in the past they will be extremely apprehensive in situations where they believe that they are again being threatened. Once the individual is removed to a safe place these 'abnormal' ideas will tend to recede if there is no true psychosis present.

Although we agree with Reid[46] that the diagnosis of schizophrenia in those with severe learning disability is not possible if standard operational criteria are applied, we believe that it is possible to diagnose patients with schizophrenia where behavioural symptoms and other observable behaviour are taken into account. In three patients in whom there was no direct evidence of a disorder of thought or perception there were marked changes in behaviour, with flattened affect, fearfulness and incongruity associated with withdrawal, deteriorating self-care, catatonic posturing and excitement and self-injury.[47] All three of these patients responded well to antipsychotic drugs but a slow reduction of medication led to a recurrence of symptoms. It was a gradual deterioration in both social functioning and personality over a period of some months, apparent anhedonia but no response to antidepressants, and catatonic behaviour which prompted the use of neuroleptic drugs, with gratifying consequences.

If there is a major change in behaviour, particularly in the absence of an acute environmental cause in a young person in their late teens or early twenties, a presumptive diagnosis of schizophrenia should be considered, especially if there is a family history of this illness. There is a good case for considering the use of antidepressant drugs if there are depressive symptoms, but if there is no response to these then the use of antipsychotic drugs should be actively considered. Adequate dosages of these drugs continued over a long period of time may be particularly advantageous in this population in whom compliance can normally be assured.

Schizophrenia Rating Scales in those with Learning Disability

Rating scales for the assessment of schizophrenia in those with learning disability are used for two main purposes:

(1) Diagnosis of schizophrenia.
(2) Assessment of course of illness over time.

More attention has been paid to development of diagnostic rating scales than to those involved in assessment and so these instruments are considered first.

Diagnostic Rating Scales

The early studies on schizophrenia in people with learning disability did not use criteria for the diagnosis of schizophrenia that would be acceptable in research carried out today. There are two main reasons for this. It is only within the last decade and a half that the diagnosis of schizophrenia has become standardized through international studies. Previously, the diagnosis of schizophrenia was made much more frequently in the United States than in Europe and was based on any evidence of eccentric behaviour associated with abnormal perceptions or beliefs.[48] Since that time there has been enormous effort, particularly in the United States, towards establishing clear operational criteria for the diagnosis of schizophrenia and these are now much more stringent than those previously operating.[49]

Until relatively recently it was acceptable for experienced psychiatrists to say that they had diagnosed a particular condition on the basis of their training and experience. If the person putting forward this judgement was eminent and distinguished it was accepted that the diagnosis must be accurate. Nowadays there is scepticism of *ex cathedra* statements and objective measures are now *de rigeur* in accurate diagnosis. Thus, in an early study examining psychotic illness in people with learning disability by Payne the only diagnostic criteria for the use of psychosis was stated by the author as 'who I regard to be psychotic'.[5] Even later authors have not used standard criteria in many cases. The widely quoted papers of Reid[6] and Heaton-Ward[7] described their diagnostic measures using 'usually accepted clinical criteria'.

Over the past two decades there have been increasing attempts to define the diagnosis of schizophrenia in the learning disability population. Studies that have been carried out in the early part of this period have used schedules that were developed on a population of those with normal intelligence. Corbett used the *International Classification of Diseases*, 8th edition (ICD-8), to examine the prevalence of psychiatric illness in a community setting.[9] This schedule did not provide a comprehensive definition of schizophrenic illness, although succeeding editions have significantly improved the reliability and validity of this questionnaire.

Hucker *et al.* used a modified version of the Feighner *et al.* (1972) criteria for the diagnosis of schizophrenia.[50] This was done in order to provide 'a wider definition of schizophrenia in order to include those patients whose symptomatology were otherwise felt to be sufficient to justify the diagnosis'. The authors divided the symptoms up into two groups, an A group consisting of five first-ranked symptoms and a B group of less reliably rated schizophrenic features, e.g. formal thought disorder, incongruity of affect. Although the main aim of this classification was to exclude affective or autistic features, this procrustean technique is not unreasonable in view of the difficulties in diagnosing schizophrenia in those with more severe impairment. It is important to note that only three group B symptoms were sufficient to make the diagnosis. As these symptoms include features such as 'behaves as if hallucinated' and 'blunting of affect', reliability was not always good. It was because of the problem of applying criteria used in the diagnosis of those with normal intelligence to those with learning disability that alternative instruments have been developed. These will be considered in chronological order.

Clinical Interview Schedule

The Clinical Interview Schedule was developed as a screening instrument for psychiatric illness in those with learning disability.[51] This schedule is based on a previous one that was designed for use in community surveys in the standard population.[52] It is divided into four sections: an unstructured record of the present and past medical history, a detailed enquiry about psychiatric symptoms that may have occurred within the previous week, an assessment of the family and personal history and, finally, a rating of abnormalities observed at interview.

   This schedule relies on information gathered by experienced clinical staff and under these conditions and with trained interviewers reliability has been shown to be good.[51] The diagnosis of schizophrenia according to this instrument depends upon the clinical judgement of the interviewer and is not one which can be made from a quantitative total of the number and type of symptoms elicited during the interview and/or by a record of the behaviours observed on mental state examination. Despite this, it is a useful screening test for adults with learning disability who have possible or presumptive evidence of mental illness.

The Psychopathology Instrument for Mentally Retarded Adults

The Psychopathology Instrument for Mentally Retarded Adults (PIMRA)[53] was developed to provide a diagnostic system for those with learning disability alone. It is structured according to the *Diagnostic and Statistical Manual of Mental Disorders*[49] and assesses seven types of psychopathology compiled from items from this manual. It is thus entirely based on a schema that is derived from a population with normal intelligence. The degree of complexity of the items has been altered so that they can be accurately comprehended by people with a learning disability. The seven questions in this schedule that are concerned with schizophrenic disorder are listed in Table 8.3.

Table 8.3 Schizophrenic disorder items in PIMRA.

1. Do you think that things around you are safe?
2. Do you hear voices that upset you?
3. Do people have trouble understanding what you say?
4. Do people know how you feel?
5. Have things been bad for you?
6. Do you like being with other people?
7. Do you like to collect unusual things like old papers or garbage?

Factor analyses were completed on every item in the scale using a principal component solution followed by varimax rotation. Factor loadings were higher for the nonpsychosis items. The first three major items in the psychosis section are not particularly illuminating, namely 'bizarre delusions', 'preoccupation with evincing behaviour of the opposite sex' and 'considered pleasant to be around', and are hardly typical of psychotic behaviour.

The internal consistency and validity of the PIMRA and schizophrenia subscale have been examined by other investigators and the initial enthusiasm of the authors for the use of their schedule has not been entirely supported. Aman *et al.* carried out an independent replication study of the psychometric properties of PIMRA shortly after its development in 160 adults living in both community and hospital settings.[54] The internal consistencies of these different measures were less impressive than the original studies,[53] although factor analysis of their data revealed the same three factors identified in the original survey: affective, somatoform and psychosis.

In a smaller study evaluating the value of PIMRA and the *Aberrant Behavioural Checklist* (ABC)[55] in 24 patients, Sturmey and Ley found that there was only modest internal consistency.[56] Cronbach's α was 0.53 with median point biserial correlation of 0.23, indicating that there is considerable overlap between the different scales of the instrument.[56] In the comparison of the PIMRA with the ABC only one factor of the five in the ABC correlated highly with the diagnosis of schizophrenic disorder – that for lethargy and social withdrawal.

Linaker and Helle have examined the schizophrenia scale of PIMRA in more detail.[57] They found that this subscale could be used for the quantitative measure of schizophrenia if the item 'Recent loss of function' was removed from the scale. This gave a Cronbach α score of 0.61 which is considered to be satisfactory for standard use, although it is not ideal if a high level of diagnostic precision is required. In a comparative study with schizophrenics of normal intelligence the authors found that those classified as having schizophrenic disorder on PIMRA had less delusions, flatter affect and more incoherent utterances.

The authors of the original scale carried out a criterion validity study of the schizophrenia subscale following this survey. An 'inter-rater' reliability of 78% for the schizophrenia checklist was obtained. However, separate analysis of variance tests comparing the scores of the schizophrenia patients on this subscale revealed considerably less discriminative power of the subscale in differentiating schizophrenia from other disorders such as depression. It also revealed a barely significant correlation between this subscale score and the diagnostic schizophrenia checklist.[58]

The PIMRA schizophrenia scale is a useful measure in assessing schizophrenia in people with learning disability. At present, however, the PIMRA is not sufficient as the only basis for diagnosis and other measures, including a test of adaptive behaviour and behavioural observations, need to be carried out before an unequivocal diagnosis can be made.[59] The scale could be improved if there was an indication of the length of illness and duration of previous symptoms. Furthermore, at present, PIMRA does not include relatively common diagnoses such as bipolar affective disorder, and this needs attention. There is the obvious problem that as the *Diagnostic and Statistical Manual*[49] goes into further versions PIMRA will need to be modified in order to take account of changing diagnostic practice.

Diagnostic Assessment for the Severely Handicapped

The Diagnostic Assessment for the Severely Handicapped (DASH) Scale[60] has been designed to assess psychopathology in those with severe learning disability. Again, the scale is based on DSM-III-R (1987) and also on DSM-IV (1994) criteria. To counter criticisms of earlier scales, the frequency, duration and severity of the symptoms are rated in this instrument. The schizophrenia subscale consists of seven items which are listed in Table 8.4.

Although the scale was tested on 506 residents in four institutions for those with severe learning disability in the United States, only 0.6% of the patients had schizophrenia and α values for the schizophrenia scale were low at 0.20, almost certainly because of the infrequent occurrence of this syndrome. The scale recognizes that in those with severe learning disability catatonic features, inappropriate mood and 'contact' with imaginary beings or things can occur in those with severe learning disability and can be rated independently.

Table 8.4 Schizophrenia subscale items in DASH.

1. Mood seems totally unrelated to what is going on around her/him
2. Stands or sits in bizarre or inappropriate positions
3. Talks with imaginary people or inanimate objects such as televisions or pictures
4. Sees things that are imaginary
5. Hears things that are imaginary
6. Experiences touch or other sensations on her/his skin that are imaginary
7. Speech is a jumble of words or ideas that makes little or no sense

Psychiatric Assessment Schedule for Adults with a Developmental Disability

The Psychiatric Assessment Schedule for Adults with a Developmental Disability (PAS-ADD)[37] is a modification of the Psychiatric Assessment Schedule (PAS)[61] which is based on items from the Present State Examination (PSE).[62] At the present time the PAS-ADD has only been reliably tested in patients with neurotic symptoms, dementia and schizophrenia.[63] The use of negative symptoms, and delusions in the diagnosis of schizophrenia in this population has been found to be questionable.

The advantage of the PAS-ADD system is parallel patient and informant interviewing which are combined to increase sensitivity. There is a three-tier vocabulary structure designed to make the interview flexible over the whole range of learning disabilities and questions are eliminated if the patient responds negatively to leading probes. This scale shows considerable promise.

Treatment of Schizophrenia in Those with Learning Disability

Although the principles of treatment of schizophrenia in those with learning disability essentially do not differ from the treatment of this condition in those with normal intelligence there are differences in emphasis which affect the practical measures that one adopts in developing a treatment programme. However, before embarking upon therapy it is important to establish a number of issues. These include:

- Is the diagnosis of schizophrenia definite?
- Have treatment options been discussed with carers and patients in appropriate language and advantages/disadvantages outlined?
- What are the risk factors for side-effects if medication is given?
- Is the patient compliant with medication?

It has been evident from what has been stated earlier in this chapter that the diagnosis of schizophrenia is difficult in those with learning disability, particularly in those with severe impairment. The term 'mental illness' is frightening to patients and carers and this applies particularly to the diagnosis of schizophrenia. The consequence of a diagnosis of schizophrenia is that in most cases medication and specialized treatment services will be required throughout life to maintain equilibrium. Unless there is definite evidence of schizophrenia it is essential that the patient and carers are not prematurely given a definitive diagnostic label. The diagnostic process, which may take many months or even years, should be discussed with them and their help enlisted in noting changes in mental state. This has to be finely balanced as relatives can understandably become over-involved. It is appropriate to test out a hypothesis that the patient may have schizophrenia, e.g. by examining the effect of neuroleptic drugs, but this is different from labelling a person as actually having this illness. It may be necessary to try different strategies at various times during the first few months of contact with the patient in order to determine the validity of the diagnosis. A reduction in antipsychotic drugs can be helpful in order to see the effect on symptoms and this helps both in establishing the diagnosis and the need for medication.

All those with learning disability who have a presumptive diagnosis of schizophrenia will need to have close contact with community health services. In the vast majority of instances this will be with a parent or carer and this usually means that compliance with drugs is assured. For this reason, it may not be necessary to give depot neuroleptic drugs, which have a higher incidence of tardive dyskinesia. However, in patients with milder degree of learning disability who do not always keep appointments depot neuroleptics may be needed.

It is vital to give as much information as possible about treatment options to the carers of a person with learning disability who has schizophrenia. Booklets published by the National Schizophrenia Fellowship (NSF) provide a number of personal accounts of schizophrenia which help other people comprehend the frightening experiences involved in this illness. It is helpful for carers to have such information as well as details of drug treatments and other measures that may protect the person against relapse. A useful leaflet on treatment with antipsychotic drugs for those with learning disability is also available.[64]

The side-effects of antischizophrenic agents can be distressing to patients and relatives especially if they have not been told about the symptoms beforehand. In particular, acute dystonic movements, including oculogyric crises (often described as 'the looky-ups' – see Acute Dystonias) can be exceedingly alarming to those who are unaware of the reason for this. There have been successful lawsuits in the United States where people with learning disability who had received neuroleptic drugs for long periods developed side-effects and were awarded compensation.[65] Akathisia, a syndrome involving a subjective feeling of restlessness associated with a compulsion to move about, is frequently found in patients treated with the older neuroleptic agents.

Antipsychotic Drugs

The mainstay of treatment of schizophrenia in those with learning disability and also in those with normal intelligence is antipsychotic drugs. These agents are most effective in reducing positive symptoms of schizophrenia but they also have some impact on negative symptoms. There is good evidence to suggest that giving antipsychotic drugs raises the threshold for the emergence of schizophrenic symptoms in sufferers but reducing adverse environmental effects also has a protective action. However, studies have shown consistently that antipsychotic drugs exert a clearly protective effect in schizophrenia and are the drugs of choice. The drugs that are used in this condition are described followed by their use in the practical management of schizophrenia.

Drugs Available

Antipsychotic drugs, otherwise known as major tranquillizers or neuroleptics, comprise several different families. The phenothiazines were the first to be synthesized (1951), closely followed by the thioxanthenes and butyrophenones. Derivatives of diphenylbutylpiperidines, e.g. pimozide, and the substituted benzamides, e.g. sulpiride, followed, together with clozapine and loxapine of the dibenzodiazepine family. A recent addition is risperidone, a benzisoxazole derivative that antagonizes central 5-hydroxytryptamine ($5HT_2$) receptors and dopamine receptors. Olanzapine and sertindole are new arrivals on the scene (see Table 8.6).

The common characteristic of all these drugs is their ability to block dopamine D_2 receptors in the limbic system and hypothalamus, although the dibenzodiazepines also affect other dopamine receptors. Risperidone blocks α-adrenoceptors and $5HT_2$ receptors. The other antipsychotic drugs also have effects on receptors and are concerned with other neurotransmitters. Their anticonvulsant activity and degree of blockade of noradrenergic receptors relate to their degree of sedation (see Table 8.5). With

Table 8.5 Relative affinities of neuroleptic drugs for receptor sites in the brain.[74,75]

	Affinity for			
	Acetylcholine (ACh) receptor	Noradrenergic (NA) receptor	Histamine H_1 receptor	$5HT_2$ receptor
Phenothiazines				
Chlorpromazine (Largactil)	++	++	+++	++
Thioridazine (Melleril)	+++	++	+++	++
Trifluoperazine (Stelazine)	0	+	+	
Fluphenazine (Modecate)	0	+	++	
Thioxanthenes				
Flupenthixol (Fluanxol)	+	+	+	++
Zucolopenthixol (Clopixol)	0	++	+++	++
Butyrophenones				
Haloperidol (Haldol)	0	++	+	+
Droperidol (Droleptan)	0	+++	+++	+
Pimozide (Orap)	+	+	0	+
Sulpiride (Dolmatil)	0	0	0	0
Clozapine (Clozaril)	+++	++	+++	++
Risperidone (Risperdal)	0	++	0	++

High affinity for ACh receptors	= Dry mouth, urinary retention, protection against extrapyramidal side-effects
High affinity for NA receptors	= Postural hypotension, tachycardia, pupillary constriction
High affinity for histamine receptors	= Sedation

0 = no affinity.
+ = some affinity.
++ = moderate affinity.
+++ = high affinity for receptor subtypes.

Table 8.6 The commonest side-effects of neuroleptics.

Neuroleptic	Side-effect								
	Dry mouth	Consti-pation	Urinary retention	Sedation	Postural hypotension	Extra-pyramidal	Agranulo-cytosis	Nasal congestion	Peripheral oedema
Chlorpromazine	+	+	+	++	+	+			
Thioridazine	+	+	+	++	+				
Trifluoperazine					+	+			
Fluphenazine					+	+			
Flupenthixol	+	+	+		+	+			
Zuclopenthixol				+	+	+			
Haloperidol				+	+	++			
Droperidol				++	+	++			
Pimozide	+	+	+		+	+			
Sulpiride	Relatively free from side-effects								
Clozapine	+	+	+	+	+		+		
Risperidone		+				+		+	
Sertindole	+				+			++	+
Olanzapine				+	+				+

Weight gain is common with almost all neuroleptics.
+ = frequent side-effect, but not usually clinically severe.
++ = frequent and severe side-effect in some patients.

all these drugs the lowest possible dose should be given to control symptoms. The main side-effects of antipsychotic drugs are shown in Table 8.6.

The majority of neuroleptics are administered by mouth but some are
given parenterally – the depot preparations. Depot neuroleptic drugs are
designed to ensure compliance with treatment. They are given by deep
intramuscular injection, usually at 2- or 3-weekly intervals, and are widely
employed in the treatment of schizophrenia.

A list of the commonly employed antipsychotic drugs is shown in
Table 8.6.

Practical Treatment of Schizophrenia in Those with Learning Disability

Acute Emergency Treatment

In an acutely agitated or violent patient the vital need is to ensure safety
for both the patient and others by adequate sedation. It is therefore appropriate to use benzodiazepines in this situation. Lorazepam 2–4 mg orally
or intramuscularly, or diazepam 5–10 mg orally or intravenously are suitable agents, although caution is needed as intravenous diazepam can cause
respiratory arrest. Alternatively zuclopenthixol acetate (Acuphase) 50–150
mg intramuscularly, or haloperidol 5–10 mg oral drops or intramuscularly
can be given. Except for Acuphase, these agents are likely to need to be
repeated every 4–8 h, depending on the response. Although the dosage of
some of these agents may occasionally be outside recommended *British
National Formulary* guidelines, it is important not to exceed these when
giving haloperidol, pimozide, fluphenazine or flupenthixol because of the

risk of sudden death.[66] If benzodiazepines are given at the same time the dose of the other agent can be lowered. Once control has been achieved a standard neuroleptic agent should be given; thioridazine is widely used in learning disability populations and has been recommended because of its sedative effects.[67] Thioridazine should not be given in a dosage of more than 600 mg daily[1] in those with learning disability because of the danger of causing retinitis pigmentosa.

Maintenance Treatment

Drugs for maintenance treatment depend upon the severity of symptoms and the likely compliance of the patient.

There are some advantages in using the substituted benzamide, sulpiride, because of its specific effects on dopamine receptors and relative lack of subsequent tardive dyskinesia. Alternative drugs are pimozide, risperidone or thioridazine. Pimozide is a specific D_2-receptor antagonist that is effective in both schizophrenia and mania but can cause potentially fatal cardiac arrhythmias in a small but significant number of people. It is now advised that an electrocardiogram (ECG) should be taken before starting this drug with subsequent monitoring of any ECG changes. Risperidone is an expensive new agent that has clear antipsychotic properties but is currently recommended only for patients who do not respond to the standard drug treatments or who have developed significant side-effects. Clozapine is licensed for the treatment of resistant schizophrenia but requires weekly monitoring of white blood cell counts because of the risk of agranulocytosis. This drug is an effective agent. An alternative dibenzodiazepine is olanzipine, which does not cause blood dyscrasias.

Following administration of neuroleptic agents there is usually a fairly rapid reduction of positive symptoms although negative symptoms are more resistant to drug treatment. Normally, additional rehabilitation strategies need to be adopted including programmes to improve social skills, education, occupation and leisure pursuits with the aim of modifying the deteriorating course that frequently accompanies a schizophrenic illness. Where indicated, more specific psychological techniques can be employed such as reducing high expressed emotion in carers.

Withdrawal of Neuroleptics

Sudden withdrawal of neuroleptic drugs leads to symptoms of dysphoria, nausea and agitation. These effects were first described in the early 1960s but are not generally recognized.[68] It is likely that a number of individuals who have been placed on neuroleptics because of a previously diagnosed schizophrenic illness may be able to have their drugs gradually withdrawn. However, in the majority of cases this is not possible. A retrospective study on individuals living in the community who had had neuroleptic drugs withdrawn showed that individuals with a psychotic disorder were significantly more likely to be restarted on neuroleptics after these had been discontinued.[69]

Side-Effects of Neuroleptics

The side-effects of the antipsychotic group of drugs are shown in both Tables 8.5 and 8.6 and have been touched upon previously. Special precautions should be taken in detecting extrapyramidal side-effects in this population, because of the inability of many subjects to accurately describe their symptoms. Extrapyramidal symptoms include three main types: Parkinsonian symptoms, acute dystonia and akathisia.

Parkinsonian Symptoms

These include bradykinesia, slowing and reduction in movements (particularly involuntary movements of expression), rigidity and tremor. Typically, affected patients can be seen entering the interview room with a masked expression, shuffling gait and loss of arm swing. These symptoms often develop early in treatment but can occur at any time during the course of therapy. It is commoner in the elderly, especially in women.

If these symptoms occur they should be treated by adding an anticholinergic drug. These agents include procyclidine (10–20 mg daily), orphenadrine, benztropine and benzhexol. These drugs block muscarinic receptors and so can cause blurred vision, dry mouth, constipation, urinary retention and erectile impotence in some cases; these effects may be enhanced by the antipsychotic drug itself. Parkinsonian side-effects do not improve quickly with these drugs and it is often necessary to wait some days before an effect occurs. However, tolerance usually develops to extrapyramidal side-effects and it is possible to reduce the dose and stop these agents in many cases, although clinicians are often reluctant to do this because of concern about the effects recurring. Anticholinergic drugs reduce the antipsychotic action of neuroleptics, and this is another reason for using them sparingly.

Acute Dystonias

Acute dystonias consist of sudden spasms of the muscles of the lips, tongue, face and throat in particular which give rise to fixed postures of the neck, face or muscles in the mouth and tongue. The best described of these dystonias is the oculogyric crisis which comprises a fixed upward or lateral gaze accompanied by spasm of the extraorbital muscles. These symptoms, often described by patients as the 'looky-ups', can be extremely alarming to those who are unaware of the reasons for these symptoms. In addition, torticollis, spasm of the muscles of the neck, and torsion dystonias of other muscle groups in this area can occur. This is more likely to occur in younger men.

Acute dyskinesias are also found. These consist of exaggerated posturing and twisting of the head, neck or jaw and also occur shortly after administration of neuroleptic drugs.

Acute dystonias and dyskinesias can be dramatically reversed by the intravenous or intramuscular injection of one of the anticholinergic drugs above.

Akathisia

Akathisia is a syndrome involving a subjective feeling of inner restlessness and agitation associated with a compulsion to move about. In mild forms there is simply shifting of the weight of the legs from one to the other, or tapping of the feet, but in more severe forms there are continuous repetitive pacing or motor movements associated with considerable anxiety. It is important to note in the learning disabled population as patients often feel very distressed and upset before the symptom develops but cannot describe the feeling. On occasions they may abscond or insist on leaving the place in which they are contained in order to move about.

The best established treatment for akathisia is propranolol at a dosage of 40–160 mg daily. Alternative drugs such as diazepam may be of help in low dosages, but should be prescribed for no longer than 2 weeks on a continuous basis. Anticholinergic drugs are not normally effective.

Tardive Dyskinesia

Tardive dyskinesia is a major problem in the use of neuroleptic drugs. It consists of orofacial and bucco-lingual involuntary movements which are the predominant features in most patients but choreo-athetoid movements of the upper and lower limbs can also occur. It is found in about one-third of patients with learning disability who receive neuroleptics for long periods. Studies of those of normal intelligence indicate that the greater the dose of the drug that blocks the dopamine D_2 receptors and the longer this dose is continued over time the more likely tardive dyskinesia is to develop.[70] There is also a greater incidence of this symptom in older people and in those with organic brain disease.

It would therefore be expected that the frequency of this symptom should be greater in a population of those with learning disability. In practice, it is rare to see patients with severe symptoms of tardive dyskinesia in institutions for those with learning disability compared with those for mental illness. This is probably because the doses of drugs used in those with learning disability are considerably lower than in those with chronic schizophrenia. However, a recent study has shown that 34% of those with a learning disability in hospital receiving neuroleptic drugs had tardive dyskinesia.[71] This is clearly, therefore, a recognized hazard of the prolonged use of these agents and it is important that they are only given with correct indications.[72] There is increasing recognition that parents and/or carers should be informed about the risk of tardive dyskinesia and it has been suggested that consent for long-term administration of neuroleptics should be sought before their employment.[65]

The treatment of tardive dyskinesia is difficult but it is often made worse by anticholinergic medication and is commonly precipitated when neuroleptic drugs are withdrawn. An increase in the dosage of these agents is of benefit but is not an appropriate treatment because the symptoms will recur and there is good evidence that they will be worse once the drug is reduced or withdrawn. However, it is important to note that in some patients who have dyskinesias on withdrawal of neuroleptics the dyskinesic symptoms may subside after a period of a few months.

It appears likely that tardive dyskinesia occurs because of dopamine receptor hypersensitivity that has been induced by the prolonged dopamine receptor blockade by the neuroleptic drugs, although this mechanism has not definitely been proven. It is good practice to reduce the dosage of neuroleptic medication very gradually in patients in whom tardive dyskinesia has been diagnosed. Alternative treatment is with a drug such as tetrabenazine, which depletes dopamine and other monoamines, and is given at a dosage of 25–50 mg daily. This is often effective in reducing abnormal movements but can cause severe depression. Benzodiazepines may have temporary effects but it is unwise to prescribe these for longer than one month on a continuous basis. Clozapine may have advantages and does not induce dopamine receptor hypersensitivity to anything like the same extent as the typical neuroleptics.

Neuroleptic Malignant Syndrome

Neuroleptic malignant syndrome is a rare but potentially fatal hazard of the use of neuroleptic drugs. This increasingly reported disorder is characterized by excessive muscular rigidity, hyperpyrexia, fluctuating blood pressure and excessive sweating. The diagnosis is confirmed by the finding of very high serum creatine kinase levels, usually over 1000 IU l⁻¹. It has been estimated that the approximate incidence of neuroleptic malignant syndrome is 1% overall and that individuals with learning disability are at greater risk from this syndrome.[73] Neuroleptic malignant syndrome may occur with any neuroleptic but haloperidol and fluphenazine have been most commonly implicated.

Once diagnosed, neuroleptics should be immediately withdrawn and specialist medical help sought. Treatment can include dantrolene and the dopamine agonist, bromocriptine or L-dopa. Anticholinergics are not effective and often make symptoms worse. Benzodiazepines may be given for sedation but in continuing acute manic or schizophrenic excitement where further neuroleptics are contraindicated electroconvulsive therapy (ECT) may be required.

Other Side-effects

In addition to blocking dopamine receptors neuroleptics are antagonists at acetylcholine, α-adrenergic and histamine H_1 receptors. The degree of affinity for the different neuroleptic drugs for these receptors is indicated in Table 8.5.

The main anticholinergic effects of the neuroleptics are blurred vision, dry mouth, tachycardia, constipation, erectile impotence and urinary retention. Delirium can also occur, particularly in those with severe organic brain damage and in the elderly.

Neuroleptics also delay cardiac conduction with S–T depression and QT prolongation on the ECG. Thioridazine and pimozide are associated with increased reports of these symptoms and the use of pimozide requires ECG monitoring, as already described. Hypotension occurs, particularly with the aliphatic phenothiazines, e.g. chlorpromazine.

Occasionally, neuroleptics can cause allergic reactions, including cholestatic jaundice, hypersensitivity rash, photosensitivity, a pigmentary retinopathy which occurs on administration of high doses of thioridazine, and occasionally agranulocytosis. They also reduce body temperature and decrease the threshold at which fits occur, which can obviously be a problem in patients who are prone to epilepsy.

Drug Interactions

The phenothiazine group of neuroleptics potentiate the central depressant actions of alcohol, benzodiazepines, antihistamines and opioid drugs. Increased anticholinergic effects occur when tricyclic antidepressants are given, particularly in those neuroleptics with high affinity for acetylcholine receptors (see Table 8.5). The combination of lithium and the neuroleptics may cause two types of interaction: increased intracellular lithium levels that has been found to occur with thioridazine and a direct neurotoxic effect, which may include neuroleptic malignant syndrome.

The phenothiazines should not be administered with antihypertensive drugs that block adrenergic neurones, e.g. guanethidine. However, hypotension can occur with angiotensin-converting enzyme (ACE) inhibitors. The anticonvulsants carbamazepine and phenytoin decrease serum neuroleptic levels because of their enzyme-inducing effects. Drugs used in the treatment of peptic ulcer such as cimetidine are enzyme inhibitors and so increase the serum levels of a number of antipsychotics because of reduced metabolic breakdown. In the same way, concurrent administration of tricyclic antidepressants and neuroleptics can lead to increased serum levels of tricyclic antidepressants and fluoxetine can increase serum neuroleptic levels. Propranolol also increases many neuroleptic levels and may explain why this agent is effective in schizophrenia when given with neuroleptic drugs.

The latest edition of the *British National Formulary* (Appendix I) gives a list of current important interactions of all drugs and should be consulted for currently recommended doses, interactions and warnings given by the Committee on Safety of Medicines.

Nonpharmacological Treatments for Schizophrenia in Learning Disability

Over 30 years ago, following the seminal work of Brown *et al.*[76] it was established that life events contributed to the onset of acute schizophrenic relapse. It was shown that major life events were associated with an increased incidence of schizophrenic relapse within a period of 3 months of the event. Furthermore, it was shown that the environment in which the schizophrenic patient was living was a major factor in determining likelihood of relapse. An environment in which relatives and carers are critical, hostile or emotionally over-involved with the schizophrenic relative or charge is associated with a greater frequency of relapse into psychosis. The term 'expressed emotion' (EE) was first used by Brown and Rutter[77] to describe such environments. It has now been shown in a large number of separate studies in Western countries that patients living in high EE environments have a significantly greater relapse rate than those patients for whom relationships are more harmonious.[78]

While it has been shown that in people with normal intelligence major life events, living in an environment with high expressed emotion and social isolation all contribute to relapse in schizophrenic illness the evidence that these factors affect outcome in those with learning disability is not yet clear.

Life Events

No well-defined study has been carried out to determine whether independent life events (i.e. those not caused by the patient) are associated with a greater risk of relapse in those with schizophrenia and learning disability. The assumption can be made that major life events are associated with relapse but no confirming data is available.

High Expressed Emotion

Again, in the learning disabled population no randomized controlled trials of family or carer interaction with the individual with learning disability and schizophrenia have been carried out. However, a study examining patients with learning disability, some of whom were receiving neuroleptic drugs, compared with a matched sample of schizophrenic patients and their families showed that the relatives of those with learning disability showed a significantly greater rate of warmth towards their affected offspring compared with the families of the schizophrenic patients ($P = <0.01$). There was also a greater rate of emotional over-involvement

(P = <0.05) in the relatives of the learning disabled group.[79] These results are not surprising as, in most cases, those with learning disability are treated more affectionately than individuals with normal intelligence who have schizophrenia. It is debatable whether this is due to the different way in which people with learning disability and schizophrenia tend to be treated, i.e. as a handicapped 'child' or as an adult with a frightening mental illness, or whether it is a response to the social isolation frequently sought by those with schizophrenia.

Social Isolation

It has been shown in schizophrenia that an unstimulating social environment can increase social withdrawal and apathy. Although the effects of increasing social contact and social skills in schizophrenic patients with learning disability has not been shown in controlled studies there is evidence that social skills training enables those with learning disability to relate better to others[80,81] and this may help to prevent relapse in schizophrenia in this population.

Cognitive Behavioural Therapy

In schizophrenic patients of normal intelligence, cognitive behavioural interventions have been found to be helpful in reducing the intensity of delusional beliefs and in giving patients some control over hallucinatory experiences.[82] To date, there is no study of similar work in the learning disabled population. Although it might be thought that such work is not possible in those with intellectual impairment two case reports have been published of successful cognitive behavioural therapy using a modified technique for severe depressive symptoms in patients with mild learning disability.[83] Cognitive behavioural strategies may be helpful in improving social skills, assertiveness and problem-solving behaviour. While these do not specifically target schizophrenic symptoms they can increase coping abilities and have been found to be of use in the learning disabled population.[84] In addition to reducing maladaptive behaviour and consequent social difficulties these strategies are important in the rehabilitation of the chronic schizophrenic patient. If the impact of environmental and interpersonal stressors is modified the likelihood of a further schizophrenic breakdown being precipitated may be reduced.

Conclusion

The field of schizophrenia in those with learning disability is one in which few controlled studies have been carried out although there are a number of questions which are germane to developing greater knowledge of this psychotic illness. Is the early development of schizophrenia in those with learning disability due to a neurodevelopmental disorder that presents early because of the degree of cerebral damage? Is the increased incidence of schizophrenia in this population related to greater vulnerability of those with learning disability or is this associated with organic cerebral damage? What is the relationship between schizophrenia and autistic disorder? Investigation of these areas would help unravel the mechanisms and origins of the complex phenomenon of schizophrenia: it is a worthy challenge.

Acknowledgements

Our thanks to Margaret Cheek for her heroic typing of this manuscript.

References

1. Hurd HM (1888) Imbecility with insanity. *American Journal of Insanity* **45**, 261–9.4.
2. Tredgold AF (1903) Insanity in imbeciles. *Journal of Mental Science* **49**, 19–36.
3. Kraepelin E (1919) *Dementia Praecox and Paraphrenia*, Barclay RM (transl), Robertson GM (ed). Edinburgh: Livingstone.
4. Kallman FJ, Barrera SE, Hoch PH & Kelly DM (1940–41) The role of mental deficiency in the incidence of schizophrenia. *American Journal of Mental Deficiency* **45**, 514–39.
5. Payne R (1968) The psychotic subnormal. *Journal of Mental Subnormality* **14**, 25–34.
6. Reid AH (1972) Psychoses in adult mental defectives. *British Journal of Psychiatry* **120**, 205–18.
7. Heaton-Ward WA (1977) Psychosis in mental handicap. *British Journal of Psychiatry* **130**, 524–33.
8. Wright EC (1982) The presentation of mental illness in mentally retarded adults. *British Journal of Psychiatry* **141**, 496–502.
9. Corbett J (1979) Psychiatric morbidity and mental retardation. In Snaith P & James FE (eds) *Psychiatric Illness and Mental Handicap*, pp. 11–25. Ashford: Headley Brothers.
10. Gostason R (1985) Psychiatric illness among the mentally retarded: a Swedish population study. *Acta Psychiatrica Scandinavica* (Suppl. 318), 1–117.
11. Lund J (1985) The prevalence of psychiatric morbidity in mentally retarded adults. *Acta Psychiatrica Scandinavica* **72**, 563–70.
12. Menolascino FJ, Gilson SF & Levitas AS (1986) Issues in the treatment of mentally retarded patients in the community mental health system. *Community Mental Health Journal* **22**, 314–27.
13. Davison K & Bagley C (1969) Schizophrenia-life psychoses associated with organic disorders of the central nervous system: a review of the literature. In Herrington RN (ed) *Current Problems in Neuropsychiatry*, pp. 113–84. Ashford: Headley Brothers.
14. Odegaard O (1972) In Kaplan NAR (ed) *Genetic Factors in Schizophrenia*, pp. 256–75. Springfield: Thomas.
15. Jablensky A (1987) Multicultural studies and the nature of schizophrenia: A review. *Journal of the Royal Society of Medicine* **80**, 162–7.
16. Gottesman II (1991) *Schizophrenia Genesis*. New York: W.H. Freeman.
17. Murray RM, Lewis SW & Reveley AM (1982) Towards an aetiological classification of schizophrenia. *Lancet* **i**, 1023–6.
18. Hafner H, Haas S, Pfeifer-Kurda M, Eichhorn S & Michitsuji S (1987) Abnormal seasonality of schizophrenic births. A specific finding? *European Archives of Psychiatry and Neurological Sciences* **236**, 333–42.
19. Daniel DG, Goldberg TE, Gibbons RD & Weinberger DR (1991) Lack of a bimodal distribution of ventricular size in schizophrenia; a Gaussian mixture analysis of 1056 cases and controls. *Biological Psychiatry* **30**, 887–903.
20. Bruton CJ, Crow TJ, Frith CD, Johnstone EC, Owens DGC & Roberts GW (1990) Schizophrenia and the brain: a prospective clinico-neuropathological study. *Psychology and Medicine* **20**, 285–304.

21. Helmsley DR (1992) Cognitive abnormalities and schizophrenic symptoms. *Psychology and Medicine* **22**, 839–42.
22. Crow TJ, Ball J & Bloom SR (1989) Schizophrenia as an anomaly of development of cerebral asymmetry. A postmortem study and a proposal concerning the genetic basis of the disease. *Archives of General Psychiatry* **46**, 1145–50.
23. Clementz BA, Iacorno WG & Beiser M (1994) Handedness in first-episode psychotic patients and their first degree biological relatives. *Journal of Abnormal Psychology* **103**, 400–3.
24. David AS (1993) Spatial and selective attention in the cerebral hemispheres in depression, mania and schizophrenia. *Brain and Cognition* **23**, 166–80.
25. Filteau MJ, Pourcher E, Bouchard RH, Baruch P, Mathieu J, Bedard F, Simard N & Vincent P (1991) Corpus callosum agenesis and psychosis in Andermann syndrome. *Archives of Neurology* **48**, 1275–80.
26. Abbott MH, Folstein SE, Abbey H & Pyeritz RE (1987) Psychiatric manifestations of homocystinuria due to cystathionine beta-synthase deficiency: prevalence, natural history, and relationship to neurological impairment and vitamin B$_6$-responsiveness. *American Journal of Medical Genetics* **26**, 959–69.
27. Reiss AL, Hagerman R, Vinogradov S, Abrams M & King J (1988) Psychiatric disorder in female carriers of the fragile X chromosome. *Archives of General Psychiatry* **45**, 25–30.
28. Gustavson KH, Modrzewska K & Wetterberg L (1986) Mental retardation in a North Swedish isolate. *Clinical Genetics* **30**, 374–80.
29. Jankovic BD (1985) Neural tissue hypersensitivity in psychiatric disorders with immunologic features. *Journal of Immunology* **135** (2 Suppl.), 853–7.
30. Plioplys AV, Thibault J, Bouchard JP, Cockburn C & Hawkes R (1987) Anti-CNS antibodies in neurological and psychiatric disorders. *Journal of Neurology, Neurosurgery and Psychiatry* **50**, 1514–21.
31. Yannitsi SG, Masoussakis MN, Mavridis AK, Tzioufas AG, Loukas SB, Plataris GK, Liakos AD & Moutsopoulos HM (1990) Factors related to the presence of autoantibodies in patients with chronic mental disorders. *Biological Psychiatry* **27**, 747–56.
32. King DJ, Cooper SJ, Earle JA, Martin SJ, McFerran NV, Reima BK & Wisdom GB (1985) A survey of serum antibodies to eight common viruses in psychiatric patients. *British Journal of Psychiatry* **147**, 137–44.
33. Pomeroyu JC (1980) Klinefelter's syndrome and schizophrenia. *British Journal of Psychiatry* **136**, 597–9.
34. Reiss S & Szyszko J (1983) Diagnostic overshadowing and professional experience with mental retarded persons. *American Journal of Mental Deficiency* **87**, 396–402.
35. Sovner R (1986) Limiting factors in the use of DSM-III criteria with mentally ill/mentally retarded persons. *Psychopharmacology Bulletin* **22**, 1055–9.
36. Eaton LF & Menaloscino FJ (1982) Psychiatric disorders in the mentally retarded: types, problems, and challenges. *American Journal of Psychiatry* **139**, 1297–1303.
37. Patel P, Goldberg DP & Moss SC (1993) Psychiatric morbidity in older people with moderate and severe learning disability (mental retardation) Part II The prevalence study. *British Journal of Psychiatry* **163**, 481–91.
38. Matson JL, Gardner WI, Coe TA & Sovner R (1991) A scale for evaluating emotional disorders in severely and profoundly mentally retarded persons. *British Journal of Psychiatry* **159**, 404–9.
39. Meadows G, Turner T, Campbell L, Lewis SW, Reveley MA & Murray RM (1991) Assessing schizophrenia in adults with mental retardation. A comparative study. *British Journal of Psychiatry* **158**, 103–5.
40. Penrose LS (1991) Survey of cases of familial mental illness. *European Archives of Psychiatry and Neurological Sciences* **240**, 315–24.
41. de Sanctis S (1906) Sopra alcune varieta della demenza precoce. *Revista Sperimentale de Freniatria* **32**, 141–65.
42. Heller R (1908) Uber dementia infantilis. *Zeitschrift für die Erforschung und Behandlung des Jugendlichen Schwachsinns* **2**, 17–28.
43. Hare H (1974) The changing content of psychiatric illness. *Journal of Psychosomatic Research* **18**, 283–9.
44. Gillberg C (1993) Autism and related behaviours. *Journal of International Disease Research* **37**, 343–72.
45. Vanstraelen M & Tyrer SP (1997) Rapid cycling bipolar affective disorder in the mentally retarded. *Journal of Intellectual Disability Research* (in press).

46. Reid AH (1989) Schizophrenia in mental retardation: clinical features. *Research into Developmental Disabilities* **10**, 241–9.
47. Dunstan J & Tyrer SP (1997) Presentation of schizophrenia in those with moderate learning disability. *Journal of Intellectual Disability Research* (in press).
48. Cooper JE, Kendell RE, Gurland BJ, Sharp EL, Copeland JRM & Simon R (1972) *Psychiatric Diagnosis in New York and London*. London: Oxford University Press.
49. American Psychiatric Association (1994) *Diagnostic and Statistical Manual for Mental Disorders*, 4th edn. Washington: APA Press.
50. Hucker SJ, Day KA, George S & Roth M (1979) Psychosis in mentally handicapped adults. In James FE & Snaith RP (eds) *Psychiatric Illness and Mental Handicap*, pp. 27–35. London: Gaskell Press.
51. Ballinger BR, Armstrong J, Presley AJ & Reid AH (1975) Use of a standardised psychiatric interview in mentally handicapped patients. *British Journal of Psychiatry* **127**, 540–4.
52. Goldberg DP, Cooper B, Eastwood MR, Kedward HB & Shepherd M (1970) A standardised psychiatric interview for use in community surveys. *British Journal of Preventative and Social Medicine* **24**, 18–23.
53. Matson JL, Senatore V & Kazdin AE (1984) Psychometric properties of the Psychopathology Instrument for Mentally Retarded Adults. *Applied Research in Mental Retardation* **5**, 81–9.
54. Aman MG, Watson JE & Singh NN (1986) Psychometric and demographic characteristics of the Psychopathology Instrument for Mentally Retarded Adults. *Psychopharmacology Bulletin* **22**, 1072–6.
55. Aman MG & Singh NN (1987) *The Aberrant Behaviour Check List*. East Aurora, New York: Slossen.
56. Sturmey P & Ley T (1990) The Psychopathology Instrument for Mentally Retarded Adults. Internal consistencies and relationship to behaviour problems. *British Journal of Psychiatry* **156**, 428–30.
57. Linaker OM & Helle J (1994) Validity of the schizophrenia diagnosis of the Psychopathology Instrument of Mentally Retarded Adults. *Research in Developmental Disabilities* **15**, 473–86.
58. Swiezy NB, Matson JL, Kirkpatrick-Sanchez S & Williams DE (1995) A criterion validity study of the Schizophrenic Subscale of the Psychopathology Instrument for Mentally Retarded Adults (PIMRA). *Research in Developmental Disabilities* **16**, 75–85.
59. Singh NN, Sood A, Sonemklar N & Ellis CR (1991) Assessment and diagnosis of mental illness in persons with mental retardation. *Behavior Modification* 419–43.
60. Matson JL, Gardner WI, Co DA & Sovner R (1991) A scale for evaluating emotional disorders in severely and profoundly mentally retarded persons. Development of the Diagnostic Assessment for the Severely Handicapped (DASH) scale. *British Journal of Psychiatry* **159**, 404–9.
61. Dean C, Surtees P & Sashidharan SP (1983) Comparison of research diagnostic systems in an Edinburgh community sample. *British Journal of Psychiatry* **142**, 247–56.
62. Wing JK, Cooper JE & Sartorius N (1974) *The Measurement and Classification of Psychiatric Symptoms*. Cambridge: Cambridge University Press.
63. Moss S, Prosser H & Goldberg D (1996) Validity of the schizophrenia diagnosis of the Psychiatric Assessment Schedule for Adults with Developmental Disability (PAS-ADD). *British Journal of Psychiatry* **168**, 359–67.
64. Bazire S & Branch S (1996) *Neuromedicines – Any Questions?* Norfolk Mental Health Care NHS Trust.
65. Intagliata J & Rinck C (1985) Psychoactive drug use in public and community residential facilities for mentally retarded persons. *Psychopharmology Bulletin* **21**, 268–78.
66. King PJ (1995) Neuroleptics and the treatment of schizophrenia. In King PJ (ed.) *Clinical Psychopharmacology*, pp. 259–327. Glasgow: Gaskell.
67. Menolascino FJ, Wilson, J, Golden CJ & Ruedrich SL (1986) Medication and treatment of schizophrenia in persons with mental retardation. *Mental Retardation* **24**, 277–83.
68. Tyrer SP (1997) The management of aggression. *Journal of Psychopharmacology* (in press)
69. Pary RJ (1995) Discontinuation of neuroleptics in community-dwelling individuals with mental retardation and mental illness. *American Journal on Mental Retardation* **100**, 207–12.
70. McClelland HA, Metcalfe AV & Kerr TA *et al.* (1991) Facial dyskinesia: a 16-year follow-up study. *British Journal of Psychiatry* **158**, 691–6.
71. Sachdev P (1992) Drug-induced movement disorders in institutionalised adults with mental retardation: Clinical characteristics and risk factors. *Australian and New Zealand Journal of Psychiatry* **26**, 242–8.

72. Wressell SE, Tyrer SP & Berney TP (1990) Reduction in antipsychotic drug dosage in mentally handicapped patients: A hospital study. *British Journal of Psychiatry* **157**, 101–6.
73. Boyd RD (1992) Recurrence of neuroleptic malignant syndrome via an inadvertent rechallenge in a women with mental retardation. *Mental Retardation* **30**, 77–9.
74. Snyder SH, Banerjee SB & Yamamura HI (1974) Drugs, neurotransmitters and schizophrenia. *Science* **184**, 1243–53.
75. Peroutka SJ & Snyder SH (1980) Relationship of neuroleptic drug effects at brain dopamine, serotonin, alpha-adrenergic, and histamine receptors to clinical potency. *American Journal of Psychiatry* **137**, 1518–22.
76. Brown G & Birley J (1968) Crises and life changes at the onset of schizophrenia. *Journal of Health and Social Behaviour* **9**, 203–14.
77. Brown GW & Rutter M (1966) The measurement of family activities and relationships: a methodological study. *Human Relations* **19**, 241–63.
78. Cavanagh D (1992) Recent developments in expressed emotion and schizophrenia. *British Journal of Psychiatry* **160**, 601–20.
79. Clerici M, Beltz J & Bertrando P (1993) Mental retardation and family environment: role of emotional factors. *Minerva Psichiatrica* **34**, 163–72.
80. Brady JP (1984) Social skills training for psychiatric patients, II: Clinical outcome studies. *American Journal of Psychiatry* **141**, 491–8.
81. Stavrakakl C & Klein J (1986) Psychotherapies with the mentally retarded. *Psychiatric Clinics of North America* **9**, 733–43.
82. Berris C & Skagerlind L (1994) Cognitive therapy with schizophrenia patients. *Acta Psychiatrica Scandinavica* **89** (Suppl 382), 65–70.
83. Lindsay WR, Howell L & Pitcaithly D (1993) Cognitive therapy for depression with individuals with intellectual disabilities. *British Journal of Psychology* **66**, 135–41.
84. Nezu CM & Nezu AM (1994) Outpatient psychotherapy for adults with mental retardation and concomitant psychopathology: research and clinical imperatives. *Journal of Consultative and Clinical Psychology* **62**, 34–42.
85. Russell AT & Tanguay PE (1981) Mental illness and mental retardation: cause or coincidence? *American Journal of Mental Deficiency* **85**, 570–4.

9

Affective Disorders

C. Barbara Ballinger

Introduction

Affective disorder, in which the basic disturbance is of mood state which may be abnormally depressed or elated and often accompanied by increased anxiety, is probably under-diagnosed and inadequately treated in people with learning disability. Depressive illness is one of the commonest mental disorders in the general population but in those with a learning disability the presenting symptoms and signs may be atypical. In addition, the presence of the intellectual disability may reduce the likelihood of a separate diagnosis of abnormal mood state being made and appropriate treatment being instigated, all the presenting symptoms being attributed to the learning disability *per se*. This phenomenon was demonstrated in a study by Reiss *et al.*[1] and described as diagnostic overshadowing.

The recognition of the concept of affective disorders in people with learning disability has developed relatively slowly with doubt being expressed, particularly in the psychoanalytic literature, about the ability of such individuals to experience the full range of emotions and emotional conflict.[2] Individual cases of affective disorder in learning disability have been reported in the literature and in 1972 Reid[3] described the clinical features of 21 patients with manic depressive psychosis and learning disability and suggested it was possible to make the diagnosis on the usual clinical grounds in those with an IQ of 20 or above and modified criteria for those with IQ below 20. Since then attempts have been made to improve the understanding of the epidemiology, clinical features and management of affective psychosis in individuals with learning disability but the relevant literature is still quite scarce compared with the literature on affective disorders in general.

Epidemiology

Epidemiological research in affective disorders in people with learning disability has been inhibited by the lack of standardized case identification procedures and the selected nature of many of the population groups studied, e.g. long-term residents in institutions. These two factors account for much of the difficulty in making useful comparisons between studies but a third complication is that of nonspecific behaviour disorders and the relationship of these disorders to formal psychiatric diagnosis in general and affective disorders in particular.

In 1985 Lund[4] reported a community survey of 302 adults with a learning disability identified through the case register of the Danish National Service for the Mentally Retarded. The MRC Handicaps Behaviour and Skills schedule was used for case identification and an overall prevalence rate of psychiatric disorder of 27% was reported, 10.9% being behaviour disorder, 1.3% schizophrenia and 1.7% affective disorder. The figure of 1.7% represented five individuals, of which two were depressed and three had bipolar disorders.

Jacobson[5] used the Developmental Disabilities Information System (DDIS) in New York to survey the distribution of psychiatric disorder based on DSM-II (1968) diagnoses in 42 474 individuals registered on DDIS. He noted that the rates of affective disorder were relatively lower than the diagnoses of schizophrenic and other psychotic disorders compared with general population studies where affective disorders were more common. He suggested that this difference in the relative prevalence of affective and schizophrenic psychosis between learning disabled and normal populations was related to phenomena such as diagnostic overshadowing and problems in the application of DSM diagnostic criteria to individuals with learning disability.

Surveys of patients in institutional care have, understandably, demonstrated higher prevalence rates for psychiatric disorder, including affective disorders, than those reported for community surveys. Wright[6] reported a prevalence rate of 2.8% for affective disorders in 1507 adult residents in an institution but if atypical affective disorders were included the rate rose to 5.5%. The atypical illnesses were said to be superimposed on some form of early childhood psychosis with major impairments of social interaction. In the same study the prevalence rate for schizophrenia was reported as 1.8%.

As the life expectancy of people with learning disability has increased there has been more interest in the prevalence of psychiatric disorders in middle-aged and older people with learning disability in both institutional and community settings. In 1985 Day[7] reported a study of 357 long-stay hospital residents aged 40 years and over and 250 new admissions over a 7-year period to a psychiatric unit for those with learning disability. Neurotic disorders were more common in the admission group and behaviour disorders in the long-stay group. The prevalence of affective disorders was 5.3% in the long-stay group and 2.3% in the admission group. The majority of the 24 cases of affective disorder were said to suffer from cyclical mood swings or hypomania and five individuals had rapid short-cycle psychoses. It is unclear whether depression was more difficult to diagnose in this group or more likely to be included in the diagnosis of neurosis rather than psychosis.

A survey of 124 hospital residents aged 60 years or over was reported by Sansom *et al.*[8] and prevalence rates of 12.9% for dementia, 6.5% for schizophrenia and 8.9% for affective disorder were noted. DSM-III-R (1987) diagnostic criteria were used in this study and of the 11 cases with affective disorder four were acutely ill and seven in remission. The rates of psychiatric disorder in general and affective disorder in particular were higher than those reported by Day in 1985[7] but this may reflect differential discharge of individuals without psychiatric disorder and an increasing concentration of individuals with psychiatric disturbance in long-term institutional care, as demonstrated in other studies.[9]

A community survey of psychiatric disorder in people with learning disability over 50 years of age was reported in 1993 by Patel *et al.*[10] A sample of 105 people with learning disability was screened using the Psychiatric Assessment Schedule for Adults with a Developmental Disability (PAS-ADD), as described by Moss *et al.*[11] In total, 16 cases were identified giving an overall prevalence rate of 15%. Seven individuals were identified as having affective disorder with or without other diagnoses and this gives a prevalence rate of 6.7% for affective disorders. One individual was said to have dysthymia related with paranoid personality disorder, two had bipolar affective disorders and four had depressive illnesses and in one individual this was associated with dementia. The relatively high prevalence of affective disorder in this sample compared with Lund's study[4] may be related to the relative sensitivity of the screening method to depressive illnesses compared with previous studies. It was notable in the study reported by Patel *et al.*[10] that although the two patients with bipolar disorder were on effective treatment, only one of the patients with a depressive illness was on antidepressant medication and that was at low dosage.

The prevalence of affective disorder in general and depressive illness in particular, in individuals with learning disability, is probably underestimated both in epidemiological studies and clinical practice.

Clinical Features of Affective Disorder in Individuals with Learning Disability

The clinical presentation of affective disorder in individuals with learning disability includes changes in mood, cognition, behaviour and physical function, as in mainstream psychiatric practice. The main difference from assessment methods in mainstream psychiatric practice is the decreased reliance on verbal information from the individual and increased reliance on reports from informants who know the individual well and observational information on changes in behaviour and vegetative function. Reid[3] noted in 1972 that affective disorder could be diagnosed on the usual clinical criteria in people with mild to moderate learning disability but in nonverbal individuals with severe or profound learning disability, longitudinal observations from informants who knew the individual well were required. The ability of individuals with mild and moderate learning disability to describe and report their feelings has probably been underestimated in the past. The stability and consistency of self-assessment of mood state in people with mild to moderate learning disability was assessed in a recent study[12] using a variety of self-assessment scales for depression and anxiety. These included the Zung Self-Rating Anxiety

Scale, the Zung Depression Scale and the General Health Questionnaire. There was a high level of convergent validity in the responses, suggesting that self-report of emotional state in this population was both reliable and valid. In addition, there was a high correlation between measures of anxiety and depression emphasizing the close relationship between these two symptoms.

Depression of mood may be misdiagnosed or missed more frequently than hypomania or bipolar disorder in people with learning disability. The onset of depression tends to be more insidious and the changes less dramatic, often being attributed to the underlying learning disability or even the onset of the dementia rather than symptoms of a depressive illness. The symptoms of depression include weepiness and social withdrawal but irritability may be much more marked and of more concern to carers, resulting in referral for assessment. Meins[13] noted that approximately half of a group of 32 depressed patients exhibited irritable mood rather than classical depression of mood and irritability became the preponderant expression of depression with increasing severity of learning disability. Psychomotor agitation was also more common in the more disabled group whereas reduced energy and fatigue were more likely to be reported in the individuals with mild to moderate learning disability.

Vegetative changes of depression in individuals with learning disability include changes in appetite and sleep pattern. Increased appetite with weight gain was reported in just under one-third of the group reported by Meins[13] and decreased appetite with weight loss in just over one-third. Insomnia was much more common than hypersomnia, particularly in those with more severe learning disability.

A wide variety of behavioural symptoms associated with depressive illness was reported by Meins.[13] The most prominent were aggression, self-injurious behaviour, stereotypies, screaming, temper tantrums, incontinence and vomiting. It was felt that these symptoms were quite specifically related to the depressive illness and it is this type of symptom that is most likely to be attributed to the learning disability rather than any superimposed mental illness and lead to misdiagnosis and denial of appropriate treatment to the individual.

Hypochondriacal symptoms may be prominent in the presentation of depressive disorder in individuals with learning disability and Reid[3] reported symptoms such as headache, abdominal pain and vomiting. Other individuals may present with a generalized deterioration in their social and self-care skills and Helsel and Matson[14] demonstrated a high correlation between ratings for depression and social skills. Where deterioration in skills is a prominent feature there is a risk, particularly for older patients with Down's syndrome, of a diagnosis of dementia being made and appropriate treatment being withheld. This issue was addressed in a study of five patients with Down's syndrome, referred for evaluation of dementia, who were found to have a major depression.[15] All these individuals had shown deterioration in behaviour and cognitive skills but responded well to antidepressants and electroconvulsive therapy (ECT).

The complex relationship between dementia and depression in older individuals with learning disabilities was explored in a study by Harper and Wadsworth.[16] They found that decrease in cognitive ability was associated with increases in reported behavioural problems and higher rates of observed depression. The main problem behaviours were self-harm and aggression and cognitive decline was more common in those who initially had more severe learning disability. The authors noted that it is difficult to ascertain whether the mood disturbance is a transient feature or part of an organic dementia or related to the generally deteriorating physical state of the older group. Burt *et al.* also noted an association between depression and dementia but this was only true for individuals with Down's syndrome and 43 adults with learning disability from other causes did not show this association.[17] With the increasing longevity of individuals with learning disability this is an important issue in clinical practice.

Hypomania

The clinical features of hypomania in learning disability include an increase in motor activity, as in the majority of hypomanic patients, but mood is less likely to be euphoric and infectious and more likely to be irritable and accompanied at times by aggression. Pressure of speech may be present but more complex verbal symptoms such as flight of ideas and clang associations are rare. Grandiose ideas and delusions may be expressed but in quite simple forms and hallucinatory experiences are rarely reported. In very severe cases catatonia and stupor can occur.

Rapid Cycling Bipolar Disorder

This type of affective disorder with four or more episodes of affective illness in any one year is associated with severe behaviour problems in individuals with learning disabilities. Reid and Naylor[18] described this condition in patients with learning disability in institutional care and in 1992 Lowry and Sovner[19] emphasized the importance of this condition in relation to cyclical changes in severe behavioural problems and in particular to self-injurious behaviour.

Glue[20] described 10 individuals with rapid cycling affective disorder in a hospital population of 100 patients and suggested that the relatively high prevalence of the condition in this patient group may be related to admission policies. The severe behavioural disturbance that accompanied rapid fluctuations in mood and the relative resistance of the condition to treatment would greatly increase the chances of being admitted to hospital care. Although in general population terms this is a relatively uncommon condition, it has considerable implications for future service provision for individuals with learning disabilities.

Affective Disorder in Severe and Profound Learning Disability

The assessment of affective disorder in people with severe or profound learning disability is complicated by the lack of verbal skills required to express feeling tone in the presence of other sensory and motor deficits in multiple handicap. However, King et al.[21] considered the diagnosis of affective disorder to be fairly straightforward, even in profound learning disability, based on reports from carers of a change in behaviour such as recent onset of emotional lability, weepiness, irritability or elevation of mood. Corroborative information came from biological features such as changes in activity level, sleep patterns, appetite and sexual behaviour. King et al.[21] also noted that anxiety may be expressed in the form of avoidance behaviour or by the autonomic features of anxiety in relation to specific situations. In addition, some individuals would cling to staff in a way that suggested anxiety about separation.

Affective Disorders in Autism

Three recent studies[22-24] have explored a possible association between affective disorders and autism. Kurita and Nakayasu[22] reported a single case of an individual with severe learning disability, autism and seasonal affective disorder. The diagnosis of affective disorder was based on information received from the main carer and one of the presenting symptoms was recurrent trichotillomania. Lainhart and Folstein[23] reviewed 17 published cases of affective disorder in individuals with autistic symptoms and concluded that making a diagnosis of affective disorder was particularly difficult against a background of autistic symptoms and that a deterioration in cognition, language, behaviour or activity was more likely to be presented than a specific change in mood. The importance of establishing the patient's baseline was also emphasized as was any change in behaviour such as increased self-injury, echolalia or handflapping. Smalley et al.[24] reported a study of the prevalence of affective disorder in the families of 36 autistic children compared with the families of 45 control probands. Elevated rates of both major depression and social phobia were found among parents and siblings in the families with an autistic child and 64% of parents affected with major depression had the first attack before the autistic child was born. They concluded that their findings in relation to affective disorders supported the view that major depression and autism may share a genetic predisposition.

Affective Disorders and Aggression

Aggression is a common symptom in affective disorders in people with learning disabilities. Meins[13] observed aggressive behaviour towards objects in one-third of his sample of 32 depressed adults with learning disability and aggression towards people in approximately one-third of the sample but the degree of overlap between these two groups was no specified. He also noted that aggression was significantly associated with increasing severity of learning disability in the depressed group. Reiss an Rojahn[25] reported a study of the relationship between aggression an depression in 528 adults. Ratings of anger were significantly associated with ratings of aggression, as would be expected, but also with ratings of depression. In addition, depression was four times more likely to be iden ified in aggressive subjects than in non-aggressive subjects.

Benson and Ivins[26] noted that self-report assessments of anger, depression and self concept in 130 adults with learning disability living in the con munity showed a negative correlation between self-esteem and depression There was a positive correlation between self-assessment and informat assessment of depression but not of anger and the less disabled group wer more likely to report anger than the more disabled. It was suggested tha the reluctance to report anger on the self-assessments could be related to social desirability response bias, with subjects feeling that it was not accep able to express anger or other negative emotions.

Aggression against self, objects or other people has been reported bot in hypomania[3] and in short cycle bipolar disorders.[19] Lewis *et al.*[27] reporte the rhythmical fluctuation of aggression and self-injurious behaviour i a group of 12 institutionalized individuals with learning disability an concluded that these two behaviours fluctuated in discreet cycle: suggesting that these may relate to biological rhythms. However, they di not explore the possibility of an association with a cyclical mood disorde

The association of affective disorders and aggression in people wit learning disability is of great practical importance. Aggressive behaviou tends to produce negative responses from carers and services and muc less sympathetic responses than those produced by obvious expressions c depression or distress. This reduces the possibility of the behavioura change being identified as an affective disorder and treated appropriatel Where aggression occurs it will dominate the presentation, and carers an professional personnel are less likely to identify other features suc as vegetative changes and dysphoria which may suggest a diagnosis c affective disorder. This can lead to the individual being subjected to inap propriate management strategies.

Case Identification Techniques and Rating Scales for Affective Disorders in Individuals with Learning Disability

In order to improve both the understanding and the management of affec tive disorders in people with learning disabilities, reliable and valid tech niques for detection of mood disorders in the learning disabled populatio are required. In addition, if therapeutic trials are to be carried out the reliable and valid rating scales which are responsive to change in moo state in this population group are necessary. The development of suc screening techniques and rating scales has tended to follow two distinc routes, the first being the modification of standard rating scales and screening interviews for mood disorders in adult psychiatric practice and the second being the modification of such scales developed initially for use with children.

By definition, individuals with a learning disability will have problems with written material so all rating scales have to be administered orally. This technique has been shown in some studies to be both reliable and valid. Lindsay *et al.*[12] reported a successful modification of the Zung Self-rating Depression Inventory[28] for use with people who had a mild to moderate learning disability but who could express themselves verbally. The necessary modifications were described by Lindsay and Michie[29] in relation to the Zung Self-rating Anxiety Scale. They noted that items were rephrased to ensure understanding and response presentations were altered to ensure reliability. The standard response presentations gave a range of response for each symptom from 'present a good part of the time' to 'sometimes' and 'quite a lot of the time', to 'most of the time'. In the modified form the response was simplified to presence or absence of the symptom and this appeared to be reliable on retesting after 6 months whereas reliability was unacceptably low with the standard response presentation. In addition to looking at test–retest reliability Lindsay *et al.*,[12] using a test battery including the Zung Self-rating Anxiety Scale and the Zung Depression Inventory, the General Health Questionnaire and the Eysench–Withers Personality Test, demonstrated a great deal of convergent validity in the responses relating to emotional experiences and feelings.

The Beck Depression Inventory[30] is widely used in psychiatric practice and consists of 21 items with a choice of one response out of four for each item. In view of the findings of Lindsay *et al.*[29] this would seem to be of doubtful value for use with people with learning disability. Kazdin *et al.*[31] reported on the use of the modified form of the Beck Depression Inventory as part of a battery of measures which showed a significant level of correlation with each other and a consistent relationship to a clinical diagnosis of depression. However, test–retest reliability was not reported as part of this study and should be addressed before the modified Beck Depression Inventory can be recommended for general use in rating affective disorder in individuals with learning disability.

Two recent reports[32,33] concerned the use of rating scales, developed primarily for the assessment of mood in children, in people with learning disabilities. The rationale put forward for the use of these scales is the similarity of problems in assessment in terms of limited verbal skills and dependence on information from third parties. Meins[32] concluded that the informant rating version of the Children's Depression Inventory[34] showed satisfactory inter-rater reliability and acceptable validity in comparison with a clinical diagnosis of DSM-III-R depressive disorder. In addition, the scores on the Children's Depressive Inventory were independent of age and sex in the learning disabled group.

Benavidez and Matson[33] reported a study of 25 adolescents with learning disability and 25 adolescents in the normal IQ range using a Children's Depression Inventory and other measures of mood. It was concluded that convergent validity had been demonstrated by strong correlations between total scores on all measures but reliability was not tested. In contrast, Rojahn *et al.*[35] reported low levels of association between a standardized clinical research questionnaire developed specifically for children, a self-report questionnaire developed specifically for individuals with learning disability and an informants rating scale in assessing depression in a group of 38 adults with mild to moderate learning disability.

The use of rating scales devised primarily for children in studies of affective disorder in adults with learning disability needs to be viewed with caution. In clinical practice much time is spent persuading parents and carers to deal with people with learning disability as adults and, in terms of life experience and other areas of development, adults with learning disability are very different from children. More rigorous studies of both validity and reliability need to be carried out before it can be concluded that rating scales for affective disorder in children can be applied to adults with learning disability.

Sturmey *et al.*,[36] in a helpful review of assessment instruments for psychiatric disorder in individuals with learning disabilities, noted that a distinction needs to be made between diagnostic instruments for assessing the presence or absence of a specific disorder and assessment instruments for rating the severity of the particular symptom, e.g. depression. Those rating scales discussed so far belong, in the main, to the second category. Ballinger *et al.*[37] described the use of a modified psychiatric clinical interview schedule to rate psychiatric symptoms and signs, and generate an ICD diagnosis in a group of hospital residents with learning disability. A previous study[38] had shown the schedule to be both reliable and valid, suggesting that standard diagnostic criteria could be applied with some modification in the diagnosis of psychiatric disorders, including affective disorder, in individuals with learning disability.

Moss *et al.*[11] described a new psychiatric semi-structured clinical interview for use with individuals with learning disability in the community. This clinical interview was based on the Psychiatric Assessment Schedule,[39] a research diagnostic system developed for use in the community. Modifications to the PAS for use with people with learning disability included simplification of the wording, parallel patient and informant interviewing and the use of memorable 'anchor' events in the subject's life to help focus discussion on the 4 weeks prior to the interview. A standardized research diagnosis can be generated from this schedule on both the ICD-9 and DSM-III-R systems, including diagnoses for affective disorders. In the study reported by Moss *et al.*[11] inter-rater reliability was good as were other measures of reliability and it was suggested that the schedule could be updated for use with ICD-10 diagnostic criteria.

The use of ICD-10 Research Diagnostic Criteria (DCR) in individuals with learning disability is currently being assessed and an initial report[40] suggests that the DCR represent an advance on previous systems with a multi-axial classification allowing severity of learning disability, physical health problems and mental health problems to be presented separately.

This is a welcome development which should lead to a more standardized approach to the diagnosis of mental disorder, including affective disorders in people with learning disability in future with concomitant improvements in diagnostic awareness and treatment.

In view of the problems in developing valid and reliable assessment systems for the detection of affective disorder in people with learning disability, there is a great attraction in the suggestion that biological measures can be used to detect depression. The Dexamethasone Suppression Test (DST) involves the administration of oral dexamethasone to subjects in the evening followed by examination of plasma cortisol levels next day. In normal subjects ACTH is inhibited by dexamethasone and plasma cortisol levels reduced but a proportion of individuals with depressive illness show an abnormal response with failure of suppression of cortisol levels. In 1982 Carroll[41] suggested that this could be a very useful test where diagnosis of affective disorder was particularly difficult, as in differentiating between depression and the onset of dementia and diagnosing depression in children. However, Sireling[42] administered the DST to 12 individuals with learning disability and depressive illness and only one subject showed an abnormal response pattern with failure to suppress cortisol levels and Sireling considered that the DST had little to offer in the differential diagnosis of depression in patients with learning disability. Soni *et al.*[43] assessed the value of the DST in 19 individuals with learning disabilities who had clinically significant depression both before and after treatment with antidepressant medication and again concluded that the DST was of little value as a diagnostic tool for the detection of depression against a background of learning disability.

This conclusion is consistent with the findings in general psychiatry reported by Berger *et al.*[44] In this study 231 psychiatric inpatients were subjected to the dexamethasone suppression test and the test did not differentiate between patients with depressive illnesses and other psychiatric disorders. It was demonstrated that intervening variables such as stress, drug withdrawal, suicidal turmoil and weight loss enhanced the rate of abnormal DST results regardless of diagnostic classification. In conclusion, it would appear that the DST has very little to offer in the pursuit of more accurate diagnosis of affective disorder against a background of learning disabilities and there is more to be gained from the development of more appropriate rating scales and diagnostic interviews.

Aetiology of Affective Disorder in Individuals with Learning Disability

A variety of genetic, biochemical, physical and psychosocial factors have been identified as having aetiological significance in affective disorders in the general population. Subjects with learning disability are particularly vulnerable in some of these areas and may be at increased risk of affective disorder, particularly depression, compared with individuals in the normal IQ range.

Genetic factors have been studied extensively in affective disorders and with the development of molecular genetics further progress can be expected.[45] There have been no systematic studies of genetic factors in affective disorders in learning disability but Glue[20] noted that five of his 10 subjects with rapid cycling bipolar disorders had first-degree relatives with mood disorders. This finding is consistent with the evidence that genetic factors are more prominent in bipolar disorders than unipolar depression. In addition Smalley *et al.*[24] commented on the increased frequency of major depression amongst first-degree relatives of autistic probands compared with the relatives of control probands. This area certainly seems worthy of more research in relation to the genetics of affective disorders and autism.

In view of the high prevalence of brain damage associated with learning disability, particularly with the more severe degrees of learning disability, it is surprising that the role of organic factors including epilepsy in the aetiology of affective disorders has received only cursory attention. Rutter[46] noted that children with learning disability accompanied by neurological abnormalities were more likely to have psychiatric diagnoses than those without such abnormalities. Lund,[47] in a study of 300 individuals with learning disability, reported that 52% of those with epilepsy had a psychiatric diagnosis compared with 26% of those without epilepsy. These studies did not examine a specific link with affective disorder but recent reports of mood disturbance against a background of neurological disorder may be relevant to the aetiology of affective disorder in learning disability.

Cornelius *et al.*[48] described the features of organic mood syndrome as presented by 130 patients with a variety of neurological disorders including epilepsy, cerebrovascular accidents and Parkinson's disease. Symptoms seen more commonly in patients with organic mood syndrome compared with patients with major depressive disorder included self-neglect, lability of mood, hostility and violent behaviour. Some of these atypical presentations are similar to those seen in affective disorders in learning disability. EEG and CT investigations in patients with organic mood syndrome indicated that the focal EEG abnormalities were most common in the temporal lobes followed by the frontal lobes, whereas the CT abnormalities were most common in the frontal lobes followed by the temporal lobes. Cornelius *et al.*[48] concluded that the organic mood syndrome had diagnostic validity but prospective studies were required to demonstrate the consistency of the diagnosis over time.

Mendez *et al.*[49] investigated further the association between epilepsy and depression, suggesting that the association may be particularly prominent with a left hemisphere lesion. Out of 1611 patients with epilepsy they identified 272 individuals whose seizures originated from a structural brain lesion other than mesial temporal sclerosis. A total of 25 (9%) of the 272 patients were said to have sustained depressive disorder and, compared with the nondepressed patients in the same group, they were significantly more likely to have a left-hemisphere lesion; this supported the view that depression is related particularly to left hemisphere dysfunction. This work,[48,49] which is currently being pursued in neurological settings, would appear to have relevance to the aetiology of affective disorder in learning disability.

A variety of social cognitive and behavioural models of depression have been developed and many of the factors thought to contribute to an increased risk of depression are particularly relevant to individuals with a learning disability. Lewinsohn[50] proposed a model of depression based on learning theory in which he suggested that a low rate of positive interactions between the individual and the environment increased vulnerability to depression. As many individuals with learning disability are relatively less competent in all spheres than people in the normal IQ range they experience negative reactions from family, peers, educational and work settings which may well lower self-esteem and lead to an increased vulnerability to depression.

A concept from the cognitive/behavioural studies of depression that may be relevant in learning disability is that of 'learned helplessness'. This concept was introduced by Seligman[51] and he suggested that when an individual is faced with repeated failure they may perceive that they cannot change the situation for the better and assume a helpless response leading to further deterioration in problem-solving behaviour and an increased vulnerability to depression. People with a learning disability are particularly prone to be faced with failure because of basic deficits in understanding and problem-solving abilities and are therefore more likely to assume a position of learned helplessness, with further deterioration in their problem-solving abilities and an increased risk of depression.

In their book on the social origins of depression, Brown and Harris[52] emphasized the importance of threatening life events in the genesis of depression and the protective effect of an intimate relationship and social support. Individuals with learning disabilities often lack the skills to establish intimate relationships which could give some degree of protection and may be very isolated with a poor system of social support, particularly in community settings, thereby increasing their vulnerability to depression.

The life event that has been studied most intensively in relation to depression is that of bereavement. The relationship of grief and loss to depression has been explored in the psychoanalytic literature; Day[7] emphasized the difficulties for individuals with learning disability in working through the grieving process. Bereavement for an individual with a learning disability may be a particularly threatening life event in that it may result in a terrifying and rapid change in circumstances if the main carer dies. Harper and Wadsworth[53] reported the clinical aspects of grief reactions in 43 adults with learning disability and the views of care providers, social workers and clergy on the grief reactions observed. Intense reactions including self-injury were noted in 10–15% of the grief reactions and depressive symptoms were frequent, indicating the importance of bereavement as an aetiological factor in affective disorders in learning disability.

Matson and Sevin,[54] in a review of the theoretical basis of dual diagnosis, commented that developmental models, based on the premise that sequences of cognitive development are universal and proceed at a slower rate in learning disability, may offer a useful framework for understanding psychopathology in people with learning disability. They noted that pre-valence rates for depression may be high in individuals with learning disability when compared with those of the same age in the normal range of IQ but normal in relation to individuals at a similar developmental age. This hypothesis has not been tested in relation to affective disorders in people with learning disability.

In conclusion, many of the organic, social, behavioural and cognitive factors that are associated with an increased risk of affective disorder are more common among individuals with learning disability than people in the normal IQ range and this has considerable implications both for service development and the management of individuals with learning disability and superimposed affective disorder.

Management of Affective Disorder in Individuals with Learning Disability

In general psychiatric settings, affective disorder is treated with a variety of psychopharmacological and psychotherapeutic approaches including a wide range of social, cognitive and behavioural interventions. In learning disability treatment approaches are being developed as professionals become more aware of the possibility of affective disorder in this popu-lation. The general principles of management of affective disorder in learning disability are the same as those which apply to individuals in the normal IQ range but with particular emphasis on the involvement of immediate carers who may be crucial intermediaries in dealing with medication or applying broadly psychotherapeutic techniques.

A wide range of antidepressant medication, antipsychotic medication and mood-stabilizing medication is in use in general psychiatry for the treatment of major depression, hypomania and bipolar disorder respec-tively. Unfortunately, the use of psychotropic medication in individuals with learning disability has been widely criticized because of the, at times, indiscriminate use of medication for behavioural control rather than treat-ment of specific identified psychiatric disorder. In addition, psychotropic medication has been used as an alternative to a more appropriate envi-ronmental change or behavioural programme being implemented. It is therefore essential that a careful diagnosis is made of affective disorder before treatment is started and any psychotropic medication should be part of a wider multidisciplinary approach to management, with appropriate cognitive and behavioural programmes being implemented if indicated.

There have been two recent reviews of the use of psychotropic medi-cation in people with learning disability.[55,56] Bregman[55] listed 13 studies of the use of psychotropic medication in affective disorder in learning disability published between 1979 and 1993, the majority of which were open trials and involved between one and five subjects. Bregman[55] concluded his review by emphasizing the need to identify a medication responsive psychiatric disorder and target symptoms before using psychotropic medication. Deb and Fraser[56] emphasized the problems of side-effects of psychotropic medication, the unacceptability of using such medication without identifying a specific psychiatric illness and the involvement of the multidisciplinary team in discussing possible use of psychotropic medication.

There have been no prospective double-blind trials of use of anti-depressant medication in the treatment of depression in individuals with learning disability but Sovner et al.[57] reported on the use of fluoxetine in two patients with severe and profound learning disability who displayed self-injurious behaviour and were apparently depressed. In both cases a reduction in self-injurious behaviour was reported on fluoxetine treatment, with diminution in other depressive symptoms and a marked improvement in sleep pattern in one of the two patients. Langee and Conlon[58] presented a retrospective study of the use of a variety of antidepressants in 175 subjects with learning disability over a period of 10 years. They noted that the responsive symptoms were depression and psychotic symptoms and the unresponsive symptoms were aggression, agitation, tantrums, self-injurious behaviour and hyperactivity. This study again emphasizes the need for diagnosis–congruent use of medication, and depression is the symptom that responds best to antidepressant medication. Antidepressants are probably underused in psychiatric practice in learning disability because of the problems of gaining access to subjective symptoms such as depression where verbal skills are limited. However antipsychotic medication may be used inappropriately because it is the behavioural consequences of the mood change that often make more of an impact on carers and are more likely to be brought to the attention of professionals.

ECT is generally accepted as an effective and safe method of treatment for severe depressive illness, particularly when a fast response is needed. As with antidepressant medication there are no double-blind trials of ECT reported in the literature but there are case reports of individuals with learning disability and depressive illness responding well to ECT.[59,60] Warren et al.[15] described a satisfactory response to ECT in three patients with Down's syndrome and major depression who had failed to respond to antidepressant medication. Individuals with learning disability have an increased risk of epilepsy and other neurological disorders but Benbow[61] suggests that these disorders are not an absolute contraindication to ECT. McClelland[62] concludes that ECT is a useful therapeutic option in patients with learning disability and severe depressive illness who fail to respond to adequate treatment with antidepressant medication.

The main difficulty in the management of severe depression in an individual with learning disability is not the lack of effective treatment methods but that of identifying depressive illness against a background of learning disability. The difficulties in making the diagnosis and the lack of appropriate instruments for measuring treatment outcome are illustrated in a case reported by Bebchuk et al.[63]

The use of psychotropic medication in the treatment of hypomania is well established in general psychiatric practice, including the use of antipsychotic medication and lithium. In 1974 Naylor et al.[64] described a double-blind trial of long-term lithium therapy in 14 patients with learning disabilities and recurrent affective disorder. They reported that the number of weeks the patients were ill during the year on lithium therapy was significantly less than during the year on placebo. Glue,[20] in a study of 10 patients with learning disability and rapid cycling affective disorder, reported that five patients showed partial or complete improvement on lithium alone or in combination with carbamazepine and that rates of response to treatment were similar to those of patients with rapid cycling affective disorder, without learning disability.

In a review of rapid cycling affective illness in general psychiatric patients in 1984, Roy-Byrne *et al.*[65] concluded that treatment was extremely difficult, with carbamazepine emerging as an alternative to lithium or an adjunctive treatment with lithium. They also stated that long-term antipsychotics had a place in the management of this disorder but their main therapeutic effect was in reducing the intensity and possibly the frequency of manic episodes.

Kastner *et al.*[66] reported a study of the use of valproic acid in 18 subjects with learning disability and affective disorder defined by the presence of three out of four symptoms of irritability, sleep disturbance, aggression or self-injurious behaviour and behavioural cycling. Fourteen individuals responded well to valproic acid and withdrawal of antipsychotic medication was achieved in 9 out of 10 patients. A history of epilepsy or suspicion of seizures was strongly associated with a good response to valproic acid, suggesting the possibility of an organically determined mood disorder in these subjects.

In the treatment of hypomania and bipolar affective disorders in individuals with learning disabilities the main problem, as with depression, is that of making an accurate diagnosis and then instituting appropriate treatment. Antipsychotic medication can be very effective in the management of hypomania and bipolar disorder but the long-term side-effects, particularly tardive diskynesia, require careful consideration. Lithium is effective in the treatment of hypomania and the prevention of relapses in bipolar disorders but again lithium has a wide range of side-effects that require careful monitoring; effective monitoring of blood levels also requires repeated venopunctures which may be an issue with some individuals with learning disability. The use of carbamazepine and more recently valproic acid as mood stabilizers may be of particular significance in the field of learning disability because of the increased risk of associated brain damage and epilepsy and should be given careful consideration in the management of affective disorders in individuals with learning disability.

In 1986 Lund[67] reported a survey of 302 subjects with learning disability of whom 85 had a psychiatric diagnosis. The subjects were representative of all individuals with learning disability in Denmark and were living in a variety of settings. Lund concluded that psychopharmacological treatment was appropriate and consistent with current treatment approaches but more elaborate treatment methods, including psycho-therapy and behavioural therapy, were underused despite the obvious need. Reiss *et al.*[68] noted the need to improve the availability of psychotherapeutic services for individuals with learning disability who had emotional problems. They commented on the paradoxical situation where individuals with a learning disability had an increased risk of emotional disorder and adjustment problems but were less likely to be offered the appropriate psychotherapeutic services than those in the general population. Affective disorders, particularly depression, are often associated with relationship problems and a psychotherapeutic approach would be considered very appropriate for an individual in the normal IQ range in a general psychiatric setting. However, the view that average, or preferably above-average, intelligence is required to enter into psychotherapy has certainly had a negative influence on the development of psychotherapeutic services for people with learning disability. This situation appears to be changing now and Bicknell[69] gives an insight into the use of psychotherapy in a way that could be very helpful in the management of affective disorder in people with learning disability.

Lindsay *et al.*[70] demonstrated that behavioural techniques that were thought to be too complex for use with individuals with learning disability could be modified very successfully in the management of anxiety. The cognitive approach to the treatment of depression is now firmly established in general psychiatric practice but no attempt has yet been made to modify the complex concepts involved in this approach for use with individuals with learning disability.

The important relationship between social skills and depression in individuals with learning disability[14] is of therapeutic significance in that improvements in social skills can result in improvement in mood. In addition, social isolation and stigmatization are important issues in the genesis of depression in people with learning disabilities and practical measures can be applied to ameliorate these issues which are of particular importance with the further development of care in the community.

In conclusion, there is a wide range of social, cognitive, behavioural and pharmacological techniques available to be applied to the management of affective disorders in individuals with learning disability. The essential first step is the accurate diagnosis of the condition followed by a coordinated multidisciplinary approach to management involving the individual and their main carers.

Suicide and Suicidal Behaviour

Suicide is rarely reported in people with learning disability but there is some evidence to suggest reluctance on behalf of the authorities to designate sudden death as suicide in an individual with learning disability. Carter and Jancar[71] reported, in a study of sudden deaths in people with learning disability in institutional care, that five patients with a diagnosis of affective disorder died suddenly but only one of the five was labelled a suicide, although all the deaths occurred after patients had gone missing from hospital and as the result of trauma.

Suicidal behaviours including threats of suicide and self-injurious behaviour with suicidal intent have been described in several studies.

Sternlicht *et al.*[72] studied a cohort of subjects in institutional care in the 1960s and reported an attempted suicide rate of 0.9% compared with 1% for the general population at that time. However, in the general population group, women were more likely to attempt suicide than men, whereas the converse was true for the learning disability group. The majority of the learning disability group who attempted suicide were in the mild and borderline range of IQ but, unfortunately, no attempt was made to formulate a psychiatric diagnosis for those who attempted suicide.

Stocks and Scott,[73] in a study of individuals who frequently harmed themselves, reported on 42 patients who had been admitted three times in one week to the Regional Poison Treatment Centre in Edinburgh, UK, for the treatment of deliberate self-harm. Five of these 42 patients were said to have had mild learning disability which would suggest a considerable over-representation of people with mild learning disability in the repeated self-harm group. In another community study of people with learning disability, Benson and Laman[74] compared 22 suicidal referrals to an outpatient clinic for individuals with combined learning disability and additional mental health problems with 22 nonsuicidal referrals. It was concluded that the suicidal group were younger, more likely to be of borderline mental handicap and to have chronic health problems or physical disability. With increasing numbers of individuals with learning disabilities living in relatively isolated situations in the community, threats of suicide and suicidal behaviour may become a more frequent management problem.

Individuals with severe and profound learning disabilities had not been thought capable of experiencing suicidal intent. However, Walters[75] described four individuals with severe learning disability who displayed behaviour which was considered to indicate a deliberate attempt to endanger their lives. It is obviously difficult to judge intent when self-injurious behaviour is a relatively common phenomenon in individuals with severe and profound learning disability but it is possible that such behaviour is sometimes related to suicidal intent in the presence of a depressive illness, as suggested by Sovner *et al.* in a study of antidepressant medication.[57]

It is likely that both suicide and suicidal intent in relation to deliberate self-harm have been underestimated in populations with learning disability. This is of particular importance both in the management of people with mild and borderline levels of learning disability living in the community in isolated situations and individuals with severe to profound learning disability displaying self-injurious behaviour.

Conclusion

Affective disorder is almost certainly underdiagnosed and undertreated in individuals with learning disability. Diagnosis is relatively straightforward using standard diagnostic criteria, with careful assessment of information from the individual and their carers and observations of behaviour. There is a lack of good data on the prevalence of affective disorder in individuals with learning disability compared with the general population and a need for well-conducted epidemiological studies using well-designed diagnostic interviews.

Treatment of affective disorder in learning disability requires knowledge of standard psychiatric approaches and there is a dearth of properly conducted treatment trials in this group of subjects. Psychotherapeutic approaches are relatively underdeveloped and there is a need for the development of modified forms of treatment programmes based on behavioural and cognitive approaches used in general psychiatry to be applied to individuals with learning disability. Skills training and social support are probably of particular relevance in the management of affective disorders in individuals with learning disability.

There are considerable implications for service development in that people with learning disability living in a variety of settings need access to appropriate community and inpatient services for assessment and treatment of affective disorders. Staff in all residential settings will require training to increase their awareness of mental health problems in general and affective disorders in particular. Community learning disability services will need appropriate expertise in psychiatry, psychology and nursing to carry out assessments and prepare management programmes.

The most important issue is probably that of raising awareness of a possibility of affective disorder in relation to behavioural change in learning disability as, on the whole, affective disorder is an eminently treatable condition.

References

1. Reiss S, Levitan GW & Szyszko J (1982) Emotional disturbance and mental retardation: diagnostic overshadowing. *American Journal of Mental Deficiency* **86**, 567–74.
2. Winokur B (1974) Subnormality and its relation to psychiatry. *Lancet* **ii**, 270–3.
3. Reid AH (1972) Psychoses in adult mental defectives: 1. Manic depressive psychosis. *British Journal of Psychiatry* **120**, 205–12.
4. Lund J (1985) The prevalence of psychiatric morbidity in mentally retarded adults. *Acta Psychiatrica Scandinavica* **72**, 562–70.
5. Jacobson JW (1990) Do some mental disorders occur less frequently among persons with mental retardation? *American Journal of Mental Retardation* **94**, 596–602.
6. Wright EC (1982) The presentation of mental illness in mentally retarded adults. *British Journal of Psychiatry* **141**, 496–502.
7. Day K (1985) Psychiatric disorder in the middle-aged and elderly mentally handicapped. *British Journal of Psychiatry* **147**, 660–7.
8. Sansom DT, Singh I, Jawed SH & Mukharjee T (1994) Elderly people with learning disabilities in hospital: a psychiatric study. *Journal of Intellectual Disability and Research* **38**, 45–52.
9. Zigler E & Burack JA (1989) Personality development and the dually diagnosed person. *Research in Developmental Disabilities* **10**, 225–40.
10. Patel P, Goldberg D & Moss S (1993) Psychiatric morbidity in older people with moderate and severe learning disability II: The prevalence study. *British Journal of Psychiatry* **163**, 481–91.
11. Moss S, Patel P, Prosser H *et al.* (1993) Psychiatric morbidity in older people with moderate and severe learning disability I: Development and reliability of the patient interview (PAS-ADD). *British Journal of Psychiatry* **163**, 471–80.

12. Lindsay WR, Michie AM, Baty FJ *et al.* (1994) The consistency of reports about feelings and emotions from people with intellectual disability. *Journal of Intellectual Disability Research* **38**, 61–6.
13. Meins W (1995) Symptoms of major depression in mentally retarded adults. *Journal of Intellectual Disability Research* **39**, 41–5.
14. Helsel WJ & Matson JL (1988) The relationship of depression to social skills and intellectual functioning in mentally retarded adults. *Journal of Mental Deficiency Research* **32**, 411–8.
15. Warren AC, Holroyd S & Folstein MF (1989) Major depression in Down's syndrome. *British Journal of Psychiatry* **155**, 202–5.
16. Harper DC & Wadsworth JS (1990) Dementia and depression in elders with mental retardation: A pilot study. *Research in Developmental Disabilities* **11**, 177–98.
17. Burt DB, Loveland KA & Lewis KR (1992) Depression and the onset of dementia in adults with mental retardation. *American Journal of Mental Retardation* **96**, 502–11.
18. Reid AH & Naylor GJ (1976) Short-cycle manic depressive psychosis in mental defectives: a clinical and physiological study. *Journal of Mental Deficiency Research* **20**, 67–76.
19. Lowry MA & Sovner R (1992) Severe behaviour problems associated with rapid cycling bipolar disorder in two adults with profound mental retardation. *Journal of Intellectual Disability Research* **36**, 269–81.
20. Glue P (1989) Rapid cycling affective disorders in the mentally retarded. *Biological Psychiatry* **26**, 250–6.
21. King BH, De Antonio C & James BA *et al.* (1994) Psychiatric consultation in severe and profound mental retardation. *American Journal of Psychiatry* **151**, 1802–8.
22. Kurita H & Nakayasu N (1994) Brief report: an autistic male presenting seasonal affective disorder (SAD) and trichotillomania. *Journal of Autism and Developmental Disorders* **24**, 687–91.
23. Lainhart JE & Folstein SE (1994) Affective disorders in people with autism: a review of published cases. *Journal of Autism and Developmental Disorders* **24**, 587–601.
24. Smalley SL, McCracken J & Tanguay P (1995) Autism, affective disorders and social phobia. *American Journal of Medical Genetics (Neuropsychiatric Genetics)* **60**, 19–26.
25. Reiss S & Rojahn J (1993) Joint occurrence of depression and aggression in children and adults with mental retardation. *Journal of Intellectual Disability Research* **37**, 287–94.
26. Benson BA & Ivins J (1992) Anger, depression and self-concept in adults with mental retardation. *Journal of Intellectual Disability Research* **36**, 169–75.
27. Lewis MH, Silva JR & Silva SG (1994) Cyclicity of aggression and self-injurious behavior in individuals with mental retardation. *American Journal of Mental Retardation* **99**, 436–44.
28. Zung WK (1965) A self-rating depression scale. *Archives of General Psychiatry* **12**, 63–70.
29. Lindsay WR & Michie AM (1988) Adaptation of the Zung self-rating anxiety scale for people with a mental handicap. *Journal of Mental Deficiency Research* **32**, 485–90.
30. Beck AT, Ward CH & Mendelson M *et al.* (1961) An inventory for measuring depression. *Archives of General Psychiatry* **4**, 561–71.
31. Kazdin AE, Matson JL & Senatore V (1983) Assessment of depression in mentally retarded adults. *American Journal of Psychiatry* **140**, 1040–3.
32. Meins W (1993) Assessment of depression in mentally retarded adults: reliability and validity of the Children's Depression Inventory (CDI). *Research in Developmental Disabilities* **14**, 299–312.
33. Benavidez DA & Matson JL (1993) Assessment of depression in mentally retarded adolescents. *Research in Developmental Disabilities* **14**, 179–88.
34. Kovacs M (1985) The Children's Depression Inventory (CDI). *Psychopharmacology Bulletin* **21**, 995–8.
35. Rojahn J, Warren VJ & Ohringer S (1994) A comparison of assessment methods for depression in mental retardation. *Journal of Autism and Developmental Disorders* **24**, 305–13.
36. Sturmey P, Reed J & Corbett J (1991) Psychometric assessment of psychiatric disorders in people with learning difficulties (mental handicap): a review of measures. *Psychological Medicine* **21**, 143–55.
37. Ballinger BR, Ballinger CB, Reid AH & McQueen E (1991) The psychiatric symptoms, diagnoses and care needs of 100 mentally handicapped patients. *British Journal of Psychiatry* **158**, 251–4.
38. Ballinger BR, Armstrong J, Presly AS & Reid AH (1975) Use of a standardized psychiatric interview in mentally handicapped patients. *British Journal of Psychiatry* **127**, 540–4.

39. Gask L (1988) *The Psychiatric Assessment Schedule (PAS) (revised)*. Manchester: Department of Psychiatry, Manchester University.
40. Clark DJ, Cumella S & Corbett J *et al.* (1994) Use of ICD-10 research diagnostic criteria to categorise psychiatric and behavioural abnormalities among people with learning disabilities: the West Midlands field trial. *Mental Handicap Research* **7**, 273–85.
41. Carroll BJ (1982) The dexamethasone suppression test for melancholia. *British Journal of Psychiatry* **140**, 292–304.
42. Sireling L (1986) Depression in mentally handicapped patients: Diagnostic and neuro-endocrine evaluation. *British Journal of Psychiatry* **149**, 274–8.
43. Soni S, Keane V & Soni SD (1992) Dexamethasone suppression test and response to anti-depressants in depressed mentally handicapped subjects. *Journal of Intellectual Disability Research* **36**, 425–33.
44. Berger M, Pirke K-M & Doerr P *et al.* (1984) The limited utility of the dexamethasone suppression test for the diagnostic process in psychiatry. *British Journal of Psychiatry* **145**, 372–82.
45. McGuffin P, Owen MJ & O'Donovan MC *et al.* (1994) *Seminars in Psychiatric Genetics*, pp. 110–27. London: Gaskell.
46. Rutter M (1971) Psychiatry. In Wortis J (ed) *Mental Retardation: An Annual Review*, Vol 3, pp. 186–221. New York: Grune & Stratton.
47. Lund J (1985) Epilepsy and psychiatric disorder in the mentally retarded adult. *Acta Psychiatrica Scandinavica* **72**, 557–62.
48. Cornelius JR, Fabrega H & Mezzich J *et al.* (1993) Characterising organic mood syndrome, depressed type. *Comprehensive Psychiatry* **34**, 432–40.
49. Mendez MF, Taylor JL, Doss RC & Salguero P (1994) Depression in secondary epilepsy: relation to lesion laterality. *Journal of Neurology, Neurosurgery and Psychiatry* **57**, 232–3.
50. Lewinsohn PM (1974) A behavioural approach to depression. In Friedman RJ and Katz MM (eds) *The Psychology of Depression: Contemporary Theory and Research*, pp. 157–85. New York: Wiley.
51. Seligman MEP (1981) A learned helplessness point of view. In Rehm LP (ed) *Behaviour Therapy for Depression: Present Status and Future Directions*, pp. 123–42. New York: Academic Press.
52. Brown GW & Harris TO (1978) *Social Origins of Depression*. London: Tavistock.
53. Harper DC & Wadsworth JS (1993) Grief in adults with mental retardation: preliminary findings. *Research in Developmental Disabilities* **14**, 313–30.
54. Matson JL & Sevin JA (1994) Theories of dual diagnosis in mental retardation. *Journal of Consulting and Clinical Psychology* **62**, 6–16.
55. Bregman JD (1995) Psychopharmacologic treatment of neuropsychiatric conditions in mental retardation. *Child and Adolescent Psychiatric Clinics of North America* **4**, 401–33.
56. Deb S & Fraser W (1994) The use of psychotropic medication in people with learning disability: towards rational prescribing. *Human Psychopharmacology* **9**, 259–72.
57. Sovner R, Fox CJ, Lowry MJ & Lowry MA (1993) Fluoxetine treatment of depression and associated self-injury in two adults with mental retardation. *Journal of Intellectual Disability Research* **37**, 301–11.
58. Langee HR & Conlon M (1992) Predictors of response to antidepressant medications. *American Journal of Mental Retardation* **97**, 65–70.
59. Kearns A (1987) Cotard's syndrome in a mentally handicapped man. *British Journal of Psychiatry* **150**, 112–4.
60. Merrill RD (1984) ECT for a patient with profound mental retardation. *American Journal of Psychiatry* **147**, 256–7.
61. Benbow SM (1995) Safe ECT practice in physically ill patients. In Freeman CP (ed) *The ECT Handbook. The Second Report of the Royal College of Psychiatrists Special Committee on ECT*, pp. 26–9. London: Royal College of Psychiatrists.
62. McClelland R (1995) ECT in learning disability psychiatry. In Freeman CP (ed) *The ECT Handbook. The Second Report of the Royal College of Psychiatrists Special Committee on ECT*, pp. 24–5. London: Royal College of Psychiatrists.
63. Bebchuk JM, Barnhill J & Dawkins K (1996) ECT and mental retardation. *American Journal of Psychiatry* **153**, 1231.
64. Naylor GJ, Donald JM, Le Poidevin D & Reid AH (1974) A double-blind trial of the use of long-term lithium therapy in mental defectives. *British Journal of Psychiatry* **124**, 52–7.
65. Roy-Byrne PP, Joffe RT, Uhde TW & Post RM (1984) Approaches to the evaluation and treatment of rapid cycling affective illness. *British Journal of Psychiatry* **145**, 543–50.

66. Kastner T, Finesmith R & Walsh K (1993) Long-term administration of valproic acid in the treatment of affective symptoms in people with mental retardation. *Journal of Clinical Psychopharmacology* **13**, 448–51.
67. Lund J (1986) Treatment of psychiatric morbidity in the mentally retarded adult. *Acta Psychiatrica Scandinavica* **73**, 429–36.
68. Reiss S, Levitan GW & McNally RJ (1982) Emotionally disturbed mentally retarded people. An undeserved population. *American Psychologist* **37**, 361–7.
69. Bicknell J (1994) Psychological process: the inner world of people with mental retardation. In Bouras N (ed) *Mental Health in Mental Retardation. Recent Advances and Practices*, pp. 46–56. Cambridge: Cambridge University Press.
70. Lindsay WR, Baty FJ, Michie AM & Richardson J (1989) A comparison of anxiety treatments with adults who have moderate and severe mental retardation. *Research in Developmental Disabilities* **10**, 129–40.
71. Carter G & Jancar J (1984) Sudden deaths in the mentally handicapped. *Psychological Medicine* **14**, 691–5.
72. Sternlicht M, Pustel G & Deutsch MR (1970) Suicidal tendencies among institutionalised retardates. *British Journal of Mental Subnormality* **16**, 93–102.
73. Stocks R & Scott AIF (1991) What happens to patients who frequently harm themselves? A retrospective one-year outcome study. *British Journal of Psychiatry* **158**, 375–8.
74. Benson BA & Laman DS (1988) Suicidal tendencies of mentally retarded adults in community settings. *Australia and New Zealand Journal of Developmental Disabilities* **14**, 49–54.
75. Walters RM (1990) Suicidal behaviour in severely mentally handicapped patients. *British Journal of Psychiatry* **157**, 444–6.

10

Ageing and Learning Disability

Jane M. McCarthy

Introduction

The last 15 years has seen a major growth of interest in individuals with a learning disability (LD) who are ageing.[1-3] This is due in part to the increase in life expectancy of people with an LD.[4] In 1929, the life expectancy for a person with Down's syndrome was 9 years compared with over 50 years in 1980.[4] Predictors of greater life expectancy among people with LD are being female, ambulant, not having a diagnosis of Down's syndrome, having a mild LD and living in the community.[5]

For the practising clinician this means a number of issues are presenting for the first time. Specific areas of concern include the diagnosis and care of people with Alzheimer's dementia, the development of services for an ageing population and the natural history of psychiatric disorder in this group. However, clinical problems must be understood in the context of early life experiences and developmental factors for the ageing group.

Studies have focused on demographic factors, mental and physical health and service use. The definition of old age in studies has been from as low as 45 years of age to that of 60–65 years, as in the general population. The variation in age definition has depended on whether the focus is on age-related fragility or on accelerated ageing as is the case in individuals with Down's syndrome. This chapter provides a view of current knowledge and includes a discussion of diagnostic and treatment issues.

Demographic Information

There are a number of elderly people with LD residing in the institutions who have lived there for many years. Table 10.1 shows that the proportion of elderly people in the large mental handicap hospitals is increasing.[6] This is a reflection of the resettlement of the younger age groups into the community, leaving a more elderly group residing in the institutions.

The majority of older people are in contact with specialist LD services. This was shown by an epidemiological study in the urban district of Oldham, UK,[7] to define the entire population with LD over the age of 50 years living or originating from the district. The total population is about 220 000 and 122 individuals were identified; 91 (75.4%) were known to the

Table 10.1.   Elderly people with learning disability in hospital care.

Study	Age (years)	Percentage of hospital population by year	
		1970	1979
DHSS (1984)[77]	Over 65	9.9 ($n = 5513$)	13.9 ($n = 6316$)
	55–64	14.2 ($n = 7908$)	14.4 ($n = 6543$)
		(total hospital population = 55 690)	(total hospital population = 45 437)
		1969	1985
Kiernan & Moss (1990)[11]	Over 60	13.8 ($n = 415$)	34.1 ($n = 335$)
		(total hospital population = 3008)	(total hospital population = 981)

Community Mental Handicap Team and 31 (25.4%) were located through an outreach procedure of contacting various services. The age banding of the whole group was roughly equivalent to that of the general population but the proportion over the age of 70 years was greater in the latter. This reflects the higher mortality in people with an LD than in the general population. There was an overall preponderance of men: they made up 56.6% of the group. The mean age for women was 65.2 years compared with 62.1 years for men. As with the general population, the greater longevity of women is reflected in the proportion reaching advanced age; of the seven individuals who were over 80 years, six of these were women.

Functional Abilities

Historically, less disabled people were admitted to long-stay institutions and thus older cohorts of current residents may be more able. However, in an epidemiological study, individuals residing in hospital were found to have significantly lower adaptive skills scores than people living in the community. This may reflect the variation in opportunities to learn skills in different living settings.[7]

In two hospital-based studies[8,9] two-thirds and two-fifths of the elderly residents were found to be functioning in the mild to moderate handicap range, the remainder being in the profound to severe group. One study showed the great majority of the individuals could feed and wash themselves but only 13% could dress themselves without help. Just under half could do domestic work without supervision. Over two-thirds were able to communicate by speech and one-third were able to talk about their own personal experiences; 6.7% could read and 3.3% could write a short letter. The conclusion was that one-third of the group could, with preparation, be resettled into the community.[9]

Evidence from the data of 3000 people on the Wessex Mental Handicap case register[10] showed that the proportion of individuals competent in self-care skills significantly increased through the age bands from early adulthood to 70 years of age. Thereafter, there was a slight decline. The consequence of differential mortality that is the more disabled group dying in early to middle age leaving a group of able and healthy individuals surviving to old age, appears to reach its main effect by the age of 60–70 years.

Behaviour Disorders

Within the elderly LD group there is a greater prevalence of behaviour disorders compared with the general population. However, behavioural problems in this group decrease with age. Kiernan and Moss[11] undertook a cross-sectional study in 1985 of 981 people living in a large mental hospital in north-west England, half of whom were over 50 years of age. They found that behaviour disorders appeared to decline in the older age group. The authors felt that the most likely explanation for this observation is partly physiological changes and partly the fact that people gain control of their behaviour as they become older.

Day[12] compared 357 long-stay hospital residents aged 40 years and over with a retrospective survey of 215 new admissions aged 40 years and over to a psychiatric unit for the learning disabled. Behaviour disorder was the largest single diagnostic category for both groups: 50.5% for the long-stay residents and 35.7% for the admission group. Most of the cases of behaviour disorders identified proved to be long-standing and persistent.

In the Oldham community study of individuals aged 50 years and over[7] it was found that a number of individuals continued to shown serious self-injurious and aggressive behaviour. However, most showed evidence of withdrawal and so the relationship between psychological well-being and ageing requires further study.

An added problem is that those who have spent most of their lives in long-stay institutions have behavioural problems that, although appropriate in order to gain attention on unstaffed wards, are clearly maladaptive in an old people's home or the local supermarket. A group of elderly people with LD who originated from the City of Westminster in 1984 was compared with the same group in 1994. There had been significant changes in the nature of the residential provision from hospital to 'community care' with a significant increase in the proportion reported to have behaviour problems.[13] There is a small number with persistent behaviour problems who will continue to require a high level of specialist input.

Psychiatric Morbidity

Mental health is an important factor in the ability of older people in the general population to live in the community.[14] Psychiatric illness in the elderly with an LD has been little examined. Depression in the general elderly population is associated with high risk of chronicity and relapse but little is known of the natural history disorders in this population. Studies have been largely restricted to hospital populations, and standardized diagnostic instruments have rarely been used.[15] There is a problem in making comparisons with studies because different population groups and difficult diagnostic criteria have been used. For instance, Lund[16] used modified DSM-III and Feighner's criteria, Corbett[17] used ICD-8 criteria and Day[12] used diagnoses from case notes to obtain an ICD-9 diagnosis.

Corbett[17] and Day[12] suggest that the prevalence of functional psychiatric illness falls with increasing age. However the Danish epidemiological study of 302 adults, of whom 94 were aged 45 and over, found that the rate did not differ from that found in the younger age groups.[16] The onset of dementia offsets the reduction in behaviour disorders.

Moss and colleagues in Manchester have developed a semistructured clinical psychiatric interview, the Psychiatric Assessment Schedule for Adults with Developmental Disability (PAS-ADD), for use with learning disabled people.[18] The PAS-ADD is designed for use by experienced clinicians and is based on items drawn from the Present State Examination.[19] The instrument can be used with a broad range of levels of handicaps and is designed to maximize the proportion of valid responses in this population group. The current version will give an ICD-10 diagnosis.

The PAS-ADD was used to detect the prevalence of psychiatric morbidity of people aged 50 years and over with moderate and severe LD living in Oldham, UK.[20] A total of 110 people was identified and 105 agreed to participate. Using the PAS-ADD, 22 individuals (21%) received a standardized psychiatric diagnosis of functional illness or dementia. There were 12 functional psychiatric cases and 12 dementia cases; two individuals received both diagnoses. This is in agreement with the findings of Lund[16] in a subgroup aged 45 years and over in which the overall prevalence of mental disorder, excluding behaviour disorders, was 25%. The prevalence of affective disorder was 4.8%, compared with the rate of 6% found by Lund.[16] Depression arising after the age of 60 is frequently associated with loss or threat of loss of close friends and chronic physical illness.[21]

Only three of the 12 PAS-ADD detected cases (25%) were receiving treatment for a psychiatric disorder. Therefore the majority were not receiving the appropriate specialist health care because staff did not appreciate the significance of the presenting symptoms. This was particularly true for anxiety disorders.

Table 10.2 provides a summary of the main studies.[6]

Dementia

Epidemiology

The question of vulnerability to dementia is particularly important as people with LD age. The link between Down's syndrome and the premature development of dementia of the Alzheimer type is well established.[22,23] There have been few studies on dementia in elderly people with an LD of an aetiology other than Down's syndrome.

Table 10.2. Prevalence of psychiatric disorder.

Study	Population	Age (years)	Functional illness (%)	Organic illness (%)
Corbett (1979)[17] n = 110	Hospital resident/ receiving services	> 60	37.1	
Day (1985)[12] n = 357	Long-stay inpatients	> 40	27.7	2.8
n = 40	Acute admissions over 7 years	> 40	90.2	9.5
n = 115	Long-stay inpatients	> 65		6
Day (1987)[8] n = 99	Hospital inpatients	>65	14	6
Lund (1985)[16] n = 94	National register	> 45	11	14
Patel et al. (1993)[20] n = 105	Total district population	>50	11.4	11.4

Day[12] found a prevalence for senile dementia of 6%, i.e. seven cases from a population of 115 long-stay hospital residents aged 65 and over. This figure is similar to the findings of Kay,[24] Parsons[25] and Livingston et al.[26] who reported prevalence rates of 5.6%, 4.4% and 6.1%, respectively, in epidemiological studies of the general population aged 65 years and over. However, the prevalence rate for dementia in people with an LD in the epidemiological studies of Lund[16] and Patel[20] is higher, 14.4% and 11.4%, respectively. Dementia was the most prevalent mental disorder in these studies, although a relatively younger group (see Table 10.2) was used compared with the studies of the general population. In the Oldham study[20] four (44%) out of the nine individuals with Down's syndrome (DS) had dementia, reflecting the greater risk for this group.

Natural History

The natural history of dementia in people with Down's syndrome is similar to that of the general population with similar symptoms of cognitive and behavioural decline.[27] One of the main difficulties is the recognition of the early stages of the disorder. In the moderate LD group the early symptoms are of apathy, withdrawal, daytime sleepiness and loss of self-help skills. In those with severe LD, gait deterioration, myoclonus and seizures are common early findings.

In adults with intellectual disability of other aetiologies, the natural history of dementia is similar in prevalence, age of onset and progression, to that in the general population. However, there is a high co-morbidity of depression, mobility problems and sensory impairments.[28]

Dementia and Down's Syndrome

Down's syndrome

Downs syndrome is the most common cause of severe mental retardation accounting for perhaps 30% of all those affected. The live birth prevalence is 1 in 660. The extra chromosome 21 was first identified by Lejeune and colleagues in 1959.[29] About 95% of cases are due to the inheritance of the extra chromosome following nondisjunction during meiotic cell division. The nondisjunction is of maternal origin and the risk increases with maternal age. The remainder are due to unbalanced chromosome translocations which may be inherited. Mosaicism is another cause of the phenotype in which there are two populations of cells, only one of which will have a trisomy.

Despite current screening policies that are based on maternal age, the number of Down's syndrome infants that will be born in England and Wales to the year 2000 will rise to a level higher than has been seen for 20 years. With consistently increased survival, this will mean that throughout the next century the population prevalence of Down's syndrome will be higher than ever before.[30]

The physical phenotypic manifestations of Down's syndrome are well known and include abnormalities of skull, eyes, tongue and hand. None are pathognomonic. Intellectual impairment is always present, except for some individuals who have the mosaic type. In addition, the extra chromosome has a major impact on the physical health of an individual with Down's syndrome. There is an increased occurrence of congenital cardiac abnormalities, gastrointestinal anomalies, cervical spine instability, respiratory disorders and leukaemia. Physical conditions that are more common in adulthood include cataracts, hearing loss, mitral valve prolapse and hypothyroidism. One-fifth of adults with Down's syndrome screened in a hospital population suffered from some degree of hypothyroidism and most were aged over 40 years.[31] There is a strong case for the routine annual screening for thyroid disease of all Down's syndrome patients over the age of 40 and others advocate screening should start earlier from the age of 30 years.

The impact on families has been influenced by changes in services, particularly educational provision, but families have also changed. The typical 'older' mother of a Down's syndrome child in the 1960s was already the mother of several children and at the end of her child-bearing career. In contrast the typical 'older' mother of recent times is a well-educated woman who has put off child-bearing until a career and home have been established. The impression from studies is that families are coping despite considerable restrictions on daily life.[32]

The rate of psychiatric and behavioural disorders in children with Down's syndrome is 40% compared with 50% for a matched group of children with LD of other aetiologies. Conduct disorder is the most common diagnosis in the Down's syndrome group.[33] Behaviour problems occur more frequently in families where parents have problems in their relationship or with their mental health.

The vulnerability of adults with Down's syndrome to psychiatric disorder is relatively unknown. One study has shown that Down's syndrome patients are more likely to be given a diagnosis of depression and dementia compared with patients with LD of other aetiologies who are more likely to be given a diagnosis of personality disorder or schizophrenia.[34] The short-term prognosis for depression in adults with Down's syndrome appears to be poor but possibly better the earlier the age of onset.[35] The mean age of onset is 28 years for females. The symptoms, which are persistent despite treatment, include psychomotor retardation, impaired concentration and loss of confidence. Others have found a poorer outcome, as measured by adaptive skills, for those with a younger age of onset.[36] One area of psychiatric disorder that has received the greatest attention in the past 10 years has been the relationship between dementia of Alzheimer's type and Down's syndrome.[22,37] In the clinic setting the presentation of dementia and depression can be similar. Significant clinical skill is required to reach the correct diagnosis, particularly if the depression partly responds to treatment or becomes persistent. Time is the great aid to diagnosis, with dementia showing a progressive decline whereas there will be evidence of improvement in a depressive illness.

Alzheimer's Disease
An association between Down's syndrome and dementia was made over 100 years ago[38] and later by Jervis in 1948.[39] Neuropathological and neurochemical defects have been found in the brains at post-mortem of all individuals with DS, aged 40 years and over, which are virtually indistinguishable from those found in the brains of Alzheimer's patients.[40] Positron emission tomography (PET) and quantitative assisted tomography of older demented Down's syndrome subjects showed patterns of abnormality identical to those described previously in patients with Alzheimer's type dementia.[41] However, the link between clinical presentation and changes observed in the brain is still not clear.[22] The clinical expression of dementia occurs 10–20 years after the occurrence of the first lesion with an average age of onset of 54 years.[42] Between 15% and 30% of people with Down's syndrome develop Alzheimer's type dementia.[43]

The early subtle changes of dementia such as simple memory difficulties are often missed being masked by poor language skills.[37] Studies of age-related cognitive deficits show that a proportion of individuals deteriorate in later life and this has been confirmed by a number of studies.[44,45] Others have found no indication of any generalized decline in performance and that mental development has been shown to continue into the third and fourth decades of life.[46] However, the delineation between 'normal' ageing in adults with Down's syndrome and changes in Alzheimer's disease requires further study.

The explanation for the strong association is apportioned to a genetic link. Amyloid is part of the neuritic plaques seen in Alzheimer's disease. The gene for amyloid precursor protein (APP) containing amyloid β-protein is on chromosome 21 and it seems abnormalities in APP metabolism are a key event; duplication of the gene occurs in the chromosomal abnormality trisomy 21. β-Amyloidosis initiates the cascade of pathological changes leading to dementia associated with Alzheimer's disease. The underlying mechanism responsible for this is unknown. The presence of the typical neuropathology does not lead to disease. One hypothesis is that there is a threshold effect. Individuals with Down's syndrome may have a higher threshold for dementia, as measured by plaque and neurofibrillary tangle counts, and when a certain threshold is crossed clinical dementia presents.[22,40]

A second hypothesis is that individuals with Down's syndrome show premature ageing, as indicated by earlier hair loss, deterioration of skin, cataract formation and premature menopause. The increased vulnerability to Alzheimer's disease is viewed as a result of premature ageing rather than a disorder resulting from a specific abnormality of the affected neurones.

Diagnosis

One of the greatest challenges for the clinician is determining the diagnosis of cognitive decline in an individual with a pre-existing intellectual impairment. Practice guidelines on the identification and assessment of adults with mental retardation who develop dementia has been produced by an international committee.[47] Criteria and features are listed to aid diagnosis of possible or probable dementia. The guidelines also provide guidance on care management and the education of carers. It is important to remember that conditions other than dementia cause cognitive decline in individuals with LD.

Adults with LD who are at risk of Alzheimer's disease include those over the age of 50, those with Down's syndrome over the age of 40, or those with a positive family history. Regular screening of these groups may identify changes that may be indicative of pathological ageing, for example changes in behaviour, decline in adaptive skills, onset of seizures. A baseline screening should include a measure of adaptive skills using for example AAMD Adaptive Behaviour Scale Part One[48] and a neuropsychological measure of memory functioning. Screening instruments for dementia in this population are still in the early stages of being fully validated in a clinic setting[49] and tools used widely in the general population such as the Mini Mental State[50,51] have limited use with those who have a mild to borderline LD. In addition, other disorders must be tested for such as thyroid disease, hearing or visual loss. Repeated evaluations over time following the baseline measurement will increase the confidence of the diagnosis.

A full diagnostic assessment should include detailed medical and psychiatric history, physical examination and mental state examination. Evenhius[49] has modified DSM-III-R criteria for the diagnosis of dementia in this population:

(1) Demonstrable evidence of decline of original level of short- and long-term memory (observed in daily circumstances).

(2) At least one of the following (observed in daily circumstances):
    (a) disturbance of original level of spatial and temporal orientation;
    (b) aphasia (language disturbance);
    (c) apraxia (impaired ability to carry out motor activities);
    (d) personality change.
(3) The disturbances in (1) and (2) significantly interfere with work or usual social activities or relationships with others.
(4) Not occurring exclusively during the course of a delirium.

Neuropsychological assessment should involve formal cognitive testing using, for example, the Rivermead Behavioural Memory Test.[52] Laboratory tests would include thyroid function test and serum B_{12} level. An electroencephalogram (EEG) is indicated if there is a suggestion of epilepsy or abnormal brain activity. Neuroimaging (magnetic resonance imaging (MRI) or neurocomputed tomography (CT) scan) is a useful aid to diagnosis and is necessary to exclude a potentially treatable brain disorder such as a chronic subdural haematoma. A number of abnormalities of the central nervous system (CNS) in Down's syndrome have been noted during neuroimaging, including reduced brain volume, small cerebellum and basal ganglia calcification. Only cerebral atrophy and ventricular dilatation are associated with the clinical syndrome of dementia.[53] Therefore, the use of CT scanning is particularly useful in people with severe LD when neuropsychology testing is limited. Although there is nothing in the literature on the specific use of neuroimaging in the elderly group without Down's syndrome, if there is evidence of a progressive cognitive decline then further investigation is indicated. A chest X-ray and an electrocardiogram (ECG) may be required if a respiratory or vascular disorder is suspected. A full review of medication should be part of the assessment and, finally, testing of hearing and vision should be arranged. Infirmities of old age such as sensory deficits are more common in people with Down's syndrome than other individuals with LD.[54]

Management

Medical management includes the treatment of seizures, depression and behaviour disorders. Over four-fifths of individuals with Down's syndrome and dementia develop generalized tonic–clonic seizures.[42] The medication of choice would be sodium valproate starting at 300 mg and slowly increasing to a therapeutic dose, usually 1200–1600 mg. This can be given once a day in the long-acting form. Carbamazepine and lamotrogine are second-line treatments. Coexistent depression and dementia frequently occur in the general elderly population.[55] The relationship between depression and dementia in those with an LD requires further clarification. However, it has been suggested that there is a link between depression and dementia in adults with Down's syndrome.[56] It is not known whether the presence of dementia increases vulnerability to depression as in non-LD older individuals or if Down's syndrome is a risk factor for depression.

Care management would focus on the provision of support and advice to carers in the home, day and residential setting. The essential aim is for the person to stay in their own home and for support to be provided until a change of residence is necessary. The care plan requires modification over time to address diminishing self-care, communication and cognitive skills. As the individual becomes more confused and shows behavioural problems greater consideration will need to be given to environment changes. Problems giving the greatest cause for concern to carers are restlessness, loss of communication skills, urinary incontinence and wandering.[57] Later, good nursing care is essential for poor mobility, feeding difficulties, incontinence and bedsores. In addition, preparing carers and families for the demands of terminal care and legal considerations will need to be addressed.

Physical Health

There are few studies on the physical health of elderly people with an LD but this is also true for the nonhandicapped population.[1] Studies have tended to rely on analysis of existing records or mental handicap register information gathered by nonmedically qualified staff.[5,58] Studies suggest that this group develops the same age-related problems, for example sensory impairment, as the general population. Information from mental handicap registers in California, Massachusetts and New York showed that the major increases seen with increasing age are in hearing impairment, vision impairment and loss of mobility.[5]

A study was carried out on the functional abilities of approximately 300 people on the Wessex Mental Handicap Register[10] from early adulthood to 70 years of age. The prevalence of epilepsy showed a reduction from the younger to the older age bands and chronic medical conditions rose from 45 years onwards. The relationship between age and incontinence was more complicated with a peak at 40 years followed by a decline, with a second peak at 80 years. Moderate mobility problems showed a large rise after the age of 70 years, while severe mobility problems show less of an age trend, with peaks at the upper and lower ends of the adult life span. The age trend for severe visual problems is similar to that for severe mobility. Moderate and severe hearing problems were found to rise steadily with age.

Mortality is the most frequently used health outcome indicator. Increased life expectancy has brought changes in mortality patterns. Deaths from age-related conditions have shown a progressive increase, while tuberculosis and status epilepsy, formerly common causes of death in institutionalized populations, have declined.[4] A cross-sectional study was undertaken in 21 mental deficiency institutions in two provinces of the Netherlands in the period 1986 to 1988.[59] A high mortality rate was found in the severely and profoundly disabled group until the age of 30 and was mainly determined by pre- and peri-natal birth defects. The healthiest residents were found in the 30–50-year age group. Comparing the Dutch general population with the severe learning disabled in institutions, it was found that the overall mortality of individuals with severe LD is substantially higher for all age groups until the age of 70 years when the mortality risks for the two groups approach.

Use of Medication

Aman,[60] in a review of psychotropic drug use in the elderly with an LD, concluded that the pattern of drug use in this population was unknown. However, a substantial amount is known about the age-related pharmacological changes in the elderly general population.[61] In the population with LD there appear to be different prescribing patterns for different age groups. Jacobson *et al.*[5] found that those with LD under 20 years of age and over 65 years of age received significantly fewer drugs than the remaining age groups.

Walters[62] looked at the prescribing patterns for 269 LD hospital residents aged over 60 years including 31 residents aged 50 years or over with Down's syndrome. Fifty of the 269 residents (19%) were receiving no medication but the mean number of prescriptions for the remaining 219 was four. Of the total sample of 269, just under one-third (32%) were taking drugs for mental disorders, 11% were taking antiseizure drugs and 63% were on long-term drug treatments for other problems. The author concluded that the frequency of multiple prescribing was higher than that reported in general practice studies,[63] but similar to that reported in studies of prescriptions in homes for the elderly.[64]

In the general elderly population, depression is often untreated although response to physical treatment is comparable with that of younger adults.[65] Newer antidepressants, such as the selective serotonin reuptake inhibitors (SSRIs), the atypical tricyclic antidepressants, e.g. lofepramine and the reversible monoamine oxidase inhibitors, may be of more value because of the relative safety and favourable side-effect profile. The principle in prescribing is to start at a low dose and increase slowly because the ageing brain is more sensitive to the effects of medication. Lithium augmentation for refractory depression in the general elderly population is encouraging and is effective as prophylaxis in depression. The elderly are more susceptible to lithium toxicity and plasma concentrations should probably be maintained at between 0.4 and 0.7 mg l^{-1} to avoid toxicity.

Thioridazine has less of a tendency than some phenothiazines to cause extrapyramidal or hepatotoxic complications and also has a sedative action. It is probably the most useful phenothiazine for the disturbed elderly population with an organic brain disorder. A single dose of 25–50 mg may be sufficient. A higher dose given TDS may be indicated for more persistent disturbance in a dementing process. For psychotic disorders a dose of 200–300 mg a day will be required. The relatively specific D2 receptor antagonist blocking drug sulpiride is effective in small doses. Depot neuroleptics have been of limited use in the elderly population.

Services

Elderly people with an LD usually have no spouse or children; sometimes they are cared for by very elderly parents. Compared with young people with an LD, the elderly are less likely to live with their family.[66] They live in more restrictive environments than do their younger counterparts, despite the greater competence of the older cohorts.[67] They are using a variety of service settings, and the type of opportunities available is determined by the philosophy of the service. Those in contact with specialist LD services tend to receive more service support than those in services for the general elderly population.[68] However, it is not clear which factors determine the most appropriate service for an individual.

In an American study, a group of 16 people with a mild LD (mean IQ 62) was followed up at intervals at 10 and 20 years after they had been moved from a large state hospital for mentally retarded individuals in 1960.[69] At the time of the most recent ethnographic study the individuals with a mean age of 61 years had lived 30 years in the community without receiving specialist support services. The author commented that 'despite advancing years, their independence, social competence, and zest for life had increased'. They were compared with their counterparts in the hospital setting. The latter group were less independent, 'less normalised' in dress, speech and recreational activities, and had less control over their lives.

Seltzer[70] undertook a telephone survey of staff to assess the service use of all people aged 55 and over with LD who received state-supported services provided by the ageing network in Massachusetts. The study looked at age-integrated (learning disability service providing for all ages), age-specialized (learning disability service for the elderly) and generic services (services for the general elderly population). The results showed that the elderly with an LD are growing in number and use an increasing number of services. The most prominent weakness of age-integrated services was that they did not provide age-appropriate activities. The activities were too pressurized and insufficiently sensitive to clients' health needs. There was an absence of a 'retirement option'. The generic ageing services offered age-appropriate programmes but these were not suitable for individuals with an LD because they were geared at too high a cognitive level or occurred in large groups. In particular, the lack of expertise in serving individuals with an LD was seen as a problem.

The greatest numbers of strengths were identified for the age-specialized services. Retirement options were more likely to be offered to clients and the services were more likely to have expertise in both ageing and learning disability. The respondents perceived that friendships flourished in this context, although individuals may be separated from their past friends and placements. However, some respondents feared that these services were less stimulating, offered fewer choices and had lower expectations than the age-integrated services.

A different approach may be required in rural, under-served geographical areas. The local development and cross-training of existing personnel in the ageing and LD service sectors are likely to have the best impact on the hard-to-reach older individual with an LD.[71]

Carers and Support Networks

The burden on carers of the general elderly population with psychiatric illness and dementia is well documented,[72] as is the burden of care on those, usually parents, who care for younger people with an LD.[73] However little is known about the carers of older adults with an LD. It is known that carers of this group are less dependent on formal support services than are the carers of younger children.[74]

Some of the older people with LD are cared for by their ageing parents and remaining family members who also may be frail with serious health problems. A study of the Birmingham LD register found that people living with single carers are older than those residing with dual carers. Over half the single carers were aged 60 and over and 14% were aged 80 years and older.[75] This has major implications for future residential care of this group.

The role of carers, relatives, friends and visitors in the lives of this group is largely unknown, although the limited evidence suggests they have small social networks. A study of 59 residents aged 65 and over living in a large mental handicap hospital found none had a living parent but two-thirds had a living sibling.[9] For the majority there was no interaction with someone who cared about them. Three-fifths had no contact with relatives and three-quarters did not have any visits from or visited any other people during their stay in hospital.

Conclusion

The picture is one of an increasing population who will have high health and social care needs. However, older people with an LD are more physically robust than the younger age groups because of the impact of differential mortality. They share with their non-LD peers the problems of ageing, namely the age-related infirmities of dementia, sensory impairment, urinary incontinence and poor mobility. They develop psychiatric disorders but because of the diagnostic problems, particularly with the defining of dementia, they remain unrecognized and untreated. Nothing is known of the relationship between psychiatric illness and social factors, e.g. life events, support networks for this population. Active involvement in leisure and social activities is one of the best predictors of 'successful' ageing along with good health and financial security.[76]

There is insufficient information to guide which service, old-age psychiatry or learning disability psychiatry, will match the needs of an individual with the additional handicap of dementia or mental illness. A number of elderly people with mild to borderline LD will be presenting to specialist health services for the first time. At the same time a rapid change is taking place in the nature of health and social care provided for individuals with permanent disability and requiring long-term care.

Although some of the jigsaw has been put in place by the increased research over the past 15 years, there are still many more pieces that need looking at before we have a fuller picture of this group. The key areas that need to be addressed in the future include the training of carers and professionals to improve their recognition of psychiatric illness and dementia, guidelines on what type and which service will best meet their health needs, how social care will be arranged in terms of leisure, day and residential provision, more information on social networks and finally how all of these link to the quality of life for this remarkably resilient group.

References

1. Hogg J, Moss S & Cooke D (1988) *Ageing and Mental Handicap*. London: Chapman and Hall.
2. Janicki MP & Wisniewski HM (1985) *Aging and Developmental Disabilities: Issues and Trends*. Baltimore: Paul Brookes.
3. Day K & Jancar J (1995) Mental and physical health and ageing in mental handicap: a review. *Journal of Intellectual Disability Research* **38**, 241–56.
4. Carter G & Jancar J (1983) Mortality in the mentally handicapped: a fifty year survey at Stoke Park Group of hospitals (1930-1980). *Journal of Mental Deficiency Research* **27**, 143–56.
5. Jacobson JW, Sutton MS & Janicki MP (1985) Demography and characteristics of aging and aged mentally retarded persons. In Janicki MP & Wisniewski HM (eds) *Aging and Developmental Disabilities: Issues and Trends*, pp. 115–41. Baltimore: Paul Brookes.
6. McCarthy JM & Mullan E (1997) The elderly with a learning disability (mental retardation) – an overview. *International Psychogeriatrics* (in press).
7. Moss SC, Hogg, J & Horne M (1992) Demographic characteristics of a population with moderate, severe and profound intellectual disability (mental handicap) over 50 years of age: Age structure, IQ, and adaptive skills. *Journal of Intellectual Disability Research* **36**, 387–401.
8. Day K (1987) The elderly mentally handicapped in hospital: a clinical study. *Journal of Mental Deficiency Research* **31**, 131–46.
9. Kearney GM, Krishnan VH & Londhe RL (1993) Characteristics of elderly people with a mental handicap living in a mental handicap hospital: A descriptive study. *British Journal of Developmental Disabilities* **76**, 31–50.
10. Moss SC (1991) Age and functional abilities of people with a mental handicap: evidence from the Wessex mental handicap register. *Journal of Mental Deficiency Research* **35**, 430–45.
11. Kiernan C & Moss SC (1990) Behaviour and other characteristics of a mental handicap hospital. *Mental Handicap Research* **3**, 3–20.
12. Day K (1985) Psychiatric disorder in the middle-aged and elderly mentally handicapped. *British Journal of Psychiatry* **147**, 660–7.
13. Rhode J, Farmer R & McCarthy J (1995) Elderly people with learning disability: a comparison of people over the age of 61 in 1984 with those over the age of 61 in 1994. *British Journal of Learning Disabilities* **23**, 143–6.
14. Gianturko DT & Busse EW (1978) Psychiatric problems encountered during a longterm study of normal ageing volunteers. In Issacs AD (ed) *Studies in Geriatric Psychiatry*, Chichester: Wiley.
15. Cooper SA (1992) The psychiatry of elderly people with mental handicaps. *International Journal of Geriatric Psychiatry* **7**, 865–74.
16. Lund J (1985) The prevalence of psychiatric morbidity in mentally retarded adults. *Acta Psychiatrica Scandinavica* **72**, 563–70.
17. Corbett JA (1979) Psychiatric morbidity and mental retardation. In James FE & Snaith RP (eds) *Psychiatric Illness and Mental Handicap*, London: Gaskell Press.

18. Moss S, Patel P & Prosser H *et al.* (1993) Psychiatric morbidity in older people with moderate and severe learning disability I: Development and reliability of the patient interview (PAS-ADD). *British Journal of Psychiatry* **163**, 471-80.

19. Wing JK, Cooper JE & Sartorius N (1974) *Measurement and Classification of Psychiatric Symptoms: An Instruction Manual for the PSE and CATEGO Program*. Cambridge: Cambridge University Press.

20. Patel P, Goldberg D & Moss S (1993) Psychiatric morbidity in older people with moderate and severe learning disability (mental retardation). Part II: The prevalence study. *British Journal of Psychiatry* **163**, 481–91.

21. James DH (1986) Psychiatric and behavioural disorders amongst older severely mentally handicapped in-patients. *Journal of Mental Deficiency Research* **30**, 341–5.

22. Dalton AJ & Wisniewski HM (1990) Down's syndrome and the dementia of Alzheimer disease. *International Review of Psychiatry* **2**, 43–52.

23. Wisniewski KE, Dalton AJ, Crapper-McLachlan DR, Wen GY & Wisniewski HM (1985) Alzheimers disease in Down's syndrome: Clinicopathological studies. *Neurology* **35**, 957–61.

24. Kay DWK, Beamish P & Roth M (1964) Mental disorders in Newcastle-upon-Tyne. *British Journal of Psychiatry* **110**, 146–58.

25. Parsons PLO (1965) Mental health of Swansea's old folk. *British Journal of Preventive and Social Medicine* **19**, 43.

26. Livingston G, Sax K, Willinson J, Blizard B & Mann A (1990) The Gospel Oak Study stage II: the diagnosis of dementia in the community. *Psychological Medicine* **20**, 881–91.

27. Evenhius HM (1990) The natural history of dementia in Down's syndrome. *Archives of Neurology* **47**, 263–7.

28. Evenhius HM (1995) The natural history of dementia in people with intellectual disability. Oral presentation to *First Congress of the European Association for Mental Health in Mental Retardation, 13–16 September 1995*. Amsterdam, The Netherlands.

29. Lejeune J, Gauthier M & Jurpin R (1959) Etudes des chromosomes somatiques de neuf enfants mongoliens. *Comptes Rendus des Seances de L'Academie des Sciences* **248**, 1721–2.

30. Nicholson A & Albeman E (1992) Prediction of the number of Down's syndrome infants to be born in England and Wales up to the year 2000 and their likely survival rates. *Journal of Intellectual Disability Research* **36**, 505–17.

31. Mani C (1988) Hypothyroidism in Down's syndrome. *British Journal of Psychiatry* **153**, 102–4.

32. Carr J (1988) Six weeks to 21 years old, a longitudinal study of children with Down's syndrome and their families. *Journal of Child Psychology and Psychiatry* **29**, 407–31.

33. Gath A & Gumley D (1986) Behaviour problems in retarded children with special reference to Down's syndrome. *British Journal of Psychiatry* **149**, 156–61.

34. Collacot RA, Cooper SA & McGrother C (1992) Differential rates of psychiatric disorders in adults with Down's syndrome compared with other mentally handicapped adults. *British Journal of Psychiatry* **162**, 671–4.

35. Prasher VP & Hall W (1996) Short-term prognosis of depression in adults with Down's syndrome: association with thyroid status and effects on adaptive behaviour. *Journal of Intellectual Disability Research* **40**, 32–8.

36. Collacot RA & Cooper S-A (1992) Adaptive behaviour after depressive illness in Down's syndrome. *Journal of Nervous and Mental Disease* **180**, 468–70.

37. Oliver C & Holland AJ (1986) Down's syndrome and Alzheimer's disease: a review. *Psychological Medicine* **16**, 307–22.

38. Fraser J & Mitchell A (1876) Kalmuc idiocy: report of a case with autopsy with notes on 62 cases. *Journal of Mental Science* **22**, 161.

39. Jervis GA (1948) Early senile dementia mongoloid idiocy. *American Journal of Psychiatry* **105**, 102–6.

40. Mann DMA (1988) Alzheimer's disease and Down's syndrome. *Histopathology* **13**, 125–7.

41. Schapiro MB, Haxby JV & Grady CL (1992) Nature of mental retardation and dementia in Down's syndrome: Study with PET, CT and neuropsychology. *Neurology of Aging* **13**, 723–34.

42. Lai F & Williams RS (1989) A prospective study of Alzheimer disease in Down's syndrome. *Archives of Neurology* **46**, 849–53.

43. Wisniewski HM & Rabe A (1986) Discrepancy between Alzheimer-type neuropathology and dementia in persons with Down's syndrome. *New York Academy of Sciences* **477**, 247–60.

44. Zigman WB, Schupff N, Lubin RA & Silverman WP (1987) Premature regression of adults with Down's syndrome. *American Journal of Mental Deficiency* **92**, 161–8.
45. Miniszek NA (1983) Development of Alzheimer's disease in Down's syndrome individuals. *American Journal of Mental Deficiency* **87**, 377–85.
46. Berry P, Groenweg G, Gibson D & Brown RI (1984) Mental development of adults with Down's syndrome. *American Journal of Mental Deficiency* **89**, 252–6.
47. Janicki MP, Heller T, Seltzer G & Hogg J (1995) *Practice Guidelines for the Clinical Assessment and Care Management of Alzheimer and other Dementias among Adults with Mental Retardation.* Washington: American Association on Mental Retardation.
48. Nihra K, Foster R, Shelhass M & Leland H (1974) *AAMD Adaptive Behaviour Scale.* Washington: American Association on Mental Retardation.
49. Evenhius HM (1992) Evaluation of a screening instrument for dementia in ageing mentally retarded persons. *Journal of Intellectual Disability Research* **36**, 337–47.
50. Teng EL & Chui HC (1987) The modified mini-mental state (MMS) examination. *Journal of Clinical Psychiatry* **48**, 314–8.
51. Sturmey P, Reed J & Corbett J (1991) Psychometric assessment of psychiatric disorders in people with learning difficulties (mental handicap): a review of measures. *Psychological Medicine* **21**, 143–5.
52. Thames Valley Test Company (1985) *Rivermead Memory Behaviour Test.* Suffolk: Thames Valley Test Company.
53. Schapiro MB, Luxenberg JS & Kaye JA *et al.* (1989) Serial quantitative CT analysis of brain morphometrics in adult Down's syndrome at different ages. *Neurology* **39**, 1349–53.
54. Roeden JM & Zitman FG (1995) Ageing in adults with Down's syndrome in institutionally based and community-based residences. *Journal of Intellectual Disability Research* **39**, 399–407.
55. Reifler BV, Larson E & Henley R (1982) Coexistence of cognitive impairment and depression in geriatric outpatients. *American Journal of Psychiatry* **39**, 623–6.
56. Burt DB, Loveland KA & Lewis KR (1992) Depression and the onset of dementia in adults with mental retardation. *American Journal of Mental Retardation* **96**, 502–11.
57. Prasher VP & Filer A (1995) Behavioural disturbance in people with Down's syndrome and dementia. *Journal of Intellectual Disability Research* **39**, 432–6.
58. Janicki MP & MacEachron AE (1984) Residential health and social service needs of elderly developmentally disabled persons. *The Gerontologist* **24**, 128–37.
59. Maaskant MA & Haveman MJ (1990) Elderly residents in Dutch mental deficiency institutions. *Journal of Mental Deficiency Research* **34**, 475–82.
60. Aman MG (1990) Considerations in the use of psychotropic drugs in elderly mentally retarded persons. *Journal of Mental Deficiency Research* **34**, 1–10.
61. Vestal RE (1984) *Drug Treatment in the Elderly.* Melbourne: Adis Health Service Press.
62. Walters R (1988) Prescribing requirements of the elderly mentally handicapped: future demands on primary health care services. *Journal of the Royal College of General Practitioners* **38**, 317–9.
63. Law R & Chalmers C (1976) Medicines and elderly people: a general practice survey. *British Medical Journal* **1**, 565–8.
64. Weedle P & Parish P (1984) Pharmaceutical care of the elderly (Part 1). *British Journal of Pharmaceutical Practice* **61**, 352–8.
65. Rockwell E, Lam RW & Zisook S (1989) Antidepressant drug studies in the elderly. *Psychiatric Clinics of North America* **11**, 215–33.
66. Krauss MW & Seltzer MM (1986) Comparison of elderly mentally retarded persons in community and institutional settings. *American Journal of Mental Deficiency* **91**, 237–43.
67. Seltzer MM, Seltzer GB & Sherwood CC (1982) Comparison of older versus younger mentally retarded adults. *American Journal of Mental Deficiency* **87**, 9–13.
68. Moss SC & Hogg J (1989) A cluster analysis of support networks of older people with severe intellectual impairment. *Australian and New Zealand Journal of Developmental Disabilities* (special monograph edition).
69. Edgerton RB (1988) Aging in the community: a matter of choice. *American Journal of Mental Retardation* **92**, 331–5.
70. Seltzer M (1988) Structure and patterns of service utilization by elderly persons with mental retardation. *Mental Retardation* **26**, 181–5.
71. Cotten PD & Spirrison CL (1988) Development of services for elderly persons with mental retardation in a rural state. *Mental Retardation* **26**, 187–90.

72. Gilleard CJ (1984) *Living with Dementia: Community Care of the Elderly Mentally Infirmed.* London: Croom Helm.
73. Sloper PC, Turner S & Cunnigham C (1991) Factors related to stress and satisfaction with life in families of children with Down's syndrome. *Journal of Child Psychology and Psychiatry* **32**, 655–76.
74. Todd S, Shearn J, Beyer S & Felce D (1993) Careers in caring: The changing situation of parents caring for an offspring with learning difficulties. *Irish Journal of Psychology* **14**, 130–53.
75. Prasher V, Clarke DJ, Harris CRW & Hunt J (1995) Carers and people with learning disability in Birmingham, UK. *British Journal of Developmental Disabilities* **81**, 91–6.
76. Schaie KW (1983) The Seattle longitudinal study: A 21 year exploration of psychometric intelligence in adulthood. In Schaie KW (ed) *Longitudinal Studies of Adult Psychological Development*, London: Guildford Press.
77. DHSS (1984) *Helping Mentally Handicapped People with Special Problems: Report of a DHSS Study Team.* London: HMSO.

11

Consent and Learning Disability

John Finch

Consent to Treatment and Care

There is no specific legal 'right' to treatment; and, despite an assertion in *The Patient's Charter* which appears to go well ahead of the current state of English Law, there is no right to information relating to any risk which may be involved in proposed treatment, or about any alternative, prior to consenting to that treatment. Judicial decisions on the more limited right to information on risks are discussed later in this section.

There are two separate though related aspects of the law relating to treatment. The law of assault and battery, the basics of which are explained shortly, provides legal remedies for wrongdoing based on unpermitted or otherwise unwarranted physical contact. Aspects of treatment and care not involving personal physical contact, such as psychotherapy, have nothing to do with the law of assault and battery, and consent is therefore not required to make treatment lawful in that particular respect. Treatment falling below an acceptable standard of professional skill and competence may, if it causes foreseeable harm to the patient, be actionable negligence. So, too, may an unacceptable failure to explain to a comprehending person a significant risk, or adverse consequence, in proposed treatment if that risk materializes and the patient can prove that he/she would not have undergone the treatment had they known the risk: this is so-called 'informed consent'.

As such, 'informed consent' or rather more accurately the receipt of information about aspects of risks in proposed treatment which a practitioner is under a professional and legal obligation to volunteer,[1] may be relevant to treatment plans for individuals whose mild learning disability allows an informed choice on the subject of possible adverse consequences. Those with a more significant, more severe, learning disability may be less able or unable to comprehend information about potential risks and similarly unable to make a real or 'informed' choice about whether or not to proceed with the proposed treatment. There is ample judicial authority to the effect that a practitioner owes no legal duty to explain adverse consequences which might forseeably cause undue worry or concern to a patient.[2] The law relating to 'informed consent' (professional legal duty to inform on risks) requires a practitioner to take no more than reasonable steps to impart such information in a comprehensible way.

Although not a case relating to a patient with learning disabilities, the decision of the House of Lords in *Sidaway v. Bethlem Royal Hospital Governors*[3] is helpful as a principal source of guidance for the legal duty of practitioners. Lord Templeman said in that case:

> *'If the doctor making a balanced judgement advises the patient to submit to the operation, the patient is entitled to reject that advice for reasons which are rational or irrational, or for no reason. The duty of the doctor in these circumstances, subject to his overriding duty to have regard to the best interests of the patient, is to provide the patient with information which will enable the patient to make a balanced judgement.'*[4]

In the case of a person with sufficient comprehension to make an informed choice on the basis of information which has been understood, that person is free to choose not to cooperate with what is proposed, even if such lack of cooperation is, or appears to the practitioner to be, irrational or even foolish. The relationship between comprehension and irrationality or foolishness is discussed below in the context of the question of whether all the evidence indicates that the individual with learning disabilities is genuinely consenting to the physical contact involved in the proposed treatment. Although habitually referred to as giving 'informed consent', the question of basic consent to physical contact such as will avoid an action for battery is normally more conveniently referred to simply as 'consent', leaving the expression 'informed consent' to refer specifically to the practitioner's duty to explain risks to a comprehending patient.

It is worth noting the matter of whether or not a patient with reasonable comprehension specifically enquires about possible risks in the treatment proposed. The general rule is expressed by Lord Bridge in the Sidaway case (above):

> *'When questioned specifically by a patient of apparently sound mind about risks involved in a particular treatment proposed, the doctor's duty must, in my opinion, be to answer both truthfully and as fully as the questioner requires'.*[5]

Although Lord Bridge refers to a 'patient of apparently sound mind', there is no law which deprives an individual with learning disabilities of the entitlement to an explanation of the type and quality described, if the practitioner proposing treatment takes the professional view that the would-be patient has sufficient intellect and capacity to comprehend the explanation of risks. Further, although also decided in relation to the generality of patients and with no specific reference to those with learning disabilities, the decision of the Court of Appeal in *Blyth v. Bloomsbury Health Authority*[6] stands as legal authority for the sensible and just proposition that the duty to give information is not dependent on the patient's enquiry. Some individuals with learning disabilities might, for instance, be capable of understanding quite substantial details relevant to proposed treatment but might, on account of their disability, be unwilling or unlikely to put specific questions designed to elicit a response from the practitioner. The law in *Blyth* which is applicable to the generality of people may therefore, for the reasons just explained, be of particular significance to those with a mild or moderate learning disability.

Discussion in the remainder of this section concentrates on the question of capacity to make a genuine choice of whether to accept treatment (or care, involving physical contact) at all, irrespective of any further duty (breach of which is actionable in negligence and not in battery) to explain risks. Such is the range of learning disability that it will always be a question of fact in each case whether a person so affected is giving genuine consent to treatment or care involving physical contact.

There is no legal category of people who are deemed to be incompetent to understand. Even longer-term detained patients (in the case of learning disability, those with abnormal aggression or serious irresponsibility) have the option to consent to medical treatment for mental disorder, as an alternative to the 'second opinion' (appointed doctor) procedure under Part IV of the Mental Health Act 1983.[7] The second opinion procedure provides for treatment to be given where consent is refused or where a patient is clearly incapable of consenting. It also provides for a situation which may arise in the case of a detained patient with learning disabilities whose apparent agreement to proposed treatment raises a doubt in the mind of the medical practitioner in charge of treatment (Responsible Medical Officer, RMO). The RMO will implement the procedure and the appointed doctor may confirm that that apparent consent is genuine and certify that such is the case.

Kennedy & Grubb[8] lay emphasis on the need to preserve the autonomy of a person with learning disabilities in the following passage:

> *'... what are we concerned about here? The answer in short is a patient's expression of will and the question whether that expression of will ought to be respected. The customary answer given is that it ought to be respected in those circumstances where the patient is capable of acting autonomously, i.e. in exercising self-determination. It is in the words 'autonomy' and 'self-determination' that the key is to be found. These words tell us that the concern of both the law and ethics is with the individual.*
>
> *'It should follow therefore, that any notion of capacity should be individual-orientated. It should not consist in mere membership of a group to whom a general classification or status is applied, regardless of the individual's circumstances, save where the clearest reasons of public policy demand. Any notion of capacity which did not adopt such an approach would, by so doing, undermine the commitment to individual rights which it is the central concern of law and ethics to advance.'*

Because of a general lack of clarity in the present state of the law, the Law Commission in 1995 published the results of a 5-year study of decision making and mental incapacity. In its report *Mental Incapacity*[13], two concepts are fundamental to a new, integrated decision making jurisdiction which it recommends. These are *capacity*, and *best interests*.

The Commission recommends a new statutory definition of what it means to be 'without capacity' to make a particular decision. An individual should be regarded as unable to make a decision if at the material time he or she is unable by reason of mental disability to make a decision on the matter in question; or is unable to communicate a decision on that matter because he or she is unconscious or for any other reason.

'An inability to make a decision' means, for this purpose: '(1) an inability to understand or retain the information about the reasonably foreseeable consequences of deciding one way or another or of failing to make the decision, or (2) an inability to make a decision based on that information'.

The term 'mental disability' means, in the context of the Commission's recommendations, 'a disability or disorder of the mind or brain, whether permanent or temporary, which results in an impairment or disturbance of mental functioning'.

The basic law on physical contact is simple. Physical contact with the person has to be 'warranted' (meaning lawfully permitted) if it is not to be an actionable battery. Battery is intentional, unwarranted physical contact; assault is the apprehension of the immediate infliction of a battery (ruling out such invasions or threats of harm in the future).

Contrary to widespread belief there is no general rule that acting in good faith makes lawful a physical contact which could ordinarily amount to an unlawful battery on account of the absence of consent. As explained below, it may be lawful to act in the 'best interests' of a severely mentally incapacitated person unable to give any real consent to treatment involving physical contact. But other requirements are attached, notably that the treatment would attract a modicum of agreement among medical practitioners in the relevant field of practice. Moreover, acting in the 'best interests' of the person concerned imposes more significant criteria for lawful action than the amorphous concept of 'good faith'. 'Good faith' may amount to nothing more sophisticated than that the person purporting so to act simply wishes to give the treatment in question because it seems therapeutically appropriate to do so.

Until recently it was thought that, following a person's reaching the age of majority (18 years), no one, including a court, had power to authorize medical treatment on an incompetent adult, however beneficial the proposed treatment. In *Re F: F v West Berkshire Health Authority* (1989)[9] the House of Lords set out the following principles applicable to the case before them. The person with severe learning disabilities was a 36-year-old patient in a hospital and was having sexual relations with a male patient. The question before the court was whether she could lawfully be sterilized in the absence of a consent which she was clearly incompetent to give. The procedure was desired by carers not for directly therapeutic reasons (such as menorrhagia) but for the arguably beneficial outcome of not becoming pregnant and becoming severely disturbed in consequence.

Their Lordships ruled that the courts have jurisdiction to declare the lawfulness of such an operation which is proposed to be performed on the ground that it is in the best interests of the patient. In deciding whether the proposed procedure is indeed in the best interests of the patient the court should apply the test of what would be accepted as currently appropriate treatment by a reasonable body of medical opinion held by professionals skilled in the administration of that particular form of treatment. In so ruling their Lordships effectively 'medicalized' the decision as to best interests, a decision which will invariably in practice be taken, in the case of a person with learning disabilities who is being cared for by health or social services or by both, by the multidisciplinary care team and not solely by the medical practitioner in the case. Not only is the decision as to 'best interests' narrowed to the view which might be taken by one among many caring professions; the decision in *Re F*[9] is also restricted in concentrating on the lawfulness of the proposed sterilization to the exclusion of other aspects of treatment and care which it would be most unusual to find given in any but a multidisciplinary care team context.

While Lord Goff based his opinion principally on the concept of necessity to justify intervention when no other principle such as consent, or consent by another person (such as a parent), is available the other Law Lords placed greater emphasis on what has been called a 'quasi-proxy'.[10] The practical relationship between a decision made by another on behalf of the individual with learning disabilities, and the legal basis upon which it might be assumed to be made, is set out by Lord Brandon in the following passage:

> 'In my opinion, the solution to the problem which the common law provides is that a doctor
> can lawfully operate on, or give treatment to, adult patients who are incapable, for one reason
> or another, of consenting to his doing so providing that the operation or other treatment con-
> cerned is in the best interests of such patient. The operation or other treatment will be in their
> best interests if, but only if, it is carried out in order either to save their life, or to ensure
> improvement or prevent deterioration in their physical or mental health. . . . When persons lack
> the capacity, for whatever reason, to take decisions about the performance of operations on them,
> or the giving of other medical treatment to them, it is necessary that some other person or
> persons, with the appropriate qualifications, should take such decisions for them. Otherwise they
> would be deprived of medical care which they need and to which they are entitled. . . .'[11]

The decision leaves unanswered numerous questions which are outside the remit of this chapter. In particular, however, the situation of more competent patients may present elements not only of a test of lawful interventions based on the person's 'best interests' but also on a 'substituted judgement'. The question of a substituted judgement involves carers and those proposing to treat in the question as to the extent, if any, to which known or perceived views and values of the patient should figure in the decision to be made by another person, or a care team on their behalf. On the facts of *Re F*,[9] where the patient had never been competent to form a view on the intervention which was being proposed for her, the substituted judgement approach to decision making was inapplicable and was not considered by the judges. In the United States, some judicial decisions have been strangely based on purported substituted judgement for a person who had never at any time been mentally competent to form a judgement.[12] In cases where the approach is realistic on account of some mental competence of the patient, perhaps past and not present, the investigation of what a person would want or decide is a valuable exercise in the preservation of autonomy of many people with learning disabilities. In the aftermath of the decision in *Re F*[9] and the questions which it left unanswered, the Law Commission published proposals which are now consolidated into its report *Mental Incapacity*.[13]

The practical impact of the Law Commission's recommendations, which await sufficient consensus and Parliamentary time to enact them into legislation for the guidance of carers and practitioners, is to be found in the introduction to a summary of the proposals:

> 'Particular attention is drawn in the report to the continuing increase in the proportion of
> very old people in the population; the fact that many people who previously lived in an insti-
> tutional setting are now living in the community where greatly increased opportunities for

substitute decision-making arise; how advances in medical science now enable people to live longer than was previously the case often with their mental capacity impaired. These demographic, social and medical changes have taken place at the same time as a recognition by the courts that there is now no person or court in England and Wales who can lawfully take personal welfare or medical decisions on behalf of adults who lack capacity to take decisions for themselves. The Commission's study has made it abundantly clear that there is a pressing need for reform.'

While clearly falling short of recommending the substituted judgement approach and preferring an approach to decision-making based primarily on the 'best interests' test, the Law Commission makes the following recommendation for future inclusion in clarifying law reform:

'A new general rule that anything done for a person who is without capacity should be done in that person's "best interests". The expression "best interests" is not defined in the draft Bill appended to the report, but the Commission lists four factors which should be considered whenever something has to be done or a decision made on behalf of a person without capacity. These factors are:

(1) the ascertainable past and present wishes and feelings of the person concerned and the factors which he or she would consider if able to do so;

(2) the need to permit and encourage the person concerned to participate, or to improve his or her ability to participate, in anything done for and any decision affecting him or her;

(3) if it is practicable and appropriate to consult them, the views as to that person's wishes and feelings and as to what would be in the best interests of that person of:
(i) any person named by him or her as someone to be consulted,
(ii) any person (such as a spouse, relative or friend or other person) engaged in caring for or interested in the person's welfare,
(iii) the donee of a continuing power of attorney granted by him or her,
(iv) any manager appointed by the court;

(4) whether the purpose for which any action or decision is required can be as effectively achieved in a manner less restrictive of the person's freedom of action.

One of the uncertainties of the present law is what action may lawfully be taken by someone caring for a person without capacity or what medical treatment a doctor can give to such a person.

The Commission recommends that it should be lawful to do anything for the personal welfare or health care of a person who is, or is reasonably believed to be, without capacity in relation to the matter in question if it is in all the circumstances reasonable for it to be done by the person who does it and it is in the best interests of that person.

This general authority to act reasonably will extend to matters concerning the personal welfare and health care of a person who is or is reasonably believed to be without capacity. There are certain health decisions, however, which can only ever be taken by the person acting for himself or herself, for example consenting to marriage, consenting to sexual relations, and voting at an election.'

Among the many problems involved in choosing the course of action calculated to further the 'best interests' of a person with learning disabilities is the question whether or not to implement a strange or even foolish choice if there is evidence of a genuine wish to pursue such a course. The problem is more likely to arise in the case of individuals whose incompetence results, for instance, from senile dementia and who, during an earlier period of greater mental incompetence, expressed an idiosyncratic wish or decision. The problem may, however, arise in the case of people with a mild or even moderate learning disability whose past or even present clear intentions may be inconsistent with what carers would decide, were the decision to be left to them. Preservation of autonomy requires close attention to the wishes and interventions even of people with diminished mental competence. In certain cases a person may simply misperceive reality and so a wish based on such misperception could safely and ethically be ignored. However, as Kennedy and Grubb point out,[14] it is important to distinguish a case where the irrationality of a person's decision affects their understanding, from one in which understanding remains unimpaired despite surrounding irrationality.

In the case of people whose mental competence is not in doubt the law makes no requirement that decisions are reasonable and rational. The Law Commission rejected a test of capacity based on the ability to formulate rational beliefs as such a test would rob the patient of his right to their own personality which may be far more serious and distinctive than anything which could follow from the patient's decision in relation to a particular proposed treatment.[15]

The Law Commission prefers a test of whether the individual is capable of understanding information relevant to a particular decision.

Rights and Sexual Relationships

One of the personal rights authorized in Article 8 of the European Convention of Human Rights (1950) is one which guarantees respect for 'private life'. An individual with learning disabilities is entitled to be treated as 'normally' as possible by the law, consistent with their protection against harm or abuse. It could be said in general terms that an individual has a 'right' to a sex life as an integral part of their life as a whole. Equally, an individual with learning disability is entitled to the protection of the law and to the freedoms which it supports. In the case of *X and Y v The Netherlands* (1985)[16] the European Court of Human Rights ruled that a state which is a signatory to the Convention must include in its criminal law some protection against sexual assault on women with a learning disability.

A balance between the expression of a right to personal freedom, on one hand, and the protection of vulnerable people from abuse and exploitation on the other, is difficult to achieve. In some cases the criminal law provides for offences whose objective is the prevention of abuse of vulnerable individuals by those in charge of their care specifically in hospitals and residential and nursing homes. More generally, the criminal law provides for offences against 'defectives' wherever they are committed, based on lack of legal consent to an act of sexual contact which is normally dependent for its lawfulness on voluntary and genuine consent. It is in the latter context that the law experiences most difficulty in addressing itself to the protection and to the legitimate expectations and human rights of individuals with a learning disability. The difficulty in striking a balance is described by Judge Ashton thus:

> *'The manner and extent to which persons who have a mental handicap may enjoy a sexual relationship with others is one of the principal areas of uncertainty in the law. Cases reaching the courts concentrate on the issues of sterilisation and abortion, and a degree of sensitivity tends to ensure that the more day to day issues do not become the subject of legal scrutiny.*

Nevertheless, those working with and attending to the daily needs of handicapped persons need to know where they stand and where the line is drawn between behaviour on their part which is acceptable, and behaviour which is a criminal offence.'[17]

Sex and the Age of Consent

The age at which both sexes may lawfully engage in lawful, consensual sexual activity is 16 years. The Sexual Offences Act 1956 provides for two criminal offences which are committed irrespective of the mental capacity of the girl in question. It is an absolute offence (that is, an offence to which no defence of mistaking the age of the girl is allowed) for a man to have sexual intercourse with a girl under the age of 13 years. If the girl is aged between 13 and 16 the man has a defence if he can prove on the balance of probabilities (more likely than not) that he believed the girl to be more than 16 years old and had reasonable cause for that belief. The defence is available only if the man is under 24 and has not previously been charged with a similar offence. There is no special differentiation for a man with learning disabilities who is accused of committing either of these offences: the absolute offence because it is not susceptible to any defence, and the other because reasonable cause for belief that the girl was aged 16 years or over is objective. However, the Code for Crown Prosecutors stipulates that account shall be taken of whether or not any element of personal attack or corruption was involved, when deciding whether or not to institute criminal proceedings. Account is also taken of balancing the interests of the public, in prosecuting and of the particular victim in each case. The relative ages of defendant and victim are also referred to. The criminal prosecution of an individual in a hospital or mental nursing home might serve little or no purpose, especially if they are already subject to a detention made for treatment for their mental disorder. In other cases, a hospital order under Section 37 of Mental Health Act 1983 or a guardianship order made under that section would be open to the court as a therapeutic alternative to a prison sentence. Both alternatives are, in the case of people with learning disabilities, subject to medical evidence of abnormal aggression or serious irresponsibility, such as bringing the individual concerned within the category of 'mental impairment' for the purpose of Section 37.

Offences Committed with 'A Defective'

The Sexual Offences Act 1956 provides for several criminal offences which may be committed with an individual who is 'a defective'. This outmoded term is now legally defined in Schedule 3 to the Mental Health (Amendment) Act 1982, and means 'a state of arrested or incomplete development of mind which includes severe impairment of intelligence and social functioning'. Such impairment does not require the additional aggression or serious irresponsibility which form an integral part of grounds for treatment or hospital orders, or guardianship, under Parts II and III of the Mental Health Act 1983.

It is an offence for a man to have unlawful sexual intercourse with a woman who is a defective, a man to procure a woman who is a defective to have unlawful sexual intercourse, a person to take a woman who is a defective out of the possession of her parent or guardian (meaning any person who has lawful care or charge of the woman, including a registered home proprietor), and a person to make an indecent assault on a woman or a man who, being 'a defective', is unable to give such consent to the act as would prevent its being an assault. In each case it is not an offence if the person charged can prove, on the balance of probabilities (more likely than not) that they did not know and had no reason to suspect that the other person came within the definition of the term 'defective'. In each case, 'unlawful' means outside marriage, so that within a matrimonial relationship an offence is not committed irrespective of the state of mind of the person committing the act or the mental capacity of the other person.

Homosexual relationships are covered by Section 1 of the Sexual Offences Act 1967, as amended by the Criminal Justice and Public Order Act 1994. A homosexual act in private between consenting adult males aged 18 or more is not an offence. An offence is committed if more than two individuals participate because the activity is not then 'in private'. The Act provides that a man who is suffering from 'severe mental handicap' cannot in law give the necessary consent. A woman may lawfully form a homosexual relationship at age 16 years, and before that age cannot give the consent necessary to prevent the act being an indecent assault.

In relation to any form of these offences a practitioner or carer may himself be guilty of an offence by 'aiding, abetting, counselling or procuring' the commission of the offence. Attention must therefore be given to the question of when, if at all, a criminal offence is committed involving the sexual activity of someone with a learning disability, and when, if at all, those in charge of their care may be guilty of aiding and abetting such an offence.

Despite the state of the law, which may appear invidious to the interests and human rights of individuals with a learning disability as well as to the good intentions of carers wishing to integrate such people into as normal a lifestyle as possible, prosecutions are, in practice, rare in both respects. A sexual offence with 'a defective' is not committed if the individual did not know, and had no reason to know, that the woman in question was 'a defective'. Thus, two people who both fall into the category of 'defective' may lawfully have sexual intercourse if the man cannot or does not recognize the extent of his female partner's mental impairment. This statement can be made with greater certainty, the greater the degree of impairment in the male partner in such a relationship. The prosecution of a moderately impaired man will be unlikely unless he is suspected not only of knowledge or suspicion of the woman's impairment but also of exploitation of a more vulnerable partner to the relationship. While there is no specific defence of 'lack of exploitation' if a prosecution is in fact brought, such absence of exploitation is likely, in practice, not only to protect the parties to the sexual relationship but also, very importantly, practitioners and carers. Given that it is a criminal offence to aid and abet unlawful intercourse with a defective, the absence of exploitation and the intention to act in the best interests of the disabled person is likely to make it acceptable in practice for carers to assist a woman even with a severe learning disability to have sexual intercourse. As Gunn pointed out,[18] if it is unlikely that the man is to be prosecuted, it is also unlikely that the member of staff or carer will be prosecuted unless he or she has acted in some way improperly.

The offence of knowingly suffering a woman who is a defective to resort to or be on premises for the purpose of having unlawful sexual intercourse, which is discussed below, is subject to exactly the same practical and professional considerations.

Specific Prohibitions

Section 27 of the Sexual Offences Act 1956 makes it a criminal offence for the 'owner, occupier or anyone who has or acts in the management or control of any premises to induce or knowingly suffer a woman who is a defective to resort to or be on those premises for the purpose of having unlawful sexual intercourse with men or a particular man'. The act must be 'unlawful' and therefore no offence is committed by the owner, occupier or other such person if the couple involved are married, nor is the act unlawful if it falls within the context of activity described in the preceding part of this chapter, given such relevant factors as lack of knowledge and good faith.

A broad category of individuals may commit this offence, including not only the owner or occupier of the premises but also any person who is involved in the management or control of those premises. Most members of staff will be involved in the general running of the establishment in some way apart, possibly, from those engaged in purely routine or medical tasks. It seems likely that Section 27 will be interpreted, should a case ever arise on the point, to mean that the person accused must be in some way involved with the disordered person's activities on the premises. This would, for instance, include a care assistant but exclude a security guard, although both are involved in the management and control of the premises. Of greater practical difficulty in compliance with the provisions of Section 27 is the element to 'knowingly suffer' the act in question to take place. Possible interpretations of the expression are analysed by Gunn thus:

> 'The requirement that the member of staff must 'knowingly' allow a defective woman to be on the premises for the purpose of unlawful sexual intercourse is unlikely to be of much significance except in the case of casual relationships. Knowledge is satisfied by the staff either being fully aware of such relationships taking place through actual knowledge or shutting their eyes to the obvious. It is possible that the courts might interpret the phrase 'knowingly suffer' to mean cause or encourage. Since most situations are ones where staff know what is happening, but do not actively encourage it, this possible interpretation could be quite important. However, other courts have taken the view that, in other offences, "suffer" simply means failing to act and permit means doing something to allow the activity to happen.'[19]

Practical difficulties facing staff in hospitals and care homes are to a considerable extent reduced by the fact that, despite doubts surrounding legal interpretation, the existence of good relations between the person involved, parents or other carers, and the police make it unlikely that an offence will be alleged. Even if an offence is alleged and is investigated and a report sent to the Crown Prosecution Service, a prosecution will only be brought if it serves a useful purpose and if there is sufficient evidence for conviction. In the absence of exploitation, convictions or even allegations of criminality are, in practice, most unlikely.

In any event the inconsistency between the wide prohibition contained in Section 27 of the 1956 Act and modern approaches to the 'normalisation' of people with a learning disability is noted by Gostin:

> 'This provision makes it particularly difficult for hospital and residential care staff to operate a progressive policy of normalisation by allowing, where appropriate, a mentally handicapped man and woman to meet in private. There is a strong case for reform of the law to bring it into line with modern attitudes towards mentally handicapped people.'20

Section 128 of the Mental Health Act 1959 (still in force, as amended by the Sexual Offences Act 1967) makes it an offence for a male member of staff or manager of a hospital or mental nursing home to have unlawful sexual intercourse with a woman, or to commit an act of gross indecency with a male patient, who is 'for the time being receiving treatment for mental disorder.' The section also applies to people attending the hospital or the home as outpatients. It is also an offence for a man to commit such an act with a mentally disordered patient who is subject to guardianship or otherwise in his custody or care under the Mental Health Act 1983, or in National Health Service premises, premises falling within Part III of the National Assistance Act 1948, or in a residential home (including a nursing home) for the mentally disordered.

Any doubts relating to the 'unlawfulness' of the acts in question, such as might be raised in the context of acts between patients or residents themselves in a hospital or home, and which are permitted to happen by a person in charge of management or control of premises, will not in practice arise here. Section 128 of the Mental Health Act 1959 is specifically directed to the prohibition of exploitation of patients or residents by those caring for them with knowledge of their learning disability.

Sales, Purchases and 'Commercial Dealings'

Sale and Purchase

The law relating to commercial transactions, even of a simple type, by individuals affected by a learning disability attempts to strike a balance between that person and the other party to the transaction. Purchases by a learning disabled person may be for what the law terms 'necessaries', or they may be for other items. 'Necessaries' in this context mean goods which are suitable to the condition of life, or lifestyle, of the learning disabled person and which are necessary to that person's actual requirements at the time of sale and delivery. The person's purchase of necessaries is governed by Section 3(2) of the Sale of Goods Act 1979. This provides that 'where necessaries are sold and delivered ... to a person who by reason of mental incapacity . . . is incompetent to contract, he must pay a reasonable price for them'. The necessary items must, of course, have been supplied by the other contracting party with an intention that payment be made for them.

The practical significance of the provision is that, in cases where the contract is unenforceable because the supplier of the necessary goods knew the other to be affected by mental incompetence to enter into a contract, the supplier may legally recover a price which is a 'reasonable' and not the price which (if higher) was specified in the purported agreement. If the supplier of the goods did not know or ought to have known of the other's mental incapacity to enter into a contract, the contract is enforceable in the normal course and the full contract price is payable.

If an individual lends money to another affected by learning disability, the whole amount is recoverable if the lender has no reasonable cause to know of the incapacity. If the lender is aware of the incapacity and nevertheless lends money, and if the money is spent, only so much of the amount lent as has been spent on necessary goods (as defined above) may be recovered.

The general principle applicable to contracts for the supply of goods and services other than those which are necessary is more indulgent. The contract is binding unless two things are proved by or on behalf of the disabled person. First, that they did not understand what they were entering into, on account of their incapacity, and second, that the other party was aware (or ought to have been aware) of the incapacity. It is for the disabled person (or someone on their behalf) to prove both these things if liability under the contract is to be avoided.

As in the context of medical treatment, so here also the competence (or otherwise) to enter into contracts and agreements requires attention to both mental capacity and actual understanding. The understanding and mental competence required to uphold the validity of the contract depends upon the nature of the transaction. There is no fixed standard of competency; for each transaction the party must have an understanding of the general nature of what they are doing.[21] Where the subject matter and value of the contract are trivial, the degree of understanding required may be low; and where the value to the person is great, the degree of understanding may be high.[22] The simple existence of learning disability is not enough to demonstrate incompetence to contract. Again, the same principle is applicable here as to incompetence to agree to treatment or other physical contact: the more grave the consequences of the proposed course of action for the learning disabled person, the greater the need in law to demonstrate a genuine understanding.

Powers of Attorney

It will, in the nature of things, be rare for a person affected by learning disability to be involved in the execution of a power of attorney. A power of attorney is a type of agency and it allows the individuals to whom the power is granted to act, in the circumstances specified in the written document creating the power, on behalf of the person wishing their property and affairs to be managed by the other. Prior to the Enduring Powers of Attorney Act 1985 the common law position was that a power of attorney was automatically revoked by the supervening mental incapacity of the person creating it. This caused great practical difficulty in cases where the power was granted to another in prospect of the possible mental incapacity of the donor (for example on account of senility), for such a person was disallowed from acting on behalf of the mentally incapacitated person at the very time the latter most needed such assistance.

An enduring power of attorney which is executed in accordance with the requirements of the 1985 Act, and of the Court of Protection (Enduring Powers of Attorney) Rules 1994[23] and the Enduring Powers of Attorney (Prescribed Form) Regulations 1990,[24] is not rendered invalid by supervening mental incapacity. Nor is the execution of such a power invalid because, at the time it was executed, the mental incompetence of the donor rendered them incapable of managing their affairs. The power is valid if, at the time of its execution, the donor understood the nature of the power (what it was for) and its intended practical effects. For the execution of the power to be valid the donor must understand that the attorney (agent) will take control of those affairs or arrangements which are specified in the formal document, and, again subject to the terms of the document, that the attorney will be able to do anything with the donor's property which the donor himself could have done.

The practical significance of an enduring power of attorney in the case of people affected by learning disabilities may, in practice, be small. However, given the requirement is that the nature and effect of the power be understood, not that the person concerned be able to do the things which the other is authorized to do, this leaves the execution of such a power a practical possibility in appropriate cases.

Making a Will

To be able to make a valid will a person must be of sound mind, memory and understanding. A person seeking to make a will must be able to understand the nature and effect of making a will, and to appreciate the extent of the property sought to be made the subject of the will.[25] Any alteration to or revocation of a will is governed by the same principle. A will is not legally revoked simply by reason of later mental incapacity. Case law relating to the competence, in the sense of the lucidity, of people seeking to make a will is centred principally on the question of whether mentally disordered people were capable, during a particular interval, of understanding the implications of what they were doing. As such, the case law is largely irrelevant to individuals affected by learning disability. The test for the validity of a will is not the same as that affecting a valid contract: 'In addition to passing the ordinary test of *understanding* the testator must also pass a *memory* test and show a sufficient *awareness* of moral obligations'.[26] In the case of a learning disabled person seeking to make a will, the elements of understanding, memory and awareness are likely to remain unchanged for some time and unlikely to change in the future. If any doubt exists as to the testamentary capacity of a learning disabled person, it is prudent to obtain a written medical opinion on capacity. It would also be wise to arrange for the medical practitioner providing such evidence to witness the will.

A will does not have to be signed in writing by the testator. It is legally sufficient if a mark (such as a cross) is made and acknowledged as such by the people who, in the presence of the testator and of each other, must sign as witnesses. If the testator cannot read it has to be established, preferably by some documentary evidence accompanying the will, that he knew and understood its contents before signing.

An individual with substantial assets but incapable of making a will may have a statutory will made by the Court of Protection. The Court of Protection has power under Section 91 (1) (e) of Part VII of the Mental Health Act 1983 to execute a will for a person as if they were not affected by learning disability.

Court of Protection

Part VII of the Mental Health Act 1983 provides for wide powers exercisable by the Court of Protection. The Court may exercise its jurisdiction over individuals who are incapable, by reason of mental disorder or incapacity, of managing and administering their own property and affairs. An individual who is amenable to the jurisdiction of the Court is referred to in Part VII of the Act as a 'patient'. It is not necessary for the individual concerned to be an inpatient in a hospital, nor is it every disordered or incapacitated individual who is a 'patient' for this purpose, incapability to manage affairs being the essential (additional) requirement. Medical evidence must establish the relationship between the two.

The Court, despite its name, is not a judicial body as such, but an office of the Supreme Court established in London.

The 'mental disorder' from which a person must suffer to fall within the jurisdiction of the Court need be no more specifically defined. In other words, the grounds of aggressive or seriously irresponsible behaviour which a learning disabled person must exhibit to be sectionable under much of Part II or III of the Mental Health Act 1983 need not be established. There must, however, be specific evidence that the patient is incapable of managing by reason of disorder. There is no particular form in which such medical evidence needs to be presented, and the Court can decide to exercise its jurisdiction on the basis of a single medical report without the practitioner furnishing it being required to give oral evidence. The medical practitioner providing the report is not in law required to have any special knowledge or experience in the diagnosis or treatment of mental disorder. In practice, the Court will wish to satisfy itself as to the quality and reliability of the medical evidence provided.[27]

If an individual does not have the mental capacity to execute a valid enduring power of attorney (see the previous section), but has money or property which they are incapable of managing, an application to the Court of Protection to appoint a receiver is advisable. The situation is likely to arise in the case of a learning disabled individual in at least five situations, as follows: first, when that individual has inherited money by way of a will or intestacy; second, where financial compensation (including notably damages for personal injury) has been awarded in litigation or by way of an out-of-court settlement; third, in any other case where the individual has come by substantial moneys and there are no trustees to administer it; fourth, where there is reason to believe or suspect that the money or property of that individual is being, or may be, misused or misappropriated by another; and fifth, if the mental disability is likely to become more significant as they become older and to make them less able to manage property and affairs than they are (if at all) at present.

The practical legal adviser's approach to application to the Court of Protection for the appointment of a receiver is expressed by District Judge Ashton:

> 'Traditionally, lawyers have advised that such application be avoided whenever possible but this may no longer be the correct approach and it may be in the best interests of a handicapped person for a Receiver to be appointed. The Court can be helpful and provides a degree of supervision which can be valuable and may not exist with other forms of delegation, but the principal disincentive is still the formality, delay and cost involved'.[28]

The jurisdiction of the Court of Protection extends to minors (under 18 years). However, in practice it will not be exercised if the property of the minor is already adequately protected and regulated in another suitable way, such as by the appointment of trustees. In a case in which a learning disabled minor is approaching the age of majority and will, on reaching that age become entitled to money or property, the Court will normally accept jurisdiction over the incompetent person's affairs.

The Receiver is appointed by a judge of the Court. Section 99 (2) of the Mental Health Act 1983 provides that the person appointed as Receiver 'shall do all such things in relation to the property and affairs of the patient as the judge ... orders or directs him to do and may do any such thing in relation to the property and affairs of the patient as the judge, in the exercise of those powers, authorizes him to do'. In acting for the benefit of the patient the Court of Protection has regard to much wider matters than material benefit, although that is of course included. Section 95 (1) provides that that judge may, with respect to the property and affairs of the patient, do or secure the doing of all such things as appear necessary or expedient for the maintenance or other benefit of the patient, for the maintenance or other benefit of the patient's family, for making provision for other persons or purposes for whom or which the patient might be expected to provide if they were not mentally disordered, and otherwise generally for administering the patient's affairs.

The wide range of specific orders and authorizations which the court may instruct the Receiver to carry out is listed in Section 96 (1) of the Act:

(a) the control (with or without the transfer or vesting of property or the payment into or lodgement in the Supreme Court of money or securities) and management of any property of any patient;

(b) the sale, exchange, charging or other disposition of or dealing with any property of the patient;

(c) the acquisition of any property in the name or on behalf of the patient;

(d) the settlement of any property of the patient, or the gift of any property of the patient to any such persons or for any such purposes as are mentioned in paragraphs (b) and (c) of Section 95 (1) above;

(e) the execution for the patient of a will making any provision (whether by way of disposing of property or exercising a power or otherwise) which could be made by a will executed by the patient if he were not mentally disordered;

(f) the carrying on by a suitable person of any profession, trade or business of the patient;

(g) the dissolution of the partnership of which the patient is a member;

(h) the carrying out of any contract entered into by the patient;

(i) the conduct of legal proceedings in the name of the patient or on his behalf;

(j) the reimbursement out of the property of the patient, with or without interest, of money applied by any person either in payment of the patient's debts (whether legally enforceable or not) or for the maintenance or other benefit of the patient or members of his family or in making provision for other persons or purposes for whom or which he might be expected to provide if he were not mentally disordered;

(k) the exercise of any power (including a power to consent) vested in the patient, whether beneficially, or as guardian or trustee, or otherwise.

The Public Trust Office in London publishes a free explanatory handbook for the guidance of anyone becoming involved with receivership matters. The initial application to the Court for the application of a receiver to carry out any or all of the functions listed above is normally made through a solicitor. The receiver, once appointed, may give instructions to the solicitor, but if the solicitor were to perceive any conflict between the interests of his learning disabled client and the instructions given by the receiver, the solicitor must, in the best interests of his client, refer the matter to the Court of Protection for directions. In cases of extreme urgency where, for instance, there is reason to believe that the individual's money or property is being misappropriated and immediate intervention appears to be necessary for that person's interests to be protected, the Court of Protection may be telephoned to enquire whether an emergency application for the appointment of a receiver is appropriate. Directions may be given directly to the solicitor, or an interim receiver may be appointed with limited powers to deal with the problem. Both of these courses of action may be adopted before the medical evidence normally required for the appointment of a receiver is furnished to the court. In cases of urgency when the necessary medical evidence has already been supplied to the Court but no receiver yet appointed, an order giving the solicitor interim directions may be made. The solicitor making the application for receivership must write to the Court explaining what is required and why it is required urgently. Such situations could include, for instance, the making of a significant necessary purchase or the payment of fees to a residential or nursing home.

Neither the Court nor an appointed receiver may lawfully direct where a learning disabled person shall live. That could be achieved in the case of a minor by a residence order, being one of the Section 8 orders made under the Children Act 1989; or in the case of an adult, by a guardianship order under Sections 7 and 8 of the Mental Health Act 1983. In the latter case, however, the order could only be made if the learning disability were associated with abnormal aggression or serious irresponsibility sufficient to bring the individual concerned within the category of 'mentally impaired' for the purpose of that Act. Jurisdiction over the learning disabled person is limited to the management of property and affairs and, as is also the case with an enduring power of attorney, does not extend to personal management in the sense of care and treatment.[29] Specifically, the powers of the Court have been held not to extend to deciding whether an individual with learning disabilities may be sterilized for therapeutic reasons.[30]

There are certain cases in which, even though an individual with learning disabilities may be incapable of managing their property and affairs, it is unnecessary to go to the lengths of appointing a receiver to deal with them. If the individual's affairs are uncomplicated as in the case of a specific aspect of a patient's financial affairs, or if the value of property and money to be administered does not exceed £5000, the Court may make an order under Rule 9 of the Court of Protection Rules 1994[31] directing any suitable person (usually, the person making the application) to use the assets in a specified way for the benefit of the individual with a learning disability.

Appointeeship

The Department of Social Security has power under Regulation 33 of the Social Security (Claims and Payments) Regulations 1987 to appoint a person to exercise, on behalf of a claimant with a learning disability who is 'unable to act', any right which that person has to social security benefits. The appointee may be authorized not only to collect the social security benefit but also to deal with it and spend it on behalf of the individual who is unable to act for themselves. Standard forms are available from social security offices on which the person seeking to become an appointee must apply in writing to receive the money due to the disabled claimant. Only one appointment is required in respect of all the benefits available. Members of the disabled individual's family, or a suitable solicitor acting on his behalf, should take heed of the reservation expressed by District Judge Ashton in his discussion of the practical working of appointeeship:

> 'The appointee must apply in writing to receive the money due to the claimant, and staff at the local DSS office are instructed to satisfy themselves as to the claimant's inability to manage his affairs and as to the suitability of the proposed appointee. This usually involves seeing the claimant or receiving medical evidence and interviewing the appointee but time pressures upon officers may result in only limited enquiries being made and the procedures are not adequate for dealing with conflicts of principle'.[32]

The policy followed by the Department of Social Security is that a close relative who lives with, or someone else who cares for, the disabled claimant is normally the most suitable person to act as appointee.

Judge Ashton comments, from his practical experience of the working of appointeeship, that 'whilst this relatively informal procedure is helpful, appointment of a parent or carer could have the effect of trapping a claimant within the family through financial control when independence or freedom is desired'.

If the claimant lives in a residential care home or nursing home it is normally desirable that the proprietor of the home become appointee only as a last resort, and not merely as a matter of administrative convenience, if the independence of the disabled person is to be supported as far as is practicable.

The legal powers of the appointee under the terms of the appointment cover only the receipt and handling of the social security benefit. If other assets are involved, other appropriate approaches to managing them on behalf of the disabled individual such as appointment of trustees, or an application to the Court of Protection, should be pursued.

In cases where for any reason appointeeship is inappropriate, another person may be authorized simply to collect the social security benefit for the disabled individual, with the obligation to hand it to them. In practice, there may be an agreed or at least implicit authority to the agent to handle the money in either general or specific ways on behalf of the disabled person. If, however, that individual is or becomes legally incapable by reason of mental incapacity of managing their own affairs, agency is not appropriate. This is because agency depends for its legal validity on the intentional delegation by the principal (in this case the person with learning disability) to the agent. An individual with learning disability may in fact be sufficiently mentally competent to delegate powers to an agent in this way, but great care must be taken to ensure that there is a genuine intention to delegate based on sufficient mental capacity to form that intention. As in the case of the much wider-ranging enduring power of attorney, so here, the mental competence of the disabled individual to express wishes and intentions is crucial. Unlike the enduring power of attorney, however, the much less formal arrangement of simple agency ceases whenever the disabled individual ceases to be able to form the genuine intention to delegate.

Consent and Daily Living

There is no specific set of legal rules or principles applicable to the management and care of people with a learning disability in their daily living.
Needless to say, they should be free from harassment and any interference
which is not necessary for proper care and safety. An individual with
learning disabilities is as entitled to personal dignity as anyone else. In
seeking to maintain adequate safety in daily living, however, carers
(whether in a domestic or an institutional setting) have a legal duty to
provide such care and should preserve against foreseeable danger. Risks
of danger, and in particular of bodily injury, could derive from another
person unused to the ways of the person concerned and unable to react
in a way wholly consistent with that individual's well-being. The risk of
injury could also reside in the person themselves in the form, for example,
of an inability to use a sharp knife safely or to cross a road using adequate
precautions.

Article 8 of the European Convention on Human Rights guarantees the
right to a private life. This right aims to preserve the individual against
unwarranted interference, but it is subject in practice to the legal duty of
care owed to people over whom care responsibilities are exercised. The
integration of people with learning disabilities into 'ordinary' daily living
may carry risks. In the case of those more substantially disabled who may
formerly have been in institutional care but are now, following progressive institutional closures, living in the community, a different type of care
programme may be in place compared with a formerly more restrictive
programme and setting.

While always mindful of professional negligence by practitioners and
carers who fall below a (very basic) level of skill and competence in their
practice, the courts of the UK are wary of becoming involved in allegations
involving lack of care provision by a service as a whole. For instance,
an allegation that a carer in a residential home negligently allowed an
individual with a learning disability to scald themselves as a result of
inadequate supervision is, in general terms, much more likely to succeed
in the courts than an allegation that a particular social services department
failed to provide sufficient day centres in its area to teach individuals with
learning disabilities safety in basic domestic skills.[33]

If, however, an institution (including a hospital, a day centre or a residential home) were to fall short of the standard of care it offers to patients,
clients or residents, a negligence action could be brought directly against
the managers, without an injured person having to prove negligence on
the part of a particular practitioner or staff member.[34] In other words, the
legal duty to take reasonable care not to injure the person concerned is
owed directly to that individual by the institution or organization.

For example, if staffing levels in a group home were inadequate to
provide for the safe care of learning disabled residents, and if a resident
were to come to harm as a result of inadequate surveillance resulting from
the level of staffing, action would lie directly against the proprietors of the
home. The injured resident would not need to prove negligence on the

part of a particular practitioner or carer. If such lack of care could, however, be proved in a particular member of staff, the employer (or employing authority) would be vicariously liable to the injured resident. It is possible for the organization to be legally liable for injury to a resident in both ways, as for instance by an inadequate system for appointing members of staff, one of whom subsequently causes injury to a resident. Each is judged by the level of practice that is reasonable to provide in the particular context of activity in question.

In addition to negligence by practitioners and carers, it is necessary briefly to consider the law of assault and battery as it may affect the daily living of a person with learning disabilities. Battery is the intentional and unlawful physical contact with the person's body, and assault is the reasonable apprehension of the immediate infliction of a battery. Physical difficulties caused to others in daily living by an individual with learning disabilities may lawfully be met by reasonable physical force or contact. The legal principle is that no more than reasonable firmness should be used. Firm but gentle contact such as moving limbs, assisting the person in a particular direction or assistance in sitting or standing, are of course perfectly permissible, despite the fact that an individual with significant learning disabilities might not be able to form the consent which is normally required for such types of contact to be lawful.

In the event of an individual with learning disability presenting challenging behaviour, the proportionality principle is equally applicable,[35] with the result that force or violence offered may carefully be met with sufficient force to preserve the safety of that person and of any other(s), including staff or carers, who may foreseeably be affected by it. In the case of intervention by practitioners and carers the legal principle allows challenging behaviour to be anticipated and preventive action to be taken. Failure to exercise normal care, especially in the case of a trained professional, could amount to actionable negligence in the event of injury. Participation in games, sports and similar activities involving physical contact may involve playful physical contact greater than ordinary firmness. The general rule is provided that such contact is not 'hostile'[36] it is permissible, and there is no reason to believe the rule to be any different in the case of genuine physical activities with individuals whose learning disability might call into question their capacity to consent positively to the level of physical contact involved. Much will in practice depend on the experience and professionalism of carers in forming a reasonable assessment of the wishes and the reasonable tolerance of those in their charge.

Physical contact by way of care and treatment, including for example dental treatment and physiotherapy, and even simple bathing and general personal hygiene, present particular problems. Not only may evidence of positive consent be lacking but actual dislike or resistance may be encountered. Such cases are discussed in the first section of this chapter devoted to consent in care and treatment. Attention in this section has so far been devoted to wrongs which may befall a disabled person. The remainder of this section examines the impact on daily life of some principal services

Psychiatry in Learning Disability

which people with learning disabilities are legally entitled to receive, and their rights in relation to them.

In practice, many individuals with learning disabilities will be supported in their daily life by one of the services (such as social, housing, education) provided by their local authority. Authorities are responsible for ensuring that individuals in their area with learning disabilities receive the care they need in the community. The objective, says Gostin,[37] 'is to help people live normally in a home-like, non-segregative, environment where they can receive an array of medical, nursing and social services'.

Plans relating to personal care of people with learning disability ('care packages') are the legal responsibility of local social service authorities. Section 47(1) of the National Health Service and Community Care Act 1990 provides that:

> 'where it appears to a local authority that any person for whom they may provide or arrange for the provision of community care services (that is, living in their area) may be in need of any such services, the authority (a) shall carry out an assessment of his needs for those services; and (b) having regard to the results of that assessment, shall then decide whether his needs call for the provision by them of any such services'.

This general duty on local authorities is made specific with regard to individual cases following the requirement imposed on authorities by Section 4 of the Disabled Persons (Services, Consultation and Representation) Act 1986. Referring to that provision, Section 47(2) of the 1990 Act provides that:

> 'If at any time during the assessment of the needs of any person ... it appears to a local authority that he is a disabled person, the authority (a) shall proceed to make such a decision as to the services he requires as is mentioned in section 4 of the Disabled Persons (Services, Consultation and Representation) Act 1986 without his requesting them to do so under that section; and (b) shall inform him that they will be doing so and of his rights under that Act'.

Section 4 of the 1986 Act was enacted in response to the fact that local authorities were not carrying out assessments either consistently or regularly. The Act imposed a duty to assess the needs of people for 'welfare' services at the request of the disabled person or of any person providing a substantial amount of care on a regular basis. Welfare services are identified in Section 2 of the Chronically Sick and Disabled Persons Act 1970 as including:

(a) practical assistance in the home;
(b) provision of, or assistance in obtaining, wireless, television, library or similar recreational facilities;
(c) provision of facilities of lectures, games, outings or other recreational facilities outside the home or assistance in taking advantage of educational facilities;
(d) provision of facilities for, or assistance in, travelling to and from home for the purpose of participating in services;
(e) assistance in arranging for the carrying out of any works of adaptation in the home or the provision of any additional facilities designed to secure greater safety, comfort or convenience;
(f) facilitating the taking of holidays, whether at holiday homes or otherwise and whether provided under arrangements made by the authority or otherwise;

(g) provisions of meals, whether in the home or elsewhere;
(h) provision of, or assistance in obtaining, a telephone and any special equipment necessary for its use.

Under the 1990 Act, the legal responsibility of local authorities goes further. They must assess an individual who in their view needs 'community care services', without being requested to do so, and must then decide on the extent and type of provision (if any) to be made. 'Community care services' are services which a local authority may provide or arrange under any of the following legal provisions: National Assistance Act 1948, Part III; Health Services and Public Health Act 1968, Section 45; National Health Service Act 1977, Section 21 and Schedule 8; and Section 117 of the Mental Health Act 1983.

Under Section 21(1) of the National Assistance Act 1948 the authority must make arrangements for providing such residential accommodation for persons who by reason of age, illness, disability or any other circumstances are in need of care and attention which is not otherwise available to them. In making such arrangements, Section 21(2) provides that local authority must have regard to the welfare of all persons for whom accommodation is provided and, in particular, to the need for providing accommodation of different descriptions suited to the various needs of such persons. This is commonly known as 'Part III accommodation', and may typically be used in the support of individuals with a learning disability either from elsewhere in the community or, following the progressive closure of large institutions, on transfer from them.

Schedule 8 to the National Health Service Act 1977 provides:

> 'A local social services authority may with the Secretary of State's approval and, to such extent as he may direct, shall make arrangements for the purpose of the prevention of illness and for the care of persons suffering from illness and for the after-care of persons who have been so suffering'.

Such approval from the Secretary of State is found in Appendix 3 to Department of Health Circular LAC (93) 10. Local authorities are directed to provide:

> 'centres (including training centres and day centres) or other facilities (including domiciliary facilities, whether in premises managed by the [local authority] or otherwise, for training or occupation of persons suffering from or who have been suffering from mental disorder'.

Section 117 of the Mental Health Act 1983 imposes a duty on local authorities, jointly with their health authority counterparts, to provide 'after-care services' for any individual to whom the section applies, until such time as they are jointly 'satisfied that the person concerned is no longer in need of such services'. The mentally disordered individuals to whom the section applies are a relatively narrow group consisting of people who have been detained in hospital under what may broadly be termed one of the 'longer-term' sections of the Mental Health Act (typically, a treatment order under Section 3 or a hospital order made by a court under Section 37) and who are discharged from section into the community.

As to the respective legal significance of, and precise relationship between, this provision and the duty under Schedule 8 of the National Health Service Act 1977 (above), Jones comments[38] that the view 'that this section duplicates the provisions of the 1977 Act is not entirely correct because while the 1977 Act directs local authorities and health authorities to provide for the after-care of the *generality* of mentally disordered persons, this section places a duty on local authorities and health authorities to consider the after-care needs of each individual to whom the section applies'. The enforceability of the individualized duty under Section 117 was considered in *R v Ealing District Health Authority, ex parte Fox*[39] in which a Mental Health Review Tribunal decided to discharge a detained patient into the community. Medical practitioners, including in particular the consultant general psychiatrist for the patient's home area, were not optimistic about the patient's prospects in the community and were unwilling to support a care scheme. The court held that the duty imposed jointly on the local authority and the health authority is enforceable by the individual. The duty (even prospective) to provide after-care services for individuals falling within the ambit of Section 117 was held by Mr Justice Otton to be a continuing duty to the individual which is 'triggered' by that individual's discharge from hospital. The duty to make appropriate provision of services has, since 1993, been consequent on the duty to assess need under Section 47 of the National Health Service and Community Care Act, 1990. This Act by implication includes the services referred to on page 274.

The enforcement of the duty is by administrative law remedies. The judge quashed the local authority's decision (based on its psychiatrists' opinions) not to put in place an after-care package for the patient in question, by an order of *certiorari*. He declined, however, to make a further order of *mandamus* to enforce the local authority's legal duty because this would have committed them to a specific package of care before they had a reasonable opportunity to devise and establish such a package.

In general, however, duties of local authorities and health authorities towards individuals with a learning disability are not enforceable by the aggrieved individual but only on a broader front. There is a general power of the Secretary of State to declare local authorities in default if they fail to comply with their social services duties,[40] and similar powers in respect of health authorities are provided by Section 85 of the National Health Service Act 1977. The procedure is that the Secretary of State calls upon the authority to account for failure to exercise its functions and may direct the authority to comply; alternatively, in very rare instances, the Secretary of State may appoint commissioners to take over and exercise the defaulting authority's functions. If, short of this final step, directions are given but are not complied with, they may be enforced by an order of *mandamus* from the High Court. Legal action under such a procedure is brought on behalf of ('ex parte') an aggrieved individual, as distinct from that person commencing legal proceedings directly as an individual.

If the issue concerns the level of financial, human and other resources (such as accommodation or day centres), these default powers may be the only legal remedy available. As stated earlier, even in cases of individual hardship or pain and suffering the courts are unwilling to become involved in directions which would effectively amount to the management of a service, be it local authority or health.[41]

References

1. Sidaway v. Bethlem Royal Hospital Governors (1985) 1 All ER 643.
2. See Lord Templeman, ibid, at pp. 665–666.
3. (1985) 1 All ER 643.
4. Ibid at p. 666.
5. Ibid at p. 661.
6. (1993) 4 Med. LR 151.
7. Section 58, relating to treatment to which Part IV of the Act applies.
8. Kennedy & Grubb (1994) *Medical Law-Text with Materials*, 2nd edn. p. 107. London: Butterworths.
9. (1989) 2 All ER 545.
10. Kennedy & Grubb, op. cit. p. 282.
11. Re F: F v West Berkshire Health Authority (1989) 2 All ER 545, at p. 551.
12. Superintendent of Belchertown State School v. Saikewicz 370 NE 2d 417 (1977)
13. Law Comm. No. 231, *Report on Mental Incapacity* HMSO (1995); HC 189.
14. Kennedy & Grubb, op. cit. p. 142.
15. And see Kennedy & Grubb. op. cit. pp. 137–140.
16. March 26, 1985; appl 16/1983/72/110.
17. Ashton (1992) *Mental Handicap and the Law*, p. 115. London: Sweet & Maxwell.
18. Gunn (1991) *Sex and the Law*, 3rd edn. Family Planning Association; p. 27.
19. Gunn (1996) *Sex and the Law*, 4th edn. Family Planning Association; p. 27.
20. Gostin, *Mental Health Services – Law and Practice*, para 25.08.3. London: Shaw & Sons.
21. Gibbon v. Wright (1954) 91 CLR 423.
22. Gostin, op. cit. para. 23.26.1.
23. S.I. 1994 No. 3047.
24. S.I. 1990 No. 1376.
25. Gostin, op. cit. para. 23.28.
26. Ashton, op. cit. p. 32; and see Law Commission Report No. 231 *Mental Incapacity* (1995).
27. Gostin, op. cit. para. 23.03.3.
28. Ashton, op. cit. p. 547.
29. Ashton, op. cit. p. 551.
30. T. v. T. (1988) 1 ALL ER 613; Re F. (a Minor) (1989) 1 All ER 1155 (CA).
31. S.I. 1994 No. 3046.
32. Ashton, op. cit. p. 565; and see S.I. 1987 No. 1968.
33. For an account of the law relating to legal proceedings for negligence, see *Speller's Law Relating to Hospitals*, 7th edn, chs 5 & 6 (1994). London: Chapman & Hall.
34. See Wilsher v. Essex AHA (1986) 3 All ER 801 (CA).
35. Albert v. Lavin (1981) 3 All ER 878 (HL); and see Gostin, op. cit. para. 21.09.
36. Wilson v. Pringle (1986) 2 All ER 440; though Lord Goff in Re F (reference 1, Supra) doubted the correctness of 'hostile' in many contexts, including that of medical treatment.
37. Gostin, op. cit. para. 4.02.
38. Jones R (1996) *Mental Health Act Manual*, 5th edn, para. 1–706. London: Sweet & Maxwell.
39. (1993) 3 All ER 170. And see reference 38 at p. 315 for explanation of the relationship between duty to assess under Section 47 National Health Service and Community Care Act 1990, and duty to provide under Section 117 Mental Health Act 1983.
40. See Ashton, op. cit. p. 230 and reference 32.
41. R. v. Secretary of State for Social Services, ex parte Hincks (1980) 1 BMLR 93 (CA).

12

Sex Offenders with Learning Disabilities

Kenneth Day

Introduction

Sex offenders comprise the largest group of learning disabled offenders. They are more likely than non-disabled sex offenders to receive a custodial sentence and account for between a one-third to one-half of all admissions to specialist treatment units. Considering their importance, they have been surprisingly neglected. Recently, however, changing policies for the care of individuals with learning disability have stimulated interest in this small but important group of patients and there is now an expanding research literature and service base. The aim of this chapter is to present what is currently known about learning disabled sex offenders with a particular focus on treatment.

Prevalence

The overall prevalence of offending by learning disabled people is low. Epidemiological studies give a point prevalence of 0.5–1% and a lifetime risk of 3–5%.[1] Data on sex offending is limited: 3% of learning disabled men in a large metropolitan area in the USA were found to present severe sexual aggression problems[2] and a literature review suggested that 10–15% of all sex offences are committed by the learning disabled.[3] Studies of learning disabled offenders consistently reveal an over-representation of sex offences with an incidence 4–6 times that in the non-disabled offenders.[4–9] Richardson and colleagues,[10] in a follow-up study of learning disabled children to age 22 years, found that 12.5% of the males had been involved in sexual misconduct (although not necessarily prosecuted) compared with only 1% of matched controls. Higher detection and prosecution rates have been advanced as an explanation[3,11] but this has been disputed[12] and in a recent study of learning disabled sex offenders rates for nondetection and nonprosecution were found to be comparable to those for nonretarded sex offenders.[13] Knowledge that a sex offender has a learning disability has also been found to be an important factor influencing the decision not to report or prosecute.[13–15] A higher risk for sex offending in the learning disabled is not surprising in view of their impaired cognitive and adaptive behaviour skills and, until recently, society's repressive and restrictive attitude towards their sexuality.[1]

Clinical Features and Offence Behaviour

Sex offending is essentially a male phenomenon (there is no record in the literature of sex offending by learning disabled females) and invariably a solitary activity. Learning disabled sex offenders share many features in common with nonretarded sex offenders. The profile in Table 12.1 is typical. The bulk of offences are committed by youths and young men functioning in the mild to borderline intellectual range who show a high incidence of adjustment problems at school, delinquency, other behaviour problems, psychiatric illness, organic brain damage, family psychopathology and psychosocial deprivation.[3,13,16–19]

While the overall pattern of offending is similar to that of nonretarded sex offenders (Table 12.2) there are a number of significant differences which provide important clues to psychopathology:

- Learning disabled sex offenders commit a high percentage of minor or nuisance offences and are much less likely to be convicted of a serious offence than nonretarded sex offenders: offences involving physical violence are rare (Mein R (1959) *A Survey of Mentally Defective Sex Offenders in Harperbury Hospital*, unpublished report, Table 12.2.[4,6,13,17,19,20]
- Learning disabled sex offenders show far less specificity for age and sex of victim and type of offence committed than nondisabled sexual recidivists.[13,17,19,21,22] In a recent study of 47 learning disabled sex offenders two-thirds of the recidivists had committed more than one category of sex offence, 20% both homosexual and

Table 12.1.   Psychosocial profile of 47 male learning disabled sex offenders (from Day[13]).

Average Age	23.9 yrs (range 15–63)
Average IQ	59.5 (range 43–82)
Brain Damage – definite history	8 (17%)
Brain Damage – suggestive history	12 (25%)
Chromosome Abn.	2 (4.25%)
Distinctive Physical Disability	24 (51%)
PH Psychiatric Illness	15 (32%)
Psychosocial Deprivation	23 (48%)
FH Delinq/Criminality	10 (23%)
Delinq Neighbourhood	16 (30%)
PH Behaviour Problems	32 (66%)
PH Conviction for Nonsex Offenders	22 (47%)
PH Residential Care	27 (56%)
Sexual Naivety	12 (25%)
Relationship Difficulties	29 (63%)
Sexual Inexperience	28 (58%)
Immature, isolated	30 (63%)
Sociopathic Personality	18 (38%)

heterosexual offences and 50% offences against both children and adults.[13] Adolescents with a learning disability have also been found to be less discriminating in their sex play – engaging in both homosexual and heterosexual activity, and to have a wider spread of victim characteristics than non-learning disabled adolescent sex offenders.[17] These findings suggest that circumstance and opportunity rather than sexual preference or orientation are the overriding factors in the choice of victim and type of offence committed in the vast majority of cases and point to sexual immaturity and inexperience as important causative factors.

- The majority of female victims are under the age of 16 and a substantial proportion under 11 years[13,19] in contrast to non-disabled sex offenders who offend mainly against adult women; this is a reflection of sexual immaturity, difficulties in developing adult heterosexual relationships, the easier accessibility of child victims and a lack of awareness of social norms rather than paedophilic tendencies. The sex of a child victim is similarly most often a matter of chance than sexual preference.
- Offences against adult women rarely occur in the context of an established or developing relationship and the majority of victims are unknown to the offender,[13,17] compared with nondisabled sex offenders where the victim is known in 80% of cases and consensual in one-fifth.[21] This is a further reflection of poor sociosexual skills and the lack of opportunities for and, until recently, active discouragement of sexual relationships between the learning disabled people. Failure to appreciate the more subtle aspects of relationships and misinterpretations of kindliness and concern occasionally lead to inappropriate sexual advances being made to professional carers, neighbours, acquaintances or family friends.[3,13,22]
- True sexual deviancy is rare. The learning disabled lack the intellectual sophistication and cognitive and imaginative capacity to develop and feed some of the more extreme paraphilias. It is a mistake to conceptualize all sex offending behaviour in the learning disabled as aberrant, as is sometimes done. The majority of cases of indecent exposure, for example, are crude expressions of frustrated sexual feelings and sometimes an invitation to further sexual activity rather than true exhibitionism.[13] Attention has been drawn to the possible role of poor sociosexual skills and social isolation in the genesis of autoerotic fetishism and transvestism in the learning disabled.[23]

Psychopathology

Modern theories of causation emphasize the multifactorial nature of sex offending and distinguish predisposing and triggering factors.[24,25] A statistically significant association has been demonstrated between unstable upbringing and the presence of behaviour disorder and criminal

Table 12.2. Sexual offences committed by learning disabled men (adapted from Day)[13].

Offence/incident	Day (1994)[13] (n = 47, 191 offences)	Milner (1949)[117] (n = 54, 65 offences)	Mein (1959), unpublished report (n = 83, 83 offences)	Criminal Statistics (1988)[118] (offenders found guilty or cautioned for indictable offences)
Indecent exposure	47 (24.6%)	13 (20%)	29 (35.7%)	–
Heterosexual	106 (55.5%) [67%]	37 (56.7%)	32 (39.6%)	6515 (64.59%)
Rape and attempted rape	1 (0.5%) [1%]	4 (6.1%)	1 (1.2%)	540 (5%)
Actual bodily harm	3 (1.5%)	–	–	–
Unlawful intercourse (<13 years)	1 (0.5%) [1%]	⎱ 5 (7.6%) (both combined)	–	214 (1.99%)
Unlawful intercourse (13–16 years)	3 (1.5%) [3%]	⎰	–	1555 (14.5%)
Indecent assault	62 (32.3%) [62%]	26 (40%)	32 (39.6%)	3961 (36.9%)
Incest	–	2 (3%)	1 (1.2%)	245 (2.2%)
Bigamy, abduction, procuration	5 (2.6%)	–	–	–
Exploiting severely mentally handicapped	1 (0.5%)	–	–	–
Associating with under-age girls	1 (0.5%)	–	–	–
Loitering with intent	–	–	–	–
Inappropriate advances/suggestions	23 (12%)	–	–	–
Following	3 (1.5%)	–	–	–
Peeping	2 (1%)	–	–	–
Obscene telephone call	1 (0.5%)	–	–	–
Homosexual	24 (12.4%) [18%]	13 (19.7%)	20 (25.7%)	3677 (35.41%)
Buggery	2 (1%) [2%]	5 (7.6%)	1 (1.2%)	412 (3.8%)
Gross indecency	2 (1%) [2%]	2 (3%)	3 (12.3%)	1496 (13.9%)
Indecency with male under 16 years	2 (1%) [2%]	–	15 (18.5%)	334 (3%)
Indecent assault on a male	12 (6.3%) [12%]	6 (9.1%)	–	736 (6.5%)
Indecent advances/suggestions	6 (3.1%)	–	–	–
Soliciting/importuning	–	–	1 (1.2%)	699 (6.5%)
Other				
Cross-dressing	8 (4.2%)	–	–	–
Stealing female underwear	6 (3.1%)	–	–	–
Bestiality	–	2 (3%)	–	–

( ) % of total offences.
[ ] % of indictable offences.

behaviour, including sex offending, in the learning disabled.[10,26] Although faulty child rearing, dysfunctional parental relationships, psychosocial deprivation and maladaptive social learning are undoubtedly key factors underlying antisocial sexual behaviour in some learning disabled sex offenders many come from warm, stable and caring families and show little evidence of significant psychopathology.[13] The key predisposing factor in the genesis of their sex offending is the restrictive and protective attitudes of society, family and carers which limits opportunities for normal sexual expression, restricts access to sociosexual information and often results in inconsistent responses to sexual behaviour or misdemeanours, with resultant sexual frustration and confused concepts.[2,15,27,28] Other important predisposing factors include:

- poor impulse control and poor anger management skills, which are frequently associated with organic brain damage[13,17,18,20,29,30]
- low self-esteem, feelings of stigmatization, isolation, loneliness, low assertiveness and high social anxiety[29,30,31]
- poor life management skills[30]
- poor interpersonal skills, difficulties in mixing with the opposite sex, poor courtship skills and a low level of pre-offence hetero-sexual experience[3,13,20,30]
- delayed development of reasoning and moral judgement and diffi-culties in internalizing social expectations due to cognitive impair-ment[32]
- serious deficiencies in sociosexual knowledge including the law and behavioural codes, age and gender appropriateness, deviant and nondeviant behaviour[3,13,20,22,28,30,33]
- cognitive distortions with sexual conservatism and stereotypic sexual beliefs about women[3,22,34]
- minor but visible physical disabilities such as speech impediment, squint or gait disturbance which reduce self-confidence and impair social interaction.[13,35]

Learning disabled people have been shown to be vulnerable to sex abuse both as children and adults[36-38] and there is evidence that this may be a causative factor in sex offending.[27,39] One-quarter of learning disabled sex offenders in one study admitted to some homosexual experience as youths and this was associated with subsequent homosexual offending,[13] and 20% of a cohort of learning disabled adolescent sex offenders had a history of sexual abuse as children.[17] In an incidence study of sex abuse in learning disabled people 50% of the males were found to display significant sexual misconduct.[34] The relationship is a complex one and, as in the nondisabled, has yet to be fully explored, in particular the distinction between those who do and those who do not go on to commit sex offences.

There is some evidence of an association between sex chromosome abnormalities in learning disabled men and sex offending but this is far from certain and more research is needed.[1,40-42]

The most commonly reported triggering events are emotional stress, cessation of active sex life, life events such as the loss of a caring relative, reduced structure and supervision and special temptations and opportunities like baby sitting or easy access to vulnerable learning disabled women.[13,30] In contrast to nondisabled sex offenders alcohol is seldom a factor[21] – a reflection not only of the low use of alcohol by learning disabled people but also the different aetiology of their sex offending behaviour.[13] A high incidence of alcohol and substance abuse, however, has been reported in one study from the USA.[43] Offending as a direct consequence of active psychiatric illness is extremely rare. In the only study to examine this, mental illness was found to be the causative factor in three out of 191 sexual incidents (a prevalence of 1.6%). There were two cases of minor indecent assault due to hypomania and one of serious indecent assault against a 6-year-old girl by a 63-year-old man with early arteriosclerotic dementia; all three men were of previously impeccable character.[13] The relationship between pornography and sex offending is a controversial issue and there is no published work on the learning disabled. Clinical experience suggests that they make little use of pornographic material; however there was one man in the author's study who had on two occasions attempted to strangle partners following consensual sexual intercourse, and later confessed that he had fantasized about this for some months after having seen *The Boston Strangler* on television.[13]

Offender Typology

Three broad categories of learning disabled offenders are suggested by the research data:[13,17,20,29]

- *Developmental.* The largest group numerically. These individuals are typically shy and immature with a limited sexual knowledge and little or no sexual experience. They usually come from warm and caring, if somewhat overprotective, families and have a low prevalence of psychosocial pathology and other antisocial behaviour. Their sex offending is essentially a developmental problem – crude attempts to fulfil normal sexual impulses in the context of lack of normal outlets, poor adaptive behaviour skills, sexual naivety, poor impulse control and social ineptness. They tend to commit less serious offences and are less likely to become recidivists, but if they do they tend to commit a broader range of sex offences than the other groups, reflecting the opportunistic and undifferentiated nature of their sexual responses. Treatment measures should focus on sex education and counselling, training in relationship and other skills and improving self-confidence and social awareness.
- *Sociopathic.* A smaller group but highly significant in terms of management and treatment needs. These are markedly damaged individuals who show a high prevalence of sociopathic personality disorder, psychosocial deprivation, brain damage and other maladaptive behaviours including nonsex offences. Their sex

284 Psychiatry in Learning Disability

offending is the consequence of a deep-seated antisocial behaviour disorder and they are more likely to commit serious offences and to become persistent offenders. They require intensive treatment and care in a structured and controlled environment.

- *Sexually deviant*. A small percentage of learning disabled men appear to engage exclusively in homosexual or paedophilic behaviour, exhibitionism, cross-dressing or other fetishisms.[13,23,44-47] They show similar characteristics to nondisabled offenders in these categories and require specific treatment interventions aimed at reducing their deviant orientation and establishing normal sexual behaviour.

To these some would add a further group, the sexually abused. These are offenders whose personal experience of sex abuse is considered to be the major aetiological factor in their sex offending and who require a treatment approach which focuses on this (B. Lutjenhuis, personal communication, 1996). This is certainly an area which merits further research both in terms of the relationship between sex abuse and sex offending in the learning disabled and treatment measures. Research in nondisabled sex offenders suggests that the relationship is complex and far from direct.[48]

Assessment and Examination

The purpose of assessment is to determine the cause of the offence behaviour, identify treatment priorities, evaluate treatment response and assess the risk of reoffending.[49,50] The aim of baseline assessment is to build as complete a picture of the offender as possible – with a particular focus on his sexual development, offence history and factors pertinent to the current offence. A systematic approach utilizing self report, other information sources, behavioural observation, physiological measurements and psychological assessment should be adopted.[50] The minimum information required is shown in Table 12.3. The history given by the patient should always be supplemented by and compared with accounts obtained from others. Information should be sought from as many collateral sources as possible, including relatives, care workers, probation and social services, the statement(s) of the offender, his victim(s) and any witnesses. Photographic and any other evidence pertaining to the current offence should always be obtained together with the previous medical, psychiatric and other records including details of all previous offences. A full physical examination should be carried out noting minor and major physical imperfections/disabilities. Psychological assessment should include IQ, educational attainments, adaptive behaviour skills, personality profile, a systematic assessment of psychosexual knowledge and a structured analysis of offence behaviour utilizing the available schedules and scales.[49,51] A routine electroencephalogram (EEG) should be carried out to exclude organic brain damage and chromosome analysis if a genosomal abnormality is suspected.

Table 12.3. Examination of sex offenders with learning disabilities.

History	
Current offence	Nature, circumstances, external and internal contextual events, e.g. life events, conflicts, pressures, temptations, level of support and supervision
Previous sex and other offence(s)	Dates, nature, disposal (including offences not prosecuted)
Sexual history	Childhood sex abuse, sexual experiences, sexual development, sexual orientation, relationships, marriage
Neuropsychiatric and medical history	Other conduct/behaviour disorders including assaultive behaviour, mental illness, epilepsy, medical problems, hospitalization
Personality features and personality type	Friends, interests, relationships, status, gang membership. Personality disorder
Current functioning	Social skills and competences
Personal history	Upbringing, family structure, schooling, employment/occupation, socio-economic status, neighbourhood
Family factors	Family history of mental illness, mental handicap, delinquency, criminality or other psychopathology. Dysfunctional family
Examination	
Mental state	Intellectual status, degree of literacy, psychiatric illness, personality disorder, fitness to plead. Sociosexual knowledge, sexual orientation and attitudes Attitude to offence, victim empathy, dangerousness and risk of further offending Attitude to treatment
Physical state	Minor and major defects
Investigations	
Psychometry	IQ, educational attainments, personality, adaptive behaviour skills, assessment of sociosexual knowledge, assessment of sexual orientation, structured analysis of offence behaviour
EEG studies	As indicated
Chromosome studies	As indicated
Phallometry	As indicated

Sex Offending Behaviour and Sexual History

The nature and circumstances of the current offence should be thoroughly explored including: the context in which it occurred, evidence of planning, the dynamics of victim selection, intensity of sexual arousal prior to offence, the use of force, any injury, sadistic behaviour and any triggering events or contributory factors including level of supervision and support at the time. A detailed sexual history should be obtained covering sexual development, history of sexual abuse, masturbatory patterns, deviant sexual fantasies and practices, heterosexual and homosexual experiences. Psychiatric examination should focus on attitude to the offence: acceptance of responsibility, denial, minimization, rationalization, understanding its seriousness and possible consequences, victim empathy, concepts of right and wrong, knowledge of sociosexual mores and the laws governing sexual behaviour and ability to discriminate deviant from nondeviant behaviour.

Sexual Orientation

If the victim is a child or a male an assessment of sexual orientation should be made. Distinguishing true paraphilia, which is comparatively rare, from deviant sexual behaviour secondary to sexual immaturity or opportunism is a key diagnostic issue which sets the treatment agenda.[52] Mitchell[53] offers some helpful clinical guidelines in relation to homosexual behaviour which can be applied more widely. Frequent homosexual behaviour accompanied by a clear emotional involvement with the victim(s) and the constant seeking out of partners of the same sex in the presence of ample opportunities for contact with, but no interest in, heterosexual appropriate partners is indicative of true homosexuality, but infrequent engagement in homosexual behaviour without emotional attachment and clear evidence of an interest in heterosexual partners but little or no opportunity for contact is strongly suggestive of situational homosexuality. A more structured approach is provided by the Sexual Interest Card Sort.[27,54] The most reliable method is penile plethysmograph which has been used successfully in the learning disabled but it is not widely available.[19,22,43,49] Pupillary response is a less intrusive and potentially useful technique which has not so far been used in the learning disabled.[41]

Risk Assessment

Assessment of dangerousness and the risk of further offending is crucial in shaping the initial treatment plan, the decision whether or not to admit to hospital, evaluation of treatment response and decisions about discharge and discontinuation of treatment. Thoroughness and persistence in data collection about dangerous behaviour and a healthy scepticism at all times is required.[55-57] Factors generally associated with a high risk of reoffending include a past history of sexual or aggressive offences, multiple paraphilias, both male and female victims, multiple victims, extrafamilial abuse and few social supports.[58-60] Additional factors relevant to the learning disabled are offender typology, impulsivity, poor understanding of the offence, vulnerable victim(s), use of physical force and a history of behaviour disorders and nonsex offences, especially fire setting and animal torture.[16,26,43] Dangerousness, defined as a tendency to inflict serious physical injury or psychological harm on others,[56] should be distinguished from risk of further offending. Prins[61] gives a helpful list of questions which should be addressed including current capacity for coping with provocation, the extent to which the patient has come to terms with what he did, the nature of the offence, responsiveness to and compliance with medication and other treatments and the level of personality disorder. The unpredictability of much sex offending by the learning disabled compounds the difficulties of risk assessment.

Psychiatric Reports to the Courts

Psychiatrists should always be mindful of the need to provide a psychiatric report for the courts. A detailed discussion of the preparation of such reports is outside the scope of this chapter and excellent guidance is available elsewhere.[62] The courts are primarily interested in the mental state of the offender and its bearing on the offence committed, his fitness to plead, dangerousness and the risk of further offending and recommendations for disposal. Psychiatric reports should be constructed around these key areas, each of which should be comprehensively addressed with supporting evidence from the history, the examination of the patient and where appropriate the research literature. A learning disabled person is fit to plead if he is able to understand the nature and possible consequence of the charge; understand the difference between a plea of guilty and not guilty; instruct counsel; follow evidence in court and challenge a juror.[63] Mildly learning disabled offenders and those functioning in the borderline range are normally fit to plead although each case must be judged individually, the greatest weight being given to an individual's ability to understand the charges he faces and the difference between a plea of guilty and not guilty.[35]

A related issue is the reliability of the statement(s) made by the offender to the police (and indeed those of the victim(s) and other witnesses should they also be learning disabled). Gudjonsson, a pioneer in this field, has shown that people with a mild learning disability are more likely than the general population to have an impaired understanding of a caution and their legal rights, to be vulnerable, acquiescent and suggestible during interrogation, and not to appreciate the potentially important consequences of making a false confession, and he has developed the Gudjonsson Suggestibility Scale to assist in the clinical assessment of the reliability of statements made by an offender.[64,65] Current UK legislation requires that a suspect thought to suffer from learning disability should be interviewed by the police in the presence of an independent 'appropriate adult' who must be either a lawyer or someone with experience in the care of the learning disabled (Police and Criminal Evidence Act, England and Wales 1984). More recently attention has been given to assisting the police in the identification of learning disabled suspects.[65]

On-going Assessment

Assessment should be a continuous and ongoing process. Progress evaluation should cover attitude to sexual behaviour: openness and honesty, acceptance of responsibility, understanding of assault cycle and risk signals, positive social interactions, general behaviour and social skills.

Treatment and Management

The aim of treatment is to prevent further sex offending and replace it with safe and acceptable sexual behaviour by assisting maturation, increasing self-control and personal responsibility, establishing acceptable social mores, instilling a sense of personal worth, improving social, occupational and educational skills and tackling specific offence behaviour. Sex offending frequently occurs in the context of a wider range of problems, including other inappropriate behaviours, all of which need to be taken into account in treatment. A holistic approach which addresses all aspects of the patient's functioning as well as offence-specific interventions is therefore required.

Treatment Setting

Treatment should be carried out in the least restrictive environment which is safe and suitable. The safety of the public is paramount. Minor offenders assessed as likely to cooperate with treatment and unlikely to reoffend can usually be managed satisfactorily at home provided that an adequate network of support and specialist services, including specific interventions for the patient's sexual problems, is available. A community residential placement may be necessary if the family is unable to cope or there is a need for more structure and support or because of ill-feeling in the immediate neighbourhood. Indications for admission to a specialist hospital unit are:

- when ordered by the court – offences serious enough to warrant a custodial sentence in the normal course of events;
- public safety – where the patient is judged to pose a significant danger to the public and likely to reoffend on the basis of the current offence and his past history;
- an in-depth assessment is required which cannot be carried out in the community;
- persistent offences which have proved unresponsive to treatment in the community even though the offences themselves have been minor in nature, e.g. repeated indecent exposure;
- inability to meet care and treatment needs in the community due to lack of specialist personnel and/or facilities or where factors unrelated to the offence such as nomadic existence, family breakdown, patient unreliable, unable or unwilling to cooperate with treatment and care, make care in the community difficult or impracticable.

Legal and Ethical Issues

Minor offenders can usually be treated on a voluntary basis in the community although the courts will often wish to impose some form of legal restraint to ensure that the treatment is properly carried out and the patient adequately supervised. In these circumstances, or if there are doubts about cooperation, a Guardianship Order under the Mental Health Act 1983 or a Psychiatric Probation Order should be considered.

Some form of legal restraint is desirable for inpatients – it protects the rights of the patient, facilitates motivation and cooperation and provides a framework for the implementation of the treatment plan. For convicted offenders this would normally be a Hospital Order (with or without restriction) under the Mental Health Act 1983 and a Civil Order (Section 3) in patients not brought before the courts. A psychiatric Probation Order with a condition of inpatient treatment is a useful alternative for those patients who do not fulfil the Mental Health Act criteria or who are judged to require only a short period of hospital care and has the added advantage of a guaranteed period of statutory aftercare following discharge.[49]

Whatever the legal framework it is important that motivation is established[49] and that the consent of the patient to all aspects of the treatment programme, particularly sex behaviour management programmes and antilibidinal medication, is obtained. However, in decisions about the treatment programme the clinician must weigh the benefits and potential risks as they influence both the patient and society.[66] Valid consent requires that the patient is able to understand the nature of the treatment and why it is proposed, its principal benefits and risks, the consequences of not receiving it and the availability or otherwise of alternative treatments.[67] Most patients functioning in the borderline and mild learning disability range are able to give valid consent provided that the explanation and accompanying advice is couched in appropriately simple terms. Judgements as to whether or not a patient is consenting should relate to the particular treatment at the particular time. Specific consent issues are addressed in later sections of this chapter.

Treatment Programme

A properly formulated treatment programme with explicitly stated goals and time scales is essential. All personnel involved in the delivery of the programme should work to an agreed strategy and meet regularly to monitor progress and review the treatment plan. The principal components of the treatment programme are listed in Table 12.4 and described below.

The precise content of the programme will depend upon the needs of the individual: not all components are required to the same extent by every patient. When the problem is essentially developmental in origin the treatment approach should reflect the wider need for social skills training and not focus too narrowly on sexual difficulties: sex education, individual counselling, training in relationship and life skills and increased opportunities for developing relationships with the opposite sex may be all that is needed. Patients whose sex offending is part of a generalized antisocial behaviour disorder or who are persistent or recurrent offenders require a comprehensive treatment programme including socialization training and offence-specific interventions, usually on an inpatient basis. Where there

Table 12.4. Treatment programme for sex offenders with learning disabilities – key components.

General	Life skills training
	Treatment of psychiatric and medical problems
	Counselling and supportive psychotherapy
	Relaxation therapy and anger management
	Socialization programmes
	Family and carer support
Offence-specific interventions	Sex education programmes
	Sociosexual skills training
	Sex behaviour management programmes
	Antilibidinal medication
	Treatment for sexually deviant behaviour
Rehabilitation, aftercare and relapse prevention	

is clear evidence of deviant sexual orientation the focus should be on measures to decrease deviant sexual arousal and increase appropriate sexual arousal and the development of coping skills.

Life Skills Training

A package of personal, social, occupational, educational and recreational skills training is a key component of all treatment programmes.[16,28,43,68] Deficiencies in life skills, including educational under-achievement, contribute significantly to the lack of self-confidence and poor self-image which are often important underlying aetiological factors in sex-offending behaviour. The focus should be on those areas which develop personal competencies, increase independence and assist integration into society. It is important that activities are enjoyable, seen as relevant by the offender and provide opportunities for personal achievement. Life skills training is best carried out in peer group situations as part of a structured weekly programme. A proper balance needs to be struck between work activity, social training and further education; recreational and hobbies training should take place in the evenings and at weekends. Life skills training also provides valuable opportunities for the development of social awareness, personal responsibility and self-control, and positive use should be made of work situations, special projects and sports activities to teach about the needs and feelings of others, collaborative effort and team work and the rewards of persistence.

Medical and Psychiatric Problems

Any coexisting physical disabilities such as epilepsy, minor physical defects, obesity and perceptual defects should be thoroughly assessed. There may be scope for improvement with corrective therapy, a slimming programme, better control of epilepsy or cosmetic surgery, with a corresponding improvement in the self-confidence and well-being of the patient. Adjustment issues should be explored and addressed through individual counselling and supportive psychotherapy.

Between a one-quarter and one-third of learning disabled sex offenders have a history of mental illness and the possibility of an associated mental illness should always be explored and, if present, treated appropriately. In those few cases where active mental illness is the primary cause of the offence, treatment for that illness may be all that is required.

Management of Families and Carers

Learning disabled sex offenders understandably cause concern to their families and direct care workers. Responses vary from sympathy and understanding to shame, fear, denial, minimization, censure and rejection: long-standing adjustment problems to having a learning disabled child may resurface. Families and carers need opportunities to vent their feelings and concerns and help in understanding, accepting and adjusting to the situation. Advice and support is often needed on a range of practical problems, including how to deal with the reaction of the local community if the victim is an immediate neighbour or the offence a particularly serious one, when the whole family can become ostracized and subject to verbal and physical abuse. Family support and cooperation can be a critical factor in the success of treatment, particularly in patients living at home. Key members of the family should be kept fully informed and involved in discussions about the treatment programme and its aims and rationale from the start. Prior to commencing treatment every effort should be made to establish a consistent value system about sexual behaviour across the family, occupational and residential placements and hospital.[69]

Socialization Programmes

Socialization programmes are the bedrock of most treatment programmes and the major intervention when sex offending is part of a generalized antisocial behaviour disorder. They aim to instil a sense of personal responsibility, improve self-control and assist the internalization of behavioural standards by utilizing approaches based on token economy principles. Tokens or points, which can be exchanged for a range of benefits, are issued on a systematic basis to reinforce socially desirable behaviour, sometimes coupled with specific penalties for undesirable behaviour. A number of programmes have been developed which differ only in such details as whether all or only specific aspects of behaviour are targeted or points/tokens are awarded immediately, daily or weekly.[8,16,18,70-74] The author has found that the simple weekly incentive scheme shown in Table 12.5 is readily understood and works well for the majority of learning disabled offenders.[16,75] Those with a moderate learning disability

Table 12.5. Northgate incentive scheme (updated from Day[16]).

Grade	Social privileges	Earnings
5	Nine social activities	Up to £15.00 per week
4	Five social activities	Up to £11.00 per week
3	Two social activities	£5.00 fixed
2	One social activity	£4.00 fixed
1	No social activities	£3.00 fixed

1. Patients enter the scheme on grade 3 and normally rise or fall by one grade at a time.

2. Below grade 3 changes in grading can be achieved in 1 week. Two consecutive weeks on grade 3 are required before a rise to grade 4, and 4 weeks on grade 4 before a rise to grade 5.

3. Minor misdemeanours not warranting downgrading may result in patients remaining on their current grade for longer. Serious misdemeanours may result in a drop of more than one grade and in certain circumstances immediate downgrading to grade 1.

4. Each grade carries a range of social and monetary privileges as shown above. On grades 4 and 5 earnings are determined entirely by performance and behaviour at work. A cash bonus or its equivalent is earned after 10, 25 and 50 consecutive weeks on grade 5.

5. A social activity is any event taking place outwith of the working day and includes activities on the hospital site and in the local community and entitlement to home leave. Activities outside the hospital depend upon parole status.

6. Gradings are decided at weekly meetings attended by all staff. All aspects of behaviour are taken into account. Each patient is called into the meeting in turn to discuss his new grade which becomes immediately effective.

7. Annual Leave and Public Holidays are independent of the scheme and may be granted at the discretion of the medial and nursing staff depending upon the individual's behaviour and parole status.

respond better to a daily points scheme initially but may be able to move later to a weekly scheme.[75] Successful application requires a critical patient mass, a controlled environment, high staff ratios, highly trained and experienced nursing staff and intensive support from a multi-professional team. Socialization programmes are therefore only suitable for use in specialized residential treatment settings.

Sex Education and Sociosexual Skills

Deficient, patchy and distorted knowledge about sex and sexual behaviour is common in all learning disabled people and is an important factor underlying sex offending behaviour.[33,49,76,77] A number of scales for assessing sexual knowledge in the learning disabled are available[51] including the Sexuality Development Index,[33,38] the Socio-Sexual Knowledge Aptitude Test,[76] the Social Sexual Evaluation Profile[78] and the recently developed Sexual Knowledge Interview Schedule[77] which has the advantage of measuring both sexual knowledge and sexual experience.

The aim of sex education is to provide accurate information about sex and sexuality, correct cognitive distortions, dispel myths, teach responsible sexual behaviour and improve relationship skills. It also provides a relatively nonthreatening introduction to treatment issues.[51] The following general areas should be covered but focus should remain on the specific deficits of individual offenders:

- basic sexual knowledge – anatomy and physiology, contraception, sexually transmitted diseases;
- issues of male and female sexuality – normal sexual behaviour, sexual myths and common misconceptions;
- the laws and social codes governing sexual behaviour – values and attitudes, consensual relationships, age, gender and setting appropriateness, privacy;
- sociosexual skills – relationships, courtship skills, the progression of physical intimacy, caring and partner responsibility, interpretation of cues, appropriate and inappropriate partners, rejecting sexual contact.

A number of excellent general guides and commercial packages are available.[22,33,79–81] Charman and Clare[28] have designed a programme specifically to teach the laws and rules relating to sexual behaviour to learning disabled sex offenders. Sex education is best carried out in small groups utilizing group discussion and the sharing of personal experiences.[33] Language should be simple, terminology understandable, concrete examples used, clear messages given and depth of interpretation varied according to the cognitive abilities and perceptiveness of the group. Anatomically correct dolls, drawings, cartoons, and other visual material are invaluable teaching aids.[28,33,68] Regular assessment of the extent to which the material has been understood and retained is essential. Difficulties in relating to the opposite sex is a common antecedent of sex offending in the learning disabled[82–84] and training in sociosexual skills is therefore an essential component of any sex education programme. Videotaped vignettes of male/female interactions including clips from popular 'soaps' and role play with videotaping and playback sessions are useful teaching techniques.[3,18,68] Regular contact with female staff provides valuable opportunities for learning about the opposite sex and developing self-confidence in relating to women. A number of training packages are available including: 'Stacking the Deck'[85] which employs a board game approach, 'Life Horizons'[80] which uses slides of human interactions, and the 'Circles' treatment package[86] which uses a chart with concentric circles to teach levels of intimacy between people; they have been criticized for the emphasis they place on providing a correct response.[87] The 'Dating Skills Programme'[88] seeks to overcome this problem by using a combination of social skills training, problem solving and modelling to teach patients how to make their own decisions and provide them with coping mechanisms to deal with the diverse situations which can arise in an unfolding sexual relationship.

Transferring skills learned in group sessions into everyday life poses considerable difficulties. Opportunities to meet with an appropriate peer group of the opposite sex in social situations which facilitate the development of normal relationships are crucial but difficult to achieve.[39] There is an understandable reluctance to encourage the relationships between known sex offenders and vulnerable learning disabled women and in specialist units severely behaviourally disturbed and emotionally unstable women may be the only peer group available. Media-based stereotypes of the 'ideal woman' held by many learning disabled men not infrequently leads them to reject contact with learning disabled females.[3]

Individual Counselling and Supportive Psychotherapy

Individual counselling is an important adjunct to group work and allows more time to be spent on specific problems and needs. The initial focus should be on the index offence, past sexual history, including sexual victimization and personal relationships, and any associated family and other personal problems. As treatment progresses sessions should be used to provide back-up and support for other aspects of the programme and to tackle any problems highlighted which require more attention than can be provided in a group setting, such as confused self concepts, peer isolation, negative sexual experiences, sexuality as furtive behaviour, lack of personal power, denial and victim empathy.[30] Sessions should be focused and time limited. Explanations and language should be kept simple, and concrete examples drawn from the patient's own experience used wherever possible.

Relaxation Therapy and Anger Management

Relaxation therapy, utilizing deep breathing, progressive muscle relaxation or guided imagery and assertiveness training can help reduce social anxiety and assist an individual more adequately and appropriately to express his sexual feelings. Both techniques have been used successfully with learning disabled people.[21,87,89,90] Anger management training using verbal self statement and relaxation training is also helpful in patients displaying poor impulse control and aggressive responses.[87,91,92] It is essential that patients have some understanding of the physiological concomitants of anger and anxiety and their relationship to offence behaviour before commencing learning these techniques.

Sex Behaviour Management

Sex behaviour management programmes are indicated in serious and persistent offenders. Until recently this has been a neglected area in the treatment of learning disabled sex offenders but a number of programmes based upon the techniques used with nonretarded sex offenders have now been developed.[2,18,27,43,93–95] Most use a group approach and employ cognitive/behavioural techniques, including psychodynamic psychotherapy. They aim to:

- help the offender to recognize, acknowledge and accept responsibility for his sex offending;
- assist the offender to gain control over and modify his behaviour through an understanding of its causes, his 'offence cycle' and the development of coping strategies and alternative acceptable sexual responses;
- change the offender's attitude by dealing with denial and minimization, rectifying cognitive distortions and increasing victim empathy.

Most programmes involve a three-stage approach as follows:

- Stage 1, establishing the group: desensitizing participants to work in a therapeutic group setting, assisting effective communications, developing trust and confidence, establishing goals and guidelines for the group and engaging clients in a therapeutic alliance.
- Stage 2, cognitive restructuring: an in-depth exploration of sex offending, cognitive distortions and other personal issues using confrontation, peer group pressure, role play and feedback, the aim being to heighten awareness and increase appreciation of the moral dimensions and practical consequences of sex offending, including the effects on the victim, and to promote acceptance of personal responsibility for one's sexual behaviour.
- Stage 3, coping strategies and relapse prevention: patients are taught the cognitive, emotional and situational factors which underlie and maintain their offence cycle (getting the offender to 'walk through' his offence is a useful technique),[3] how to recognize, avoid and cope with high-risk situations in which relapse is likely by leaving the scene, engaging in some alternative activity or using verbal self statements about the legal, social and emotional consequences to themselves and the victim to interrupt sexual arousal at the earliest possible stage of the offence cycle.

Programmes usually run for 1–3 years and progression depends upon satisfactory completion of the previous stage. Patients are only admitted to Stage 3 once they have demonstrated sufficient insight into their sex offending and a genuine desire to overcome it. During this stage therapy is more individualized and based upon a detailed behavioural analysis of the offence cycle;[3] behaviour programmes addressing specific problematic sexual behaviours are introduced if necessary.[18] Once coping/escape strategies have been satisfactorily established in the treatment setting, using role play and rehearsal, they are tested and consolidated in 'real life' situations by carefully controlled and supervised exposure to potential risk situations.

Group facilitators must be skilled, sensitive and properly trained (J. Taylor, the Northgate Staff Training Programme, unpublished).[53,96] Male and female co-therapists provide a positive role model for normal adult male/female relationships, help counter male chauvinism and facilitate more open discussion of sexual issues.[2] Small groups of about 7–8 participants and short sessions (30–90 min) weekly or twice weekly are recommended. Categorical learning and labelling rather than inductive or deductive reasoning should be employed[2,68,94] and there is a need for over-learning and the constant issuing of reminders about the purpose of the group. Individual goal setting, daily journals, self charting and homework help increase self awareness, promote personal responsibility and provide verification that information has been correctly received and understood.[2,43]

Patients should be carefully selected following a realistic appraisal of their ability to participate in and benefit from such a programme. Factors to be considered are offence behaviour, level of motivation, willingness and ability to cooperate with group treatment, ability to cope with self revelation, level of verbal communication skills and predicted ability to develop alternative coping mechanisms.[2,94] A treatment contract covering terms, conditions and goals should be signed prior to commencing treatment.[2,50]

Antilibidinal Drugs

Pharmacological reduction of the intensity of the sex drive is a long-established approach in the management of sex offenders, including those with a learning disability.[97,98] The newer antilibidinal drugs with their more focused action and fewer side-effects continue to have a useful role in treatment and their judicious use may obviate the need for institutional care in some cases. The principal indications are:

- as an initial short-term measure while a detailed assessment is being undertaken and other treatment methods are being explored and implemented, or to provide additional control at times of particular stress;
- as an adjunct to other treatments to facilitate concurrent therapy and enable behavioural and socialization programmes to be more safely undertaken;
- to control sexually deviant impulses and behaviour and provide relief from intrusive fantasies in the paraphilias;
- as the principal or sole therapeutic intervention in patients who have failed to respond to other treatment approaches and who continue to pose serious problems to their own well-being and the safety of others.

The anti-androgen cyproterone acetate is currently the drug of choice. Its efficacy in reducing sexual drive and sexual response has been well demonstrated in controlled trials of sex offenders generally[97] and in learning disabled patients.[98] The usual starting dose is 25–50 mg twice daily building up to a normal maximum of 300 mg daily (up to 1000 mg is recommended by some authorities). Dosage levels should be titrated according to the desired effect. It is not always necessary to completely eliminate sex drive, the aim in most cases being reduction to a level that the patient can control and which allows participation in behavioural treatment programmes. Care should be taken to ensure orgasm can be readily achieved as serious damage to skin of the penis during masturbation can result. Because of the level of supervision generally available compliance is rarely a problem. Where it is, a depot preparation of 300 g intramuscularly every 10–14 days can be used and should be considered for patients living in or about to be discharged to the community who although willing to receive treatment are judged to be forgetful or unreliable.

Cyproterone acetate is contraindicated in patients with a history of thromboembolic disease, liver disease and severe chronic depression; it should be used with caution in patients with diabetes mellitus and should not be prescribed to males under the age of 18 years or where bone and testicular development is incomplete, as in some syndromes associated with learning disability.[97] Spermatogenesis is inhibited but returns to normal within a few months of stopping treatment. Side-effects are few but gynaecomastia, sometimes with accompanying galacturia and occasionally irreversible, occurs in about 20%. Adrenocortical and liver function, blood sugar and blood count should be checked regularly during treatment: monitoring testosterone, follicle stimulating hormone (FSH), luteinizing hormone (LH) and prolactin levels is also recommended.[98]

Cyproterone acetate is effective in about 80% of cases; where it is not, it is worth trying the butyropherone neuroleptic benperidol in a dose of 0.25–1.5 mg daily, which although a weak libido reducer can sometimes be effective.[97] The usual side-effects of the neuroleptics may occur, and occasionally gynaecomastia, and the drug should be used with caution in patients suffering from epilepsy as it may lower the convulsive threshold. Liver function and blood count should be monitored regularly during treatment.

Two other drugs with powerful antilibidinal properties are goserelin acetate and medroxyprogesterone acetate. Although neither is licensed for this purpose in the United Kingdom they should always be considered if conventional antilibidinal drugs and other treatment measures have failed and there are continuing serious problems and chemical suppression of the sex drive is judged to be the only way forward. Goserelin acetate, a hormone analogue developed for the treatment of prostatic cancer, has been used with good effect as an antilibidinal agent in the learning disabled.[97,98] Administration is by subcutaneous injection into the anterior abdominal wall at a dosage of 3.6 mg every 28 days. Medroxyprogesterone acetate (Depo-provera) is widely used as an antilibidinal agent in North America[98] and is administered by deep intramuscular injection, usually at a dose of 100–400 mg to a maximum of 1000 mg every 7–10 days. Fluid retention may occur and prolonged use can lead to gynaecomastia and hypogonadism. Medroxyprogesterone acetate is contraindicated where there is a history of thromboembolic disease or liver dysfunction and should be used with caution in diabetic patients.[98] Monitoring should be carried out as described for cyproterone acetate.

Assessment of the efficacy of antilibidinal medication depends upon patients' self reports about sexual feelings, erections, masturbatory activity and fantasies, which can be unreliable, supplemented by the observations of relatives and staff. Serum testosterone levels may fall but are not a reliable measure of efficacy,[97,98] phallometry is used in some specialist services[3,49] but is not a practical option in general clinical work and reliable therapeutic blood ranges have yet to be established. A lengthy period of treatment is usually necessary and dosage levels should be constantly monitored and modified according to global improvements in the patient's behaviour and in response to offence-specific treatments. Withdrawal should be a carefully phased process and in the case of inpatients implemented well in advance of discharge.

The use of antilibidinal drugs must always be discussed in detail with the patient and his family and, wherever possible, the written consent of the patient obtained prior to commencing treatment. In the author's experience the majority of patients are willing to undertake treatment and are capable of giving informed consent. If there are doubts about the consenting status of the patient, or goserelin or medroxyprogesterone are being considered, it is good practice to obtain an informal second opinion from a colleague. In the case of patients detained under the Mental Health Act 1983 Section 58 applies but, as a general rule, antilibidinal medication should not be given to learning disabled sex offenders against their will. A judicial review in 1988 concluded that goserelin was neither a hormone nor administered by surgical implant and could therefore be given under Section 58 of the Mental Health Act 1983.[99]

Treatment of Deviant Sexual Behaviour

A careful assessment of sexual orientation is essential before embarking on a specialist treatment programme. Much apparent deviancy is secondary to the lack of normal sexual outlets and quickly replaced by normal heterosexual behaviour once opportunities for this are available.[27,51,52] Patients showing true sexual deviancy, with the exception of homosexuality, may require treatment aimed at refocusing or inhibiting deviant sexual arousal and establishing, if possible, appropriate sexual arousal. There has been very little work in this area with the learning disabled. There are reports of the successful use of covert desensitization, aversion therapy, satiation therapy and other behavioural techniques in the treatment of paedophilia, exhibitionism and fetishism.[2,3,21,44,49,82] However, a review of 13 research reports found that they were mostly single case studies and concluded that although high success rates were reported the majority did not employ a sufficiently rigorous experimental design to permit an adequate evaluation of their findings.[82] If behavioural treatments fail or are contraindicated antilibidinal drugs should be considered. Good results have been reported in cases of paedophilia, exhibitionism and fetishism in the learning disabled.[3,44,46]

Rehabilitation, Aftercare and Follow-up

Assessment of readiness for discharge should take account of response to treatment, type of offence, risk of further offending, patient characteristics and the quality of aftercare available.[61] It is always best to err on the side of caution: premature discharge can have dire consequences both for the community and the offender. Indicators of a good response to treatment include improvements in general behaviour, self-control, personal responsibility and social awareness and evidence of a more mature understanding and approach to sexual behaviour and sexual relationships.

Planning for rehabilitation and aftercare should begin immediately following admission. Families and community personnel should be fully involved from the start. Return to the community after a period of hospital treatment should be a carefully phased process beginning with a reduction of restrictions on personal liberty within the hospital, including moves to less restricted treatment settings, and progressing through day, weekend and longer leaves to eventual discharge.[8,16,75] A period of extended or trial leave is advisable to test the patient's willingness and ability to cooperate with the aftercare programme. It also permits a quick return to hospital should the situation break down.

A comprehensive aftercare package, including domicillary support, occupational placement, residential placement (where required) and leisure activities is essential if social breakdown and further offending is to be avoided.[6,16,35,100] Regular contact should be maintained with the treatment team and patients encouraged to seek immediate help in the event of a partial relapse. 'Crisis' cards with personal stop and go statements and a telephone number to ring for help are issued in some programmes.[49] Booster sessions may be required. A key worker should be appointed to monitor the implementation of the aftercare plan and act as the main point of contact with the patient.[55] There should be a system for regular review including risk assessment.[55] Staff in community based facilities must be fully informed about the patient's problems and needs. If there is concern about the ability of the patient to cooperate a Guardianship Order under the Mental Health Act 1983 should be considered. Patients considered to be at high risk for further offending should be placed on the Supervision Register. Conditional discharge for restricted patients and the recently introduced Supervised Discharge Order (Community Care Order in Scotland) provide a further layer of supervision for those patients about whom there is special concern.[55]

Outcome and Prognosis

Recidivism is common with reported rates of 20–50% for more than one conviction for a sex offence (R. Mein, unpublished data).[4,16,20] Of the learning disabled sex offenders in the Northgate study, 85% were involved in more than one sexual incident and 38% had received one, 17% two and 17% three or more convictions during an average period of 10.3 years.[13] A total of 3500 sex offences against 250 victims had been committed by 17 learning disabled patients treated in the Oregon Programme[43] and the mean frequency for sex offences in 35 special hospital patients studied by Murrey and colleagues was 3.9.[19] A history of behaviour disorder or previous convictions for sex offences substantially increases the likelihood of further offending.[1,26,59,101,102] Reconviction for serious offences is, however, uncommon[59,100,102] and there is no evidence of a trend towards escalation from minor to serious offences.[13]

Prognosis appears to be more favourable following treatment. Swanson and Garwick[2] reported that 60% of the 15 clients admitted to their programme had not reoffended during a $2^1/_2$ year period and that only two (13%) had committed further sexual offences leading to arrest. Only one out of eight sex offenders treated in the Northgate programme was reconvicted for a sex offence during a 3–5-year follow-up.[16] In a 10-year follow-up study of 69 mentally retarded sex offenders admitted to the Oregon Programme the recidivism rate was 23%[43] and 6 out of 16 patients treated by Lund[18] did not reoffend during a mean follow-up period of 2 years. A good response to treatment, duration of institutional treatment greater than 2 years and good quality aftercare are positively correlated with a better outcome.[6,13,16,18,43,100,102]

Prevention

More enlightened attitudes towards the sexuality of learning disabled people and their rights to sexual expression, coupled with the increasing availability of sex education programmes and the normalizing of lifestyles with opportunities for developing relationships with the opposite sex in normal social settings, should have a considerable longer term impact in reducing the incidence of sex offending by the learning disabled.

Simple sensible precautions can do much to reduce or minimize the risk of sex offending. Situations which might potentially lead to anti-social sexual behaviour such as playing with small children or baby-sitting should be avoided or carefully monitored. Known sex offenders should never be placed in unsupervised situations with potential victims in community homes or multipurpose treatment units.[1] In a study of 84 sexually abused learning disabled men and women half of the perpetrators had a learning disability.[38] All care staff should be trained to understand the sexuality of learning disabled individuals and how to recognize and manage inappropriate sexual behaviours. Institutions and residential homes should have clear policies and procedures for addressing issues of sexuality, identifying and protecting potentially vulnerable individuals and dealing with incidents if they occur.[103] Positive action should always be taken at the first sign of antisocial sexual behaviour even if the incident is considered to be trivial. The all too common tendency to ignore or overlook creates a negative learning situation which can result in further incidents.[2,36] Known sex offenders should receive proper treatment and management. This requires the ready availability of skilled personnel, specialist units and specialist treatment and relapse prevention programmes.

Service Provision

It is generally agreed that offenders with learning disabilities, including sex offenders, require specialist treatment services developed as part of a Learning Disabilities Psychiatric Service.[8,16,104–107] Currently, these vary considerably in size and scope from small single units to large comprehensive services offering a range of facilities and treatment programmes.[1,8,16,71–73,107–115] Specialist treatment programmes for high-risk sex offenders have been developed in institutional[2,13,16,18,43,94] and community settings.[27,94,116]

A model comprehensive service for learning disabled offenders has been described by Day.[1] The key components are:

- community based services for treatment, aftercare and continuing care including specialist teams and specialist residential, occupational and training facilities
- treatment and assessment units with varying levels of security for more dangerous offenders
- open units for the assessment and treatment of less serious offenders and rehabilitation
- long-term secure facilities
- rehabilitation hostels
- specialist training and treatment programmes
- appropriately trained and experienced staff.

Because of the small numbers of patients involved and the highly specialized facilities required, viable specialist forensic psychiatry services can only be developed on a regional/subregional basis. All aspects of the service must be in place if it is to run effectively and a single provider is preferable to ensure continuity of care for the patient. Duration of treatment can be lengthy and this must be taken into account when calculating bed numbers. Good multi-agency cooperation is essential in the planning, development and delivery of rehabilitation and aftercare services. Experience has shown that learning disabled offenders can rarely be satisfactorily managed in regular community services for learning disabled people, which are not able to meet their continuing need for structure and supervision, and that specialized provision is required in the early stages of rehabilitation for the majority and on a continuing basis for some.[16,109]

Conclusion

The care and management of learning disabled sex offenders is a developing field in which there is still much to be learned. Further research is needed in all areas, including the characteristics of offenders, offender typology, the aetiology of offence behaviour, assessment techniques, evaluation and treatment methods. Positive action is required in the strategic planning and provision of specialist forensic services, the development of specialist treatment programmes and staff training.

References

1. Day K (1993) Crime and mental retardation: a review. In Howells K & Hollin CR (eds) *Clinical Approaches to the Mentally Disordered Offender*, pp. 111–44, Chichester: John Wiley.
2. Swanson CK & Garwick GB (1990) Treatment for low functioning sex offenders: Group therapy and interagency co-ordination. *Mental Retardation* **28**, 155–61.
3. Murphy WD, Coleman EM & Haynes MR (1983) Treatment and evaluation issues with the mentally retarded sex offender. In Greer JG & Stuart IR (eds) *The Sex Aggressor: Current Perspectives on Treatment*, pp. 22–41. New York: Van Nostrand Rheinhold.
4. Milner KO (1949) Delinquent types of mentally defective persons. *Journal of Mental Science* **95**, 842–59.
5. Tutt NS (1971) The subnormal offender. *British Journal of Subnormality* **17**, 42–7.
6. Walker N & McCabe S (1973) *Crime and Insanity in England*, Vol 2. Edinburgh: Edinburgh University Press.
7. Robertson G (1981) The extent and pattern of crime amongst mentally handicapped offenders. *Journal of the British Institute of Mental Handicap* **9**, 100–3.
8. Day K (1990) Mental retardation: clinical aspects and management. In Bluglass R & Bowden P (eds) *Principles and Practice of Forensic Psychiatry*, pp. 399–418. Edinburgh: Churchill Livingstone.
9. Hawk GL, Rosenfeld BD & Warren JI (1993) Prevalence of sexual offences amongst the mentally retarded criminal defendant. *Hospital and Community Psychiatry* **44**, 784–6.
10. Koller H, Richardson SA, Katz M & Haynes MR (1982) Behaviour disturbance in childhood and early learning adult years in populations who were and were not mentally handicapped. *Journal of Preventive Psychiatry* **1**, 453–68.
11. Schilling RF & Schinke P (1988) Mentally retarded sex offenders: fact, fiction and treatment. *Journal of Social Work and Human Sexuality* **7**, 33–48.
12. Hirschi T & Hindelang MJ (1977) Intelligence and delinquency: a revisionist review. *American Sociological Review* **42**, 471–87.
13. Day K (1994) Male mentally handicapped sex offenders. *British Journal of Psychiatry* **165**, 630–9.
14. Kiernan C & Albort A (1991) *People with Mental Handicap Who Offend*. Manchester: University of Manchester Hester Adrian Research Centre.
15. Lyall I, Holland AJ & Collins S (1995) Offending by adults with learning disabilities and the attitudes of staff to offending behaviour: Implications for service development. *Journal of Intellectual Disability Research* **39**, 501–8.
16. Day K (1988) A hospital based treatment programme for male mentally handicapped offenders. *British Journal of Psychiatry* **153**, 635–44.
17. Gilby R, Wolfe L & Goldberg B (1989) Mentally retarded adolescent sex offenders. A survey and pilot study. *Canadian Journal of Psychiatry* **34**, 542–8.
18. Lund CA (1992) Long term treatment of sexual behaviour problems in adolescent and adult developmental disabled persons. *Annals of Sex Research* **5**, 5–31.
19. Murrey JG, Briggs D & Davis MS (1992) Psychopathic disordered, mentally ill and mentally handicapped sex offenders: A comparative study. *Medicine, Science and the Law* **32**, 331–6.
20. Radzinowicz L (1957) *Sexual Offences: Report of the Cambridge Department of Criminal Science*. London: Macmillan.
21. Griffiths D, Hingsburger D & Christian R (1985) Treating developmentally handicapped sexual offenders: The York Behaviour Management Services Treatment Programme. *Psychiatric Aspects of Mental Retardation Reviews* **4**, 49–52.
22. Edmondson B, McCombs K & Wish J (1979) What retarded adults believe about sex. *American Journal of Mental Deficiency* **84**, 162–6.
23. Bowler C & Collacott R (1993) Cross-dressing in men with learning disabilities. *British Journal of Psychiatry* **162**, 556–8.
24. Wolf SC (1985) A multi-factor model of deviant sexuality. *Victimology: An International Journal* **10**, 359–74.
25. Finkelhor D (1984) *Child Sexual Abuse: New Theory and Research*. New York: Free Press.
26. Lund J (1990) Mentally retarded criminal offenders in Denmark. *British Journal of Psychiatry* **156**, 726–31.
27. Griffiths DM, Quinsey VL & Hingsberger D (1989) *Changing Inappropriate Sexual Behaviour: A Community Based Approach for Persons with Developmental Disabilities*. Baltimore: Paul H Brookes.

28. Charman T & Clare (1992) Education about the laws and social rules relating to sexual behaviour. *Mental Handicap* **20**, 74–80.
29. Gebhard PH, Gagnon JH, Pomeroy WB & Christenson CV (1965) *Sex Offenders: An Analysis of Types*. London: Heinemann.
30. Hingsburger D (1987) Sex counselling for the developmentally handicapped: the assessment and management of seven critical problems. *Psychiatric Aspects of Mental Retardation Reviews* **6**, 41–5.
31. Jahoda A, Markova I & Cattermolem M (1988) Stigma and self concept of people with a mild mental handicap. *Journal of Mental Deficiency Research* **32**, 103–15.
32. Stephens B (1974) Symposium on development gains in reasoning. Moral judgement and moral conduct of non-retarded persons. *American Journal of Mental Deficiency* **79**, 117–61.
33. Johnson ER (1984) Community based sexuality programmes for developmentally handicapped adults. In Berg JM (ed) *Perspectives and Progress in Mental Retardation*, vol. 1, pp. 313–21. Baltimore: University Park Press.
34. Carparulo F, Comte M, Gafgen J Haaven J, Kaufman K, Kempton W, Sissala L, Whitaker JM & Wilson R (1988) A summary of selected notes from the working sessions of the *First National Training Conference on the Assessment and Treatment of Intellectually Disabled Juvenile and Adult Sexual Offenders*. Ohio: Columbus.
35. Hunter H (1979) Forensic psychiatry in mental handicap. In James FE & Snaith R (eds) *Psychiatric Illness and Mental Handicap*, pp. 141–6. London: Gaskell Press.
36. Turk V & Brown H (1993) The sexual abuse of adults with learning disabilities: results of a two year incidence survey. *Mental Handicap Research* **6**, 193–216.
37. Brown H & Turk V (1994) Sexuality: towards a more balanced view. In Bouras N (ed) *Mental Health in Mental Retardation*, pp. 168–84. Cambridge: Cambridge University Press.
38. Beail N & Warden S (1995) Sexual abuse of adults with learning disabilities. *Journal of Intellectual Disability Research* **39**, 282–287.
39. Knopp FH & Lackey LB (1987) *Sexual Offenders Identified as Intellectually Disabled: A Summary of Data from 40 Treatment Providers*. Orwell VT: The Safer Society Press.
40. Green R (1973) Mental retardation and sexuality: some research strategies. In de la Cruz FF & LaVeck GD (eds) *Human Sexuality and the Mentally Retarded*. pp. 250–63. New York: Brunner/Mazel.
41. Berlin FS (1983) Sex offenders: a biomedical perspective and status report on biomedical treatment. In Greer JG & Stuart IK (eds) *The Sexual Aggressor: Current Perspectives on Treatment*, pp. 83–123. New York: Van Nostrand Reinhold.
42. Lachman M, Brzeka A, Mellan J, Hampl R, Starka L & Mojcik K (1991) Recidivous offence in sadistic homosexual pedophile with karyotype 48 XXXY after testicular pulpestomy. *Journal of Experimental Clinical Endocrinology* **28**, 171–4.
43. Haaven J, Little R & Petre-Miller D (1990) *Treating Intellectually Disabled Sex Offenders: A Model Residential Programme*. Orwell VT: Safer Society Press.
44. Myers BA (1991) Treatment of sexual offences by persons with developmental disabilities. *American Journal of Mental Retardation* **95**, 563–9.
45. Thomas PR & DeAlwis K (1995) Transvestism in a person with learning disabilities presenting with behavioural problems. *Journal of Intellectual Disability Research* **39**, 454–6.
46. Collacott RA & Cooper SA (1995) Urine fetish in a man with learning disabilities. *Journal of Intellectual Disability Research* **39**, 145–7.
47. Cooper SA, Mohamed WM & Collacott RA (1993) Possible Aspergers syndrome in a mentally handicapped transvestite offender. *Journal of Intellectual Disability Research* **37**, 189–94.
48. Jehu D (1991) Clinical work with adults who were sexually abused in childhood. In Hollin CR & Howells K (eds) *Clinical Approaches to Sex Offenders and Their Victims*, pp. 229–60. Chichester: John Wiley.
49. Clare ICH (1993) Issues in the assessment and treatment of male sex offenders with mild learning disabilities. *Sexual and Marital Therapy* **8**, 167–180.
50. Beckett R (1994) Assessment of sex offenders. In Morrison P, Erooga M & Beckett RC (eds) *Sexual Offending Against Children*, pp. 55–79. London: Routledge.
51. Taylor JT (1997) Educational approaches to treatment. In Hoghugi M, Bhate S & Graham F (ed) *Working with Sexually Abusive Adolescents*. London: Sage. (in press).
52. Hayes S (1991) Sex offenders. *Australia and New Zealand Journal of Developmental Disabilities* **17**, 221–7.

53. Mitchell LK (1985) *Behavioural Intervention in the Sexual Problems of Mentally Handicapped Individuals*. Illinois: Charles C Thomas.
54. Abel G & Becker J (1985) Sexual Interest Card Sort. In Salter A (ed) *Treating Child Sex Offenders and Victims – A Practical Guide*. Beverley Hills: Sage.
55. Department of Health (1994) *Guidance on the Discharge of Mentally Disordered People and Their Continuing Care in the Community*. HSG (94) 27. Heywood: Health Publications Unit.
56. Hamilton JR & Freeman H (1982) *Dangerousness: Psychiatric Assessment and Management*. London: Gaskell.
57. Scott PD (1987) Assessing dangerousness in criminals. *British Journal of Psychiatry* **131**, 127–142.
58. McGrath RJ (1991) Sex offender risk assessment and dispositional planning: A review of empirical and clinical findings. *International Journal of Offender Therapy Comparative Criminology* **35**, 328–50.
59. Gibbens TCN & Robertson G (1983) A survey of the criminal careers of Hospital Order patients. *British Journal of Psychiatry* **143**, 362–75.
60. Soothill KL & Gibben TCN (1978) Recidivism of sexual offenders: a reappraisal. *British Journal of Criminology* **18**, 267–76.
61. Prins H (1993) A service provision and facilities for the mentally disordered offender. In Howells K & Hollin CR (eds) *Clinical Approaches to the Mentally Disordered Offender*, pp. 35–67. Chichester: John Wiley.
62. Bowden P (1990) The written report and sentences. In Bluglass R & Bowden R (eds) *Principles and Practice of Forensic Psychiatry*, pp. 183–97. Edinburgh: Churchill Livingstone.
63. Gunn J (1979) Forensic psychiatry. In Glanville-Grossman K (ed) *Recent Advances in Clinical Psychiatry*. Edinburgh: Churchill Livingstone.
64. Gudjonsson G (1992) *The Psychology of Interrogations. Confessions and Testimony*. Chichester: John Wiley.
65. Clare ICH & Gudjonsson GH (1995) The vulnerability of suspects with intellectual disabilities during police interviews: a review and experimental study of decision making. *Mental Handicap Research* **8**, 110–28.
66. Halleck SL (1981) The ethics of anti-androgen therapy. *American Journal of Psychiatry* **138**, 642–3.
67. Department of Health & Welsh Office (1993) *Code of Practice: Mental Health Act 1983*, pp. 53–9. London: HMSO.
68. Briggs B (1994) The management of sex offenders in institutions. In Morrison P, Erooga M & Beckett RC (eds) *Sexual Offending Against Children*, pp. 129–45. London: Routledge.
69. Hingsburger D & Griffiths D (1986) Dealing with sexuality in a community residential service. *Psychiatric Aspects of Mental Retardation Reviews* **5**, 57–61.
70. Burchard KD (1967) Systematic socialisation: a programmed environment for the rehabilitation of antisocial retardates. *Psychological Record* **17**, 461–76.
71. Santamour MB & Watson PS (1982) *The Retarded Offender*. New York: Praeger.
72. Denkowski GC & Denkowski KN (1984) Community based residential treatment model for mentally retarded adolescent offenders. In Berg JM (ed) *Perspectives and Progress in Mental Retardation, Volume 1. Social, Psychological and Educational Aspects*, pp. 303–11. Baltimore: University Park Press.
73. Fidura JG, Linsey ER & Walker GR (1987) A special behaviour unit for the treatment of behaviour problems of persons who are mentally retarded. *Mental Retardation* **25**, 107–11.
74. Sandford DA, Elzinga RH & Grainger W (1987) Evaluation of a residential behavioural programme for behaviourally disturbed mentally retarded young adults. *American Journal of Mental Deficiency* **91**, 431–4.
75. Day K (1990) Treatment of antisocial behaviour. In Dosen A, Van Gennep A & Zwanikken GJ (eds) *Treatment of Mental Illness and Behavioural Disorder in the Mentally Retarded*, pp. 103–32. Leiden, Netherlands: Logan Publications.
76. Wish JR, McCombs KF & Edmondson B (1980) *The Socio-Sexual Knowledge and Attitude Test*. Wood Dale: Stoetling Co.
77. Forchuk C, Martin ML & Griffiths M (1995) Sexual Knowledge Interview Schedule: reliability. *Journal of Intellectual Disability Research* **39**, 35–9.
78. Perroncel CC (1989) *The Social-Sexual Evaluation Profile*. Connecticut: Torrington.
79. Craft A (1987) *Mental Handicap and Sexuality: Issues and Perspectives*. Tunbridge Wells: Costelloe Press.
80. Kempton W (1990) *Life Horizons*. Santa Barbara: James Stanfield.

81. Linsay WR, Bellshaw E, Culross G, Staines G & Michie A (1992) Increases in knowledge following a course of sex education for people with intellectual disabilities. *Journal of Intellectual Disability Research* **36**, 531–9.
82. Foxx RM, Bittle RG, Bechtel DR & Livesay JR (1986) Behavioural treatment of the sexually deviant behaviour of mentally retarded individuals. *International Review of Research in Mental Retardation* **14**, 291–317.
83. Robertson I, Richardson AM & Youngson SC (1984) Social skills training with mentally handicapped people: a review. *British Journal of Clinical Psychology* **23**, 241–64.
84. Matson JL & DiLorenzo TM (1986) Social skills training in mental handicap and organic impairment. In Hollin CR & Trower P (eds) *Handbook of Social Skills Training*, vol. 2, pp. 67–90. Oxford: Pergamon.
85. Foxx RM & McMorrow MR (1983) *Stacking the Deck: A Social Skills Game for Retarded Adults*. Champaign: Research Press.
86. Champagne M & Walker-Hirsch L (1988) *The Circles*. Santa Barbara: James Stanfield.
87. Benson BA & Valenti-Hein D (1997) Cognitive and social learning treatments. In Dosen A & Day K (eds) *Handbook of Treatment of Mental Illness and Behaviour Disorders in Children and Adults with Mental Retardation*. Washington: American Psychiatric Press.
88. Valenti-Hein D & Mueser K (1990) *The Dating Skills Programme: Teaching Sociosexual Skills to Adults with Mental Retardation*. Worthington, OH: IDS Publishing.
89. Linsey SAWR, Baty FJ, Michie AM & Richardson I (1989) A comparison of anxiety treatments with adults who have moderate and severe mental retardation. *Research in Developmental Disabilities* **10**, 129–40.
90. Nezu CM, Nezu AM & Arean P (1991) Assertiveness and problem solving training for mildly mentally retarded persons with dual diagnoses. *Research in Developmental Disabilities* **12**, 371–86.
91. Benson B (1994) Anger management training: a self control programme for persons with mild medical retardation. In Bouras N (ed) *Mental Health in Mental Retardation*, pp. 224–32. Cambridge: Cambridge University Press.
92. Cullen C (1993) The treatment of people with learning disabilities who offend. In Howells K & Hollin CR (eds) *Clinical Approaches to the Mentally Disordered Offender*, pp. 145–63. Chichester: John Wiley.
93. Cox-Lindenbaum D (1997) Group therapy for mentally retarded sex offenders. In Dosen A & Day K (eds) *Handbook of Treatment of Mental Illness and Behaviour Disorders in Children and Adults with Mental Retardation*. Washington: American Psychiatric Press (in press).
94. Cox-Lindenbaum D & Lindenbaum L (1994) A modality for treating of aggressive behaviours and sexual disorders. In Bouras N (ed) *Mental Health in Mental Retardation*, pp. 244–5. Cambridge: Cambridge University Press.
95. Knopp FH (1984) *Retraining Adult Sex Offenders: Methods and Models*. Orwell, VT: Safer Society Press.
96. Cox Lindenbaum D (1990) A model for staff training and clinical treatment for the mentally retarded offender. In Dosen A, Van Gennep A & Zwanikken GJ (eds) *Treatment of Mental Illness and Behavioural Disorders in the Mentally Retarded*, pp. 381–94. Leiden, Netherlands: Logan Publications.
97. Clark DJ (1989) Antilibidinal drugs and mental retardation: a review. *Medicine, Science and Law* **29**, 136–48.
98. Cooper AJ (1995) Review of the role of two antilibidinal drugs in the treatment of sex offenders with mental retardation. *Canadian Journal of Psychiatry* **33**, 42–8.
99. Dyer C (1988) Mental Health Commission defeated over paedophile. *British Medical Journal* **296**, 1660–1.
100. Craft M (1984) Should one treat or gaol psychopaths. In Craft M & Craft A (eds) *Mentally Abnormal Offenders*, pp. 384–96. London: Ballière Tindall.
101. Payne C, McCabe S & Walker N (1994) Predicting offender patient reconvictions. *British Journal of Psychiatry* **125**, 60–4.
102. Tong JE & Mackay GW (1969) A statistical follow up of mental defectives of dangerous or violent propensities. *British Journal of Delinquency* **9**, 276–84.
103. Sundrum CJ & Stavis PF (1994) Sexuality and mental retardation: unmet challenges. *Mental Retardation* **32**, 255–64.
104. Royal College of Psychiatrists (1986) Psychiatric services for mentally handicapped adults and young people. *Bulletin, Royal College of Psychiatrists* **10**, 321–2.
105. Department of Health (1989) *Needs and Responses: Services for Adults with Mental Handicap*

Who are Mentally Ill, Who have Behaviour Problems or Who Offend. London: Department of Health Leaflets Unit.

106. Department of Health & Home Office (1992) Review of health and social services for mentally disordered offenders and others requiring similar services. Final summary report. CM2088. London: HMSO.
107. Isweran MS & Bardsley EM (1987) Secure facilities for mentally impaired patients. *Bulletin, Royal College of Psychiatrists* **11**, 52–4.
108. White BL & Wood H (1988) The Lancaster County Mentally Retarded Offenders Programme. In Stark JA, Menolascino FJ, Albarelli MH & Gray BC (eds) *Mental Retardation and Mental Health: Classification, Diagnosis, Treatment, Services*, pp. 402–8. New York: Springer.
109. Murphy G & Clare I (1991) MIETS (Mental Impairment, Evaluation and Treatment Service). 2. Psychological assessments and treatment, outcome for clients and service effectiveness. *Mental Handicap Research* **4**, 180–206.
110. Murphy G, Holland A, Fowler P & Reap J (1991) MIETS: A service option for people with mild mental handicaps and challenging behaviour of psychiatric problems. 1. Philosophy, service and service users. *Mental Handicap Research* **4**, 41–66.
111. Smith J (1988) An open forensic unit for borderline mentally impaired offenders. *Bulletin, Royal College of Psychiatrists* **12**, 13–5.
112. Johnson C, Smith J & Stainer G *et al*. (1993) Mildly mentally handicapped offenders: an alternative to custody. *Psychiatric Bulletin* **17**, 199–201.
113. Mayor J, Bhate M, Firth H, Graham A, Knox P & Tyrer S (1990) Facilities for mentally impaired patients: three years experiences of a semi secure unit. *Psychiatric Bulletin: Royal College of Psychiatrists* **14**, 333–5.
114. Hoare S & O'Brien G (1991) The impact of the Mental Health (Amendment) Act 1983 on admissions to an interim regional secure unit for mentally handicapped offenders. *Psychiatric Bulletin* **15**, 548–50.
115. Cumella S & Sansom D (1994) A regional mental impairment service. *Mental Handicap Research* **7**, 257–72.
116. Hames A (1987) Sexual offences involving children: a suggested treatment for adolescents with mild mental handicaps. *Mental Handicap* **15**, 19–21.
117. Milner KO (1949) Delinquent types of mental defective persons. *Journal of Mental Science* **95**, 842–59.
118. Home Office (1990) *Statistics of Mentally Disordered Offenders, England and Wales 1988. Statistical Bulletin June 1990*. Croydon, Surrey: Statistical Department, Home Office.

13

Behavioural Approaches

Kelvin Mackrell

Introduction

Over the past three to four decades, psychological approaches have increasingly been used in understanding, managing and developing behaviour in people who have learning disabilities. During this period, a growing number of psychological models and techniques have been applied, covering a whole range of behavioural, cognitive and psychotherapeutic approaches.[1] However, the first application of psychological theory to have a major impact in the field was based on a behavioural model. Reports of behaviour modification procedures first began to appear in the research literature just prior to 1960,[2,3] and the use of these techniques became widespread during the 1960s and, in the United Kingdom, particularly in the 1970s.

Prior to this, the prevailing view among clinical psychologists (and most other practitioners) was that behavioural excesses and deficits shown by people with a learning disability were largely, if not entirely, the direct result of the underlying disabling condition rather than reflecting reduced opportunity to learn, poor teaching techniques and so on. For example, people with IQs below 20 were seen as being unable to benefit from training in toileting, dressing and feeding, whereas it was thought people with IQs of around 50 would generally eventually learn these self-help skills but be unable to recognize letters of the alphabet. People with learning disability were seen as different from the majority of the population in psychomotor ability, personality and thought processes, as well as in overall level of intelligence. Furthermore, these characteristics were seen as 'constitutional', caused by damage to the central nervous system and present throughout life. Under these circumstances, the psychologist's role was largely restricted to assessing intelligence and personality.[4]

Against this pessimistic background, the early reports of successful behavioural change from psychologists in North America created considerable interest among clinical psychologists in the UK. The apparent strength of the approach lay in its derivation from experimental analysis of behaviour in the laboratory: principles investigated initially with animals were tested out in a variety of human populations, then applied systematically in hospitals, schools and other applied settings. These experimental applications gradually came to form the basis of a set of clinically useful techniques based on the behavioural model.

In the field of learning disability, the behavioural model challenged the idea that behaviour resulted directly from underlying disabling conditions.

According to this model the underlying condition may impose limits on the range of behaviours an individual might learn and/or the speed of learning, but nevertheless specific behaviours are learned. This means that 'problem' behaviours can be unlearned and behavioural deficits can be overcome. If an individual has not learned particular skills by 'ordinary' means he or she can be taught by using highly efficient teaching methods. Unfortunately, once an individual's learning difficulties have attracted a label of 'mental handicap' (or when behaviour modification was first introduced, 'subnormality'), the expectations of that person are lowered. The result of lowered expectations is usually reduced opportunity to learn (because less effort is made to teach everyday skills). In addition, the individual may be allowed to 'get away with' behaviours that would be seen as undesirable in an 'average' child. The reduced range of opportunities offered leads to restriction of life experiences and leads to deficits in skills acquisition, which together with the acquisition of problem behaviours tends to confirm the original expectations, and so on in a 'vicious circle'. The interest in behaviour modification stemmed from the introduction of techniques to teach new skills effectively and to reduce 'problem' behaviours directly.

Initial attempts to teach new behaviours and eliminate behavioural excesses tended not to focus on causes of behaviour, instead seeking to use principles of behaviour to develop procedures to bring about behavioural change.

The principles used were derived from work on operant conditioning by Skinner[5] and others. In the 1950s the operant approach was extended in an attempt to account for human behaviour.[6,7] The practical implications were quickly recognized, and in the following decade procedures derived from operant principles were tested and evaluated in a variety of applied settings. Two programmes of research were particularly influential. First, Ayllon and his co-workers systematically applied operant principles in psychiatric wards,[2,8,9] culminating in the conception of the token economy.[10] Second, Bijou and his colleagues began applied operant work in a preschool nursery and a school for learning disabled children.[11,12] Other programmes of research followed, and by 1968 there was sufficient research being conducted to allow the establishment of a new journal, the *Journal of Applied Behaviour Analysis*, to provide a publication outlet for this body of work.

By the early 1970s, clinical psychologists in the UK were recognizing the potential importance of behavioural approaches.[13] It was further recognized that, since successful behaviour modification depended on consistent and continuous application of the procedures, nurses, teachers, parents and others in close, everyday contact with the client were in the best position to change behaviour. This led to the development of manuals, workshop plans and training programmes for such individuals,[14,15] the introduction of 'home teaching' systems to train and support parents in the use of the approach[16] and the inclusion of behavioural approaches in the nursing training syllabus.

In general, there has been an over-emphasis on teaching behavioural 'techniques' to be applied to various problem behaviours rather than on the principles of learning from which these procedures were drawn. Specifically, there has been little attention paid to teaching staff and parents to analyse behaviour in such a way as to understand the variables already affecting that behaviour, and therefore also affecting the impact of artificially arranged variables aimed at changing the behaviour. This has resulted in something of a 'cookbook' approach to behaviour modification, where techniques are applied largely on the basis that they have previously proved successful with the particular behaviour they are aimed at. The problem with this approach is that different people may perform a particular behaviour for entirely different reasons (i.e. 'topographically' similar behaviours may have different 'functions'). This means that techniques applied on such a trial-and-error basis may lack the flexibility to cope with individual and situational variability and thus are only sometimes successful with some people. Instead, attention must be paid to analysis of the functions of particular behaviours for particular individuals ('functional analysis'), and interventions must be tailored accordingly.

A second major problem of the way in which behaviour modification has been implemented is that new research findings have not always found their way into clinical practice. Many practitioners have continued to use techniques derived from early research when more recent work suggests more effective ways of understanding and overcoming a problem. This is largely because most behaviour modification practitioners have still not been taught the principles underlying the approach, and many behavioural interventions are attempted without reference to clinical psychologists who are more likely to have kept pace with developments in understanding behaviour (including nonbehavioural methods).

This present chapter provides a brief outline of operant behavioural principles, then focuses on applications of these principles to develop new skills and reduce undesired behaviour. For readers seeking more detail, two texts edited by Honig[17] and Honig and Staddon,[18] present collections of experimental work underlying the principles. Kazdin[19] reviews research into applications of the principles and Presland[20] presents a practical guide to using the approach.

Operant Behavioural Principles

Definition of Terms

The 'behavioural approach', as applied in learning disabilities, is based on theory and research into learning processes known as 'operant conditioning'.

Operant behaviours are controlled by the events that regularly precede and follow them (i.e. the 'antecedents' and 'consequences' of the behaviour). Changes in the probability of a behaviour occurring can be brought about by changing antecedents and consequences of the behaviour in question.

The use of operant conditioning principles to change behaviour is known as 'behaviour modification', while using the principles to understand precisely how prevailing contingencies are operating on a person's behaviour by carrying out a functional analysis and then designing tailor-made individual interventions based on this understanding is known as 'applied behaviour analysis' or simply 'behaviour analysis'.

Consequences

Operant behaviours are controlled largely by their consequences, in other words, by the events which are contingent upon them. For practical purposes, it is convenient to divide consequent events into two types: positive events and aversive events, roughly corresponding to events which are pleasant and rewarding to the individual and events which are unpleasant and undesirable to the individual, respectively. Events can either occur or terminate contingent upon a particular behaviour. A behaviour is made more likely either by the contingent occurrence of a positive event or by the contingent termination of an aversive event. Both contingencies are termed 'reinforcement': reinforcement refers to any action of consequences which increases the rate of a behaviour. A behaviour is made less likely either by the contingent occurrence of an aversive event or by the contingent termination of a positive event. Both of these contingencies are termed 'punishment': punishment refers to any action of consequences which decreases the rate of behaviour. Table 13.1 illustrates these types of contingency and their effects.

Reinforcement

An increase in the rate of a behaviour resulting from the contingent occurrence of a positive event is termed 'positive reinforcement'. Sometimes, events which are not obviously positive can function as positive reinforcers. Suppose a child teases his sister, and every now and then she loses her temper and gets upset, and this makes him more likely to tease her in the future. In this case, the sister's reaction has acted as a positive reinforcer for the teasing behaviour.

Table 13.1. Types of consequence and effects on behaviour.

	Occurrence contingent on behaviour	Termination contingent on behaviour
Positive event	Positive reinforcement (increases likelihood of behaviour	Punishment (decreases likelihood of behaviour)
Aversive event	Punishment (decreases likelihood of behaviour)	Negative reinforcement (increases likelihood of behaviour)

What will function as a positive reinforcer varies a great deal from individual to individual, and also from situation to situation (for example a child may find attention from a teacher positively reinforcing in the classroom but attempt to avoid attention during play-times). Access to preferred activities can also function as a positive reinforcer for behaviour it is contingent upon. If a child enjoys watching a particular television programme and he is only allowed to watch it when he has finished his homework, access to the television is likely to act as a positive reinforcer for doing homework.

An increase in the rate of a behaviour resulting from the contingent termination of an aversive event is termed 'negative reinforcement'. An aversive event is usually something unpleasant or undesirable to the individual, something that an individual seeks to escape from or avoid. Escape from an aversive situation negatively reinforces whatever behaviour leads to that escape. Termination of an aversive event increases the rate of behaviour it follows. As with positive reinforcement, what will function as an aversive event varies from individual to individual and situation to situation.

Positive and negative reinforcement interact in everyday life. A mother may give a child a lot of attention when he is having a tantrum because she knows this stops the tantrum. Her behaviour is negatively reinforced by termination of the tantrum (an aversive event to her). At the same time, the child's tantrum behaviour may be positively reinforced by the attention, and the likelihood of further tantrums may increase.

Avoiding an aversive event is negatively reinforcing also. In the above example, if the child's tantrums are always preceded by a request to be picked up and cuddled, the mother may learn to avoid tantrums by acceding to this request before the tantrum starts. In this case picking the child up has been negatively reinforced by avoidance of the tantrums.

Now suppose the child's mother does not give him attention when he cries and stamps his feet, but waits until he starts screaming. Gradually, the child will learn that it pays to start screaming earlier. Because only this aspect of the tantrum is reinforced, it is more likely to occur in the future and the nature of the tantrum is gradually changed. This process is called 'shaping'.

Punishment

A decrease in the rate of a behaviour resulting from either the contingent occurrence of an aversive event or the contingent termination of a positive event is termed 'punishment'. The technical use of the term corresponds to the everyday use except that, as with reinforcement, punishment is defined by the effect on behaviour: if the behaviour does not become less likely when a particular event follows it, punishment has not occurred and the event is not 'punishing'.

Again, what a particular person finds punishing is a very individual matter. For example, consider a child who is disruptive in school and is told off by the teacher and given 'detention'. The teacher's intention is to punish, but the intended punishment may actually positively reinforce the disruptive behaviour if being in trouble results in prestige among other class members.

Punishment and negative reinforcement are often confused with each other: however, they have opposite effects on behaviour. Generally speaking, an event which punishes behaviour it follows (i.e. an aversive event) will negatively reinforce behaviour when it is terminated contingent on the occurrence of that behaviour. Similarly, if an event positively reinforces behaviours it follows, then terminating that event contingent on behaviour will generally act as a punisher for that behaviour (this is what parents make use of when they take away a child's favourite toy when it is naughty).

Although punishment reduces the rate of the behaviour it follows, there are a number of 'side-effects' associated with it. These include 'emotional responses' on the part of the person whose behaviour is punished, aggression toward the punishing agent or toward the self, and escape and avoidance responses.

Extinction and Schedules of Reinforcement

The previous section was concerned with what happens when a behaviour is followed consistently by a particular consequence. In fact, such consistency is rare: behaviours are followed by reinforcers at some time, by punishers at others and by nothing at all at others. If a particular behaviour is not always followed by the same consequence, the pattern of behaviour is affected.

Extinction

If a behaviour which has been followed by a reinforcer is no longer reinforced, it eventually becomes less frequent and finally ceases: this is referred to as 'extinction'. Extinction results from nonreinforcement of previously reinforced behaviour. Extinction occurs if a reinforcer stops suddenly: if a reinforcer is withdrawn slowly, extinction tends not to occur (see below). At the beginning of the extinction process, the behaviour usually first increases in frequency, but as long as the behaviour continues not to be reinforced, this 'burst' of behaviour ends and the behaviour gradually decreases in frequency and finally stops.

As with reinforcement and punishment, extinction is a naturally occurring process which has an effect on behaviour and knowledge of the process can be useful in understanding why people behave as they do.

Schedules of Reinforcement

If a behaviour is sometimes followed by a reinforcing consequence and at other times has no consequence, we say it is being 'intermittently reinforced'. The pattern of reinforcement is known as a schedule, so that an 'intermittent reinforcement schedule' simply means that the reinforcer only follows the behaviour sometimes, while a 'continuous reinforcement schedule' means that the behaviour is always followed by a reinforcer. Similarly, it is possible to have 'intermittent punishment schedules'. The reinforcer (or punisher) may occur every second or third time the behaviour is performed, or at the other extreme, every one-hundredth time. The occurrence may be fixed (e.g. reinforcement follows the behaviour after every tenth response) or variable (e.g. on average every tenth response is reinforced, but the actual number of responses between instances of reinforcement varies from instance to instance). The behaviour may also be intermittently reinforced and intermittently punished at the same time or reinforced by two different intermittent reinforcers. The importance of schedules is that different schedules have different effects on behaviour. For example, some schedules lead to high-frequency, steady rates of responding and others to what is known as 'break and run' behaviour – bursts of response interspersed with pauses.

Where two or more different behaviours are reinforced over the same period of time in the same place, the behaviours are said to be maintained by concurrent schedules. These are important because people generally cannot do two things at once without one behaviour interfering with the other. Thus, altering the consequences of one behaviour affects the rate of occurrence of other concurrent behaviours as well as the behaviour that leads to the consequence. For example, when two behaviours occur simultaneously, the consequences of one have a similar effect on both: if one behaviour is reinforced, a second simultaneous behaviour will be accidentally reinforced because it has also been followed by the reinforcer. In other cases where different behaviours do not occur at precisely the same moment, reinforcing one will decrease the rate of the others.

Antecedents

Stimuli regularly present when a behaviour is reinforced are important because they come to signal that the behaviour is likely to be reinforced. As a result, these stimuli tend to trigger the behaviour in the future. Similarly, stimuli present when the behaviour is not reinforced signal that behaviour is not likely to be reinforced, so these stimuli become less likely to be followed by the behaviour. The individual responds differently to the two sets of stimuli: the behaviour is more likely to occur when stimuli previously associated with reinforcement are present than when stimuli previously associated with nonreinforcement are present. In this way, different stimuli act as antecedents for different behaviours. This is referred to as 'stimulus control'. A response may gradually come to be performed when other stimuli similar to the original signalling stimuli are present: this is known as 'generalization'.

Any stimulus or set of stimuli can function in this way. Many behaviours consist of a chain of individual responses, where the consequences for one response serve to signal the next link in the chain. In other words, the consequences for one behaviour can function as antecedents for another. Different times and places come to signal different behaviours, and the behaviour (or even just the presence) of another person can trigger certain behaviours. An individual's own behaviours, feelings and thoughts and moods also act as antecedents for other behaviours. What we say to each other and to ourselves can also exert stimulus control over behaviour: our behaviour is signalled by, encouraged or discouraged by the rules we learn to follow. Parents constantly point out what it is safe or unsafe to do, and this 'short cuts' the process of having to experience consequences in order to learn: rules specify (or imply) the consequences for certain courses of action. In addition, we have the facility to derive our own rules describing what is happening in our environment. We can solve problems by evaluating the likely consequences of particular behaviours or strategies, and choosing the course most likely to result in reinforcing consequences.

The interaction of antecedents, behaviours and consequences can be very complex, and analysing contingencies of reinforcement is rarely simple. Nevertheless, operant principles have formed the basis of a technology for understanding and changing behaviour.

Developing New Skills

Using Consequences to Change Behaviour

Reinforcement, punishment and extinction are natural processes which have been harnessed for use in changing behaviour. Much of this work has been based on early research, and more recent findings have highlighted inadequacies in behaviour modification practices, including misuse of some principles and failure to take note of others.

Applying Reinforcement

Many programmes of behaviour modification have centred on providing positive reinforcement for 'desired' behaviours. In general, this is an acceptable and appropriate use of behavioural principles, but a few words of caution are necessary.

First, the behaviour modifier may forget that behaviour is a function of contingencies operating in the individual's current environment, and the learning experiences the individual has had previously. For any particular behaviour, 'natural' reinforcers and punishers are operating in the environment. To increase or decrease the rate of any behaviour we should identify and take into account those reinforcers and punishers already operating on the behaviour, since these may override the effect of artificially arranged contingencies. Ideally, we should use natural consequences to teach behaviours. For example, if we want to teach a child to put on a warm coat when they go outside in cold weather, then giving sweets for putting on the coat may help in acquisition of the mechanical skill. However, this will not maintain the behaviour unless the child is made aware that they feel warmer as a consequence of putting the coat on. In other words, pointing out and explaining natural consequences is as important as arranging programmes of contrived reinforcement. Changing behaviour usually involves altering consequences so that natural reinforcers are rearranged to follow different behaviours: for example staff may pay attention to a client's positive behaviours rather than to the problem behaviours they had previously attended to, and this will increase the rate of positive behaviour (provided that attention is a reinforcer).

A second type of error is made by the behaviour modifier who assumes that a particular consequence is reinforcing for a particular individual because a text book has listed that consequence as a reinforcer, or a journal article has reported successful behaviour modification using that consequence as a reinforcer, or the behaviour modifier has successfully used the consequence as a reinforcer with another client or in another situation. This overlooks the fact that reinforcement is highly idiosyncratic: we cannot specify whether a stimulus is or is not a reinforcer without testing its effect on a particular person's behaviour.

Finally, there is a danger in reinforcing 'desired' behaviours if the assumption is made that the environment the person functions in is fine and it is the person who is antisocial, ill, deviant, unacceptable and so forth. We must be careful to exercise behavioural approaches for the benefit of the client, not simply to encourage compliance. Very often it is the environment which is odd rather than the person: odd environments produce odd behaviour.

Shaping

Shaping is a naturally occurring process whereby only certain aspects of a behaviour are reinforced so that the individual comes to perform those aspects of the behaviour relatively more frequently and the nature of the behaviour is gradually changed.

Behaviour modifiers have utilized this process to teach new skills, by reinforcing successive approximations to the desired behaviour. For example, if a therapist is teaching an individual to use a sign to indicate that something is wanted, at first any rough approximation to the sign is reinforced. Gradually, in a series of small steps, the criterion for reinforcement is raised so that the sign has to become more and more like the correct sign in order to gain reinforcement. Shaping is a very useful technique when used in conjunction with suitable reinforcers (see comments in the previous section) and other procedures derived from research into the effects of antecedents on behaviour.

Using Antecedents

Prompting

A simple example of the use of antecedent stimuli in behaviour modification is the procedure known as 'prompting'. Prompts are attempts to make a behaviour occur by verbal, gestural or physical means. Thus, the therapist might explain, demonstrate or use physical guidance to bring about a particular behaviour. When the behaviour is performed, it is reinforced and the prompt becomes a signal for reinforcement, which then makes the behaviour more likely to follow the prompt in the future. Prompts are usually 'faded out' gradually as the behaviour is learned.

Unfortunately, behaviour modifiers often fail to appreciate that prompts acquire stimulus control over behaviour by signalling that the behaviour is likely to be reinforced. Under some circumstances, the prompting procedure may even make the behaviour occur less frequently: if a behaviour to be prompted occurs at a low rate and the prompts involve giving attention to the client (and the client finds attention reinforcing) then, in effect, the individual will receive greater reinforcement for not performing the behaviour than for performing it. In addition, many people with learning disabilities have difficulty in attending to and organizing incoming information, and the addition of further stimuli to a situation in the form of prompts (especially when verbal, gestural and physical prompts are used together) may complicate the learning task rather than helping. Under these circumstances, the individual may give all their attention to the prompts rather than the task being taught so that when prompts are faded out, there is a sudden decrease in the level of performance.[21] This can be overcome by teaching the person to pay attention to natural stimulus features of the task itself, or by teaching strategies to enable the individual to monitor and control his or her behaviour (for example, using self statements or rules describing salient features of the task or the behaviour required).[22]

Chaining

The concept of chaining has been applied to the teaching of many skills by behaviour modifiers. Many complex behaviours consist of a chain of individual tasks. For example, dressing consists of 'putting on underpants', 'putting on trousers', 'putting on a shirt', 'putting on sock and shoes', and so on. Each of these tasks can be further subdivided into chains of smaller responses, which can then be sorted into logical order ready to be taught one at a time in sequence. This process is known as task analysis, and an illustrative task analysis for 'putting on a T-shirt' is given in Table 13.2.

When teaching the task, the last response in the chain is usually taught first (backward chaining), until the trainee performs it (and is reinforced) consistently. In the example illustrated, the last response is 'pulling the shirt down from the chest to the waist'. The teacher puts the shirt on the trainee and pulls it down as far as the person's chest. The trainee is then encouraged to pull it down to the waist and is reinforced when he or she does so. Eventually, 'having a shirt on and pulled down as far as the chest' will act as a signal for 'pulling down to the waist', and the next step (in the example, 'pulling the shirt down from the armpits to the chest') can begin. This step will not be directly reinforced by the teacher, since the response is reinforced by the shirt being in position to begin the last

Table 13.2. Illustrative task analysis.

Goal: To put shirt on.

Task Analysis
1. Trainee orientates T-shirt so that it is back uppermost with the neck away from him.
2. Trainee holds the bottom back of the T-shirt with both hands.
3. Trainee pulls T-shirt over his head.
4. Trainee puts head through neck of T-shirt.
5. Trainee puts right arm through right armhole.
6. Trainee puts left arm through left armhole.
7. Trainee pulls T-shirt down from armpits to chest.
8. Trainee pulls T-shirt down from chest to waist.

response, which can already be performed, and the trainee is reinforced on completion of this response.

Task analyses for use with chaining programmes have been produced for many behaviours, outlining possible steps toward completion of the task. One danger here is that assumptions are made about there being a 'correct' order in which to complete a task whereas in fact different people have different strategies (some people put their T-shirt on in the order shown in Table 13.2, while others put their arms in the sleeves first, and so on). The important point here is that different people working with the same trainee should be consistent.

Precision Teaching

Many teaching programmes combine reinforcement, shaping, prompting and chaining approaches. In the example of teaching a person to put on a T-shirt, the sequence of responses is taught by backward chaining, but each individual response may have to be split into even smaller steps and taught by successive approximations, and prompts may be used at all stages. This is known as 'precision teaching'. Provided that care is taken to avoid the common pitfalls outlined above, precision teaching can be a successful approach, at least in the short term. There have, however, been doubts expressed about whether gains made during training in one setting at one time generalize to other settings at a later date.[19] A key response to this problem is to build training into the client's everyday environment, and train agents in that environment to continue to use appropriate strategies.

Reducing Undesired Behaviour

Using Consequences

Punishment

Behaviour modifiers have attempted to decrease the rate of undesirable behaviours by applying aversive stimuli or events contingent upon the behaviour, and by the contingent withholding or withdrawal of positive reinforcers.

Aversive stimuli used have included physical punishment,[23] electric shock[24] and administration of disagreeably tasting substances.[25] The most commonly used aversive procedures, however, are reprimands and criticism, both in planned behaviour modification programmes and in everyday life.

Response cost refers to withdrawing positive reinforcers contingent upon a behaviour. Fines and deprivation of privileges are common examples. Time-out is a procedure where an undesired response is followed by a short period during which normally available reinforcement is withheld. Commonly this is achieved by removing the individual to a designated time-out room or area contingent upon undesired behaviour. Overcorrection typically involves requiring an individual to compensate for any damage done and to 'overcorrect' or improve on the original situation (for example, an individual who urinates on the floor may be made to clean the floor, not just where he has urinated, but over the whole room). Where such restitution is impossible, individuals have been made to engage in repetitive practice of behaviours which are incompatible with the undesired act (for example, someone who masturbates in public may be made to engage in a series of repetitive exercises). In both cases, the punishing effect is presumably achieved because the individual finds the required behaviours aversive.

As when applying reinforcement, behaviour modifiers have often failed to analyse and take account of naturally occurring contingencies when applying punishment. If a problem behaviour occurs often enough for punishment to be considered as a corrective procedure, by definition there must exist contingencies of reinforcement which maintain the behaviour at its present level. If an aversive event is introduced to decrease the rate of the behaviour without reference to the prevailing natural reinforcement contingencies, the effect is likely to be temporary at best because when punishment stops, the natural reinforcement contingencies will increase the rate of behaviour.

Behaviour modifiers have also often made prior assumptions about what will be punishing for a particular person. For example, some practitioners have assumed that a smack will always act as a punisher,[23] but for some children attention given while administering a smack is reinforcing and outweighs the punishing effect. A second instance of this type of mistake is when someone is put into a time-out room contingent upon undesired behaviour, when the individual does not like being in the situation in which the problem behaviour occurs. Performing the problem behaviour will in this case allow the individual to escape from the unpleasant situation and therefore this behaviour will be negatively reinforced rather than punished.

A major drawback with the use of punishment is that it has a number of significant undesirable effects. First, escape or avoidance behaviours are promoted (since any such response is negatively reinforced), and may cause the client simply to keep away from the situation where punishment is used. Second, emotional responses frequently occur which indicate distress on the part of the client and disrupt the training process. Third, the person being punished is likely to become aggressive, either toward themselves or toward the person doing the punishing. In particular this can lead to problems in programmes involving physical contact with the client (taking someone to a time-out area, making them 'overcorrect' and so on).

Unfortunately, because punishment initially suppresses the behaviour it is aimed at, the person applying the punishment is negatively reinforced for its use. Even if the behaviour subsequently reappears as a result of naturally occurring contingencies of reinforcement, the temptation is to apply more punishment because it proved effective at first. Perhaps because of this, many care staff and parents have placed an over-emphasis on punishment. However, since behaviour modification was first introduced, there has been increasing concern about the ethics of using techniques which can cause distress, coerce clients into behaving for the benefit of the staff rather than their own good, and so forth. Furthermore, most psychologists acknowledge that much problem behaviour has meaning, in the sense that it may provide clues that the individual has suffered (or is suffering) trauma, loss or abuse. Behaviour modification practitioners should turn away from punishment as a method of behaviour change.

Extinction and Schedules of Reinforcement

Extinction is a natural process which occurs when a behaviour which was formerly reinforced is no longer reinforced. It has been utilized by behaviour modifiers as a less coercive and more acceptable method of reducing the rate of undesirable behaviours than using aversive procedures or removing positive reinforcers.

There are a number of reasons why in practice it is difficult to apply extinction in clinical settings. First, the behaviour to be extinguished is often being maintained by complex schedules of natural reinforcement involving more than one reinforcing consequence; removing one reinforcer may not make much difference, but extinction programmes often rely on discontinuing one consequence presumed to be reinforcing the undesired behaviour. Extinction has often been translated by behaviour modifiers into 'ignoring undesirable behaviour' on the assumption that attention is a reinforcer for the behaviour. If extinction is to be effective, the true reinforcer(s) must be identified. Even if this can be achieved, it is difficult to withhold that reinforcer consistently, since the behaviour modification agent rarely has complete control over the availability of the reinforcer. Consequently, it is likely that the behaviour will be reinforced on some occasions. In other words, the behaviour is placed on an intermittent reinforcement schedule, which may be sufficient to maintain the behaviour at a relatively high rate.

A further problem with applying extinction is that by attempting to withhold reinforcement we may actually shape more undesirable behaviour. For example, suppose an individual shouts aggressively and occasionally breaks things in order to gain attention from staff in a residential home.

The staff attempt to withhold attention but, although this is possible when the person shouts, they find they have to pay attention when something is broken so that other residents are not likely to hurt themselves. This means that 'breaking things' has been differentially reinforced relative to shouting, and is more likely to be repeated.

Despite these practical difficulties, extinction is a useful procedure if it is used in conjunction with reinforcement procedures for more appropriate behaviours. This is a practical application of research into concurrent schedules. A decrease in the rate of one response is brought about by increasing reinforcement for other responses: this is known as 'differential reinforcement of other behaviour' (DRO). The effect is strengthened if behaviours physically incompatible with the desirable response are reinforced: this is called 'differential reinforcement of incompatible behaviour' (DRI). For example, a client might receive reinforcement for engaging in constructive tasks rather than sitting in a chair rocking, playing with saliva, or other similar behaviours.

Using Antecedents

There has been relatively little reported use of antecedents in programmes for the reduction of problem behaviours. If stimuli can be identified which regularly trigger undesired behaviour, it might be possible to prevent them occurring and so reduce the rate of the behaviour. Similarly, if the problem behaviour is the end behaviour in a chain, and is preceded by other behaviours which are less problematic, it may be possible to interrupt the chain before the client reaches the stage of performing the problem behaviour itself. In practice, what often happens is that a carer sees such an antecedent stimulus or behaviour occurring, and realizing what usually follows, tries to prevent the behaviour by saying 'No'. Unfortunately, such a verbal warning will soon become ineffective unless it is either associated with a reducing consequence or followed by some form of distraction procedure (given the objections raised earlier to the use of reducing consequences, the latter is generally preferable).

Many therapeutic interventions have failed to take account of the role antecedents play in controlling behaviour. For example, the conditions (time, place, etc.) under which learning occurs become antecedents for particular behaviours, while other conditions signal a different set of behaviours. Nevertheless, special units are often set up in hospitals, schools, etc., where clients undergo behaviour modification and other treatments for challenging behaviour before returning to their natural environment; it is hoped changes effected in behaviour will generalize to this environment. What happens is predictable: often the client's behaviour is successfully modified in the special unit, but when they return to their natural environment, the behaviour returns. This is because, in the unit, reinforcement is made available for desired behaviour, but when the client returns to the natural environment, different behaviours are reinforced – the very ones which led the person to be sent to the special unit. Behaviour adapts to the reinforcement contingencies in the natural environment and, if these contingencies are unchanged when the client returns, the client's behaviour re-adapts to these contingencies. Special units can be useful for assessment and for testing different methods of behaviour change, but in order to bring about long-term changes in the natural environment, contingencies in that environment must also be changed.

Constructional Approaches

As we have seen, the temptation is to focus on using reducing consequences to manage 'problem' behaviours (the author still receives referrals phrased in terms such as 'what sanctions can we use when so and so does such and such behaviour?'). Research into DRO and DRI suggests a more positive approach may be possible. Goldiamond[26] developed this theme further when he pointed out that analysis of behaviour often shows that undesired behaviours are 'unacceptable means to acceptable ends': for example, seeking to gain attention is entirely appropriate and understandable, but gaining it by hitting someone else, headbanging, screaming, and so on, is less appropriate in terms of satisfactory social adjustment. Goldiamond stressed the importance of focusing on building up more acceptable means to the ends desired by the client, rather than on eliminating problem behaviours. He suggested a reorientation towards educational strategies and specific programmes using positive reinforcement to teach alternative skills. This has become known as the 'constructional approach'. This is perhaps the least coercive behavioural approach to reducing undesired behaviours, since it aims to extend the individual's behavioural repertoire and so increase the range of options and choices open to that person.

Functional Analysis

Goldiamond[26] emphasized that behaviour has meaning in the sense that problem behaviour is generally aimed at achieving appropriate goals. Nevertheless, many behaviour modification programmes have merely arranged special contingencies to eliminate the problem, rather than taking a constructional approach to developing alternative strategies and behaviours to allow the client to attain desired goals. Behaviour analysis approaches provide the means to analyse the contingencies of reinforcement which produce problem behaviour, and to identify the consequences that particular behaviours achieve (in other words the function of the behaviour for the individual). This process is known as 'functional analysis'.

The ABC Paradigm

Consequences have the function of increasing or decreasing the rate of behaviours they follow. Antecedents function as signals for the consequences. The first step in functional analysis is therefore to draw up a list of events that precede and follow the behaviour of interest on a regular basis, with the aim of identifying the antecedents and consequences actually operating on that behaviour at that time. Table 13.3 presents an illustrative ABC chart, completed by training centre staff in an attempt to identify antecedents and consequences for tearing clothing.

The ABC chart is used to provide the necessary information to allow the behaviour analyst to answer key questions about the function of the behaviour (is the behaviour followed by a positive reinforcer; does the behaviour allow the person to escape from or avoid a 'demand' situation?) and to identify regular triggers for the behaviour. It is important to bear in mind that the same behaviour may have different functions at different times (for example, an individual may bang his or her head for attention when sitting unoccupied in a large group setting, and may at other times head-bang in order to avoid being made to do something he or she does not want to do). Analysis is further complicated by the fact that antecedents and consequences may be private events experienced by the client, but not directly observable by others. For example, head-banging may be triggered by strong emotions such as jealousy or anger, or the consequences for head-banging may be self-stimulatory.

In practice, ABC recordings often simply do not provide sufficient information to identify the function of the behaviour. In the example in Table 13.3, it would appear from the chart that the main antecedent for tearing is some aspect of the table-top activity John is involved in, but the recording is not specific enough to allow further discrimination between the effects of different aspects of that situation. It is also difficult to draw conclusions with regard to the consequences reinforcing the behaviour, since the chart shows different consequences being applied by the staff on different occasions.

Table 13.3. ABC chart for John's behaviour of tearing his T-shirt.

Occasion	Antecedent	Behaviour(s)	Consequences
1	Sat with group at table	Tearing T-shirt	Another T-shirt on
2	Engaged at table	Tearing T-shirt	Told off
3	Occupied at table	Tearing T-shirt	Removed to toilet area
4	Sat at table with equipment	Tearing T-shirt	Ignored
5	Sat at table	Tearing T-shirt	Ignored
6	Sat at table	Tearing T-shirt	Another T-shirt
7	Asked to sit at table	Tearing T-shirt	Told off
8	Asked to start activity	Tearing T-shirt	Removed to toilet
9	Sat with group at table	Tearing T-shirt	Ignored
10	Sat at table with equipment	Tearing T-shirt	Ignored
11	Engaged at table	Tearing T-shirt	Ignored
12	Finished jigsaw	Tearing T-shirt	Removed to toilet
13	Banging head with equipment	Tearing T-shirt and became distressed	Taken home early
14	Sat at table with equipment	Tearing T-shirt	Took T-shirt away
15	Sat at table	Tearing T-shirt	Took T-shirt off him
16	Sat at table	Tearing T-shirt	Another T-shirt on

Beyond ABC

In order to obtain useful information, it is often necessary to carry out more detailed observations. This may involve recording 'samples' of the client's behaviour as it occurs, noting the precise onset and cessation of the behaviour and correlating this with the onset and cessation of particular events (arrival or departure of particular staff, requests to perform certain tasks, behaviour of other people, attention or other consequences provided). In order to provide a more complete picture, it is important to analyse other behaviours occurring in the situation and to observe whether the behaviour of interest is part of a chain of behaviours. Information about more distal influences on the behaviour can also be helpful in understanding its function. The environment the person lives in may itself promote undesired behaviours. Undesired behaviours are more common when there is a 'low density' of reinforcement: when reinforcement is at a premium, people will try almost anything to obtain it. Gradually, the importance of bereavement, multiple losses (e.g. staff moving on, moving from one residential situation to another), rejection and emotional, physical and sexual abuse in causing and maintaining problem behaviour has been recognized. While these concepts are not derived from the behavioural approach, they cannot be ignored when carrying out a functional analysis, as they serve as 'setting events' for the behaviour.

Table 13.4. Functional analysis of John's behaviour in the training centre.

Proximal factors		
Antecedents	Behaviours	Consequences
On own without activity	Stereotyped behaviour	Self-stimulation ('internal' positive reinforcement)
On own with non-preferred activity	(Chain) ↓	
Preferred activity on table but finished task	Tearing T-shirt (undesired behaviour)	Removed to toilet (avoids non-preferred task – negative reinforcement
One to one with preferred activity		Intrinsic enjoyment from task (preferred activities)
One to one with non-preferred activity	Working on task ('engaged')	
On own with preferred activity	(Desired behaviour)	Attention/social contact from staff (even non-preferred activities reinforcing with one-to-one staffing)

Distal factors
1. Learning disability and sensory handicaps
2. History understimulation at home – left in room on own (correlated with development of self-stimulatory repertoire)

Table 13.4 presents the results of a fuller functional analysis of John's behaviour in the training centre. First, his tearing appears to be the terminal response in a chain of stereotyped behaviour. Antecedents for these behaviours include being asked to perform certain 'nonpreferred' activities or being left unoccupied, while on-task behaviour is occasioned by presence of staff or being given certain 'preferred' activities. On these latter occasions, staff attention and enjoyment of the task appear to positively reinforce the on-task behaviour. It seems likely that stereotyped behaviour is maintained at least partly by escape from nonpreferred tasks (by being sent to the toilet or given a new T-shirt to put on), and partly by the internal stimulation it provides for John (this view is strengthened by John's history of understimulation exacerbated by sensory handicaps). This analysis is to some extent speculative and likely to be incomplete. Any analysis of this kind should develop and become more accurate as further information is collected. Nevertheless, it provides a starting point for understanding why John tears and provides clues as to some of the requirements to be built in to constructional interventions (attempts to identify and provide a wider range of preferred activities; provision of one-to-one attention when nonpreferred activities have to be introduced; use of distraction procedures early in the chain of stereotyped behaviour, etc.).

Training Carers

Behavioural Approaches in the 'Natural Environment'

Nurses, teachers, parents and others in the 'natural environment' of the client are in the best position to change behaviour. There have been many studies demonstrating that such agents can be effective in accomplishing this.[19] Early studies described cases where non-psychologists were taught to apply behavioural procedures to a limited number of behaviours under supervision from experienced behaviour analysts. Clearly, it would be advantageous for such agents to learn to apply more general principles rather than learning specific behaviour change skills for specific problems; this would allow application of the approach to new clients and situations and assist in maintenance of change once initial interventions are completed.

Training in Behavioural Principles

There has been a proliferation of texts and teaching 'manuals' presenting behavioural principles for use by non-psychologists (for example [15]). Unfortunately, there is evidence that without structured teaching written materials are ineffective in teaching principles.[27] Furthermore, structured teaching in behavioural principles using didactic lecture–discussion methods has been shown to have little effect on the performance of individuals in the natural environment: while lectures may increase verbal skills, performance skills need to be taught by methods more directly related to these skills.[28]

Teaching Performance Skills

A number of teaching programmes in behavioural approaches have combined didactic training in principles with training in performance skills using a method based on precision teaching, where the trainee is required to perform behaviour modification skills and receives consequences, prompts and so on from the trainer.[14] Feedback is often provided via videotape and role-playing is often employed as an alternative to letting trainees practise on real clients until they have acquired some expertise. Precision teaching can be an effective method of developing performance skills but there is evidence that these skills do not always generalize to new settings, behaviours and clients, or affect the carer's performance in the natural environment.[29] Therefore, there remains a need to teach behavioural principles.

Teaching Behaviour Analysis

Just as individuals in daily contact with a client are in the best position to change behaviour, these individuals are also in the best position to gather information about the variables causing and maintaining client behaviour. Consequently, it would appear valuable to develop nurses', teachers' and parents' skills in functional analysis rather than simply providing training in the implementation of behaviour modification techniques. Some texts have emphasized these skills,[20] but functional analysis depends on knowledge of principles of behaviour analysis, and it cannot be assumed that written materials alone will be effective in teaching these principles, or that teaching by didactic lecture-based methods will affect trainees' ability to analyse behaviour in the natural environment. Consequently, the question arises of how best to teach these principles.

Alternative Teaching Methods

Training in behavioural principles can be viewed as an attempt to establish stimulus control over analytical and performance skills by constructing a set of rules to govern functional analysis and management of reinforcement contingencies. Because training in principles has not generally been effective in changing trainees' performance in the natural environment, it has generally been assumed that knowledge of principles is insufficient to alter performance. However, it may simply be that the principles have not been taught effectively.

There has long been criticism of didactic methods from a learning theory standpoint for being at odds with principles of learning. The Personalized System of Instruction (PSI) approach was developed to overcome some of the deficits of lecture–discussion approaches.[30] PSI is characterized by active learner responding (such as completing assignments which then receive feedback from tutors), mastering each unit of the course before progressing to new material, student pacing of course work and reinforcement for course work. The author has used the PSI method to teach nurses and teachers behavioural principles,[31] hypothesizing that this approach would give trainees a better grasp of the rules governing behaviour analysis and contingency management. Comparisons of PSI with conventional didactic approaches demonstrated that PSI did indeed lead to improved performance upon test of knowledge of the principles. Further studies suggested that nurses who had attended a 1-week PSI in-service training course in behavioural principles performed more effectively in behavioural interventions on a ward than did untrained nurses, and that such courses were effective in teaching functional analysis skills. These studies highlighted the importance of the training format in developing relevant skills.

Giving Psychology Away

Although it is clearly advantageous to develop carers' behaviour analysis and behaviour change skills, it must be emphasized that it is impossible for psychologists to pass on all the complexities and nuances of the behavioural approach in short courses lasting a few days or less. Attempts to pass on basic skills have necessarily led to (over)simplification of the information disseminated. This raises ethical issues concerning giving away potentially powerful psychological techniques to non-psychologists, since their understanding of the techniques is necessarily limited and therefore likely to lead to misuse and misapplication. Therefore, in order to safeguard the client it is advisable to involve psychologists in the design and implementation of programmes of behaviour analysis and contingency management whenever possible, and to develop policies regulating the use of these approaches.

Safeguarding the Client

Since behavioural approaches were first introduced, there have been many advances in understanding the causes of challenging behaviour, both in terms of 'proximal' antecedents and consequences and 'distal' traumatic events and episodes in the life of the individual. Nevertheless, there is a continued risk that behavioural approaches will be used simply to provide 'sanctions' for challenging behaviour without real regard to the underlying reasons for that behaviour, and/or without any attempt to build a repertoire of more positive skills to enhance the person's quality of life and enable them to exert more control and take more responsibility. Under these circumstances, it is good practice to develop explicit multidisciplinary policies to regulate the use of behavioural techniques.

Such a policy has been developed by the Leeds Community and Mental Health Trust Learning Disability Service (see Appendix 1). I include it here as one example of formal multidisciplinary discussion and agreement in this area, and recommend similar policies be developed in all organizations where staff are likely to use these techniques. In addition, it is essential that services develop general guidelines for the prevention and control of challenging behaviour (i.e. not just restricted to the use of behavioural techniques), and set up mechanisms to allow the necessary multi-disciplinary planning, implementation and monitoring of all behavioural programmes (e.g. the 'Behavioural Clinics' referred to in the Leeds Policy in Appendix 1).

Provided that adequate safeguards are in place, behavioural approaches still have a vital role in the understanding and management of behaviour, particularly in the field of learning disability. It is important that interventions are based on thorough functional analysis and informed by knowledge of behavioural and other psychological principles, and further, that procedures are not used simply as a method of controlling behaviour to the advantage of staff and parents at the expense of the needs and rights of the client.

Appendix I

Leeds Community & Mental Health Teaching NHS Trust Policy on the Use of Behavioural Techniques

I. Introduction

    (a) This Policy focuses on the use of specified behavioural techniques; those which attempt to control behaviour which is considered challenging. These techniques are specified as:

        (i) Those which present an **aversive stimulus**, i.e. those which present consequences which are unpleasant and disliked by the resident such as physical restraint, over-correction, seclusion.

        (ii) Those which **restrict or remove positive reinforcement**, i.e. the removal of something which the resident likes or values such as time-out, loss of cigarettes, money, treats, etc.

    (b) The above techniques are most often used to provide direct methods of managing episodes of challenging behaviour which are of such a nature that they cannot be simply disregarded. Behavioural techniques in general can be helpful when staff feel that they need extra strategies to cope with a difficult situation. Such techniques, properly used, can offer a practical framework in aiding staff. The Mental Health Act Code of Practice (revised 1993)[32] highlights the need for these techniques to be well understood and adequately supervised so as to encourage the following:

        (i) Individual development.

        (ii) Maintenance of positive relationships.

(iii) Promotion of good practice.

(iv) Prevention of further problems.

(v) Improved quality of care.

All programmes of care must be able to demonstrate all five of the above points.

This policy requires the maximum involvement of unit staff in the production of care plans which include behavioural techniques. Such care plans are produced within the guidance and supervision which are legally required.

(c) Institutional services for people with learning disabilities/mental handicap, such as hospital, have a long history of controlling patients through rules, regulations and systems of reward and punishment. In order for services to develop more humane policies which help clients to learn new skills and responsibilities and preserve their individual rights, it is recognized that many issues will need to be addressed such as resources, staff training and staff support.

(d) However, on a day-to-day basis, it is the responsibility of staff to use the skills and experience they currently possess to enable clients to develop socially appropriate ways of meeting their needs.

(e) Occasionally, staff may wish to use the techniques specified above as part of a skills teaching programme. The use of these techniques to persuade or encourage a client to learn or to use a self-care, work or other skill is **not recommended**.

(f) Where the use of behavioural techniques is defined in paragraph 1(a) above is being considered for whatever reason, then the policy and procedures detailed below must be implemented.

2. Policy

(a) The first consideration is always to try to understand the causes of behaviour and to take positive steps to prevent it occurring through environmental change, skill teaching, etc. All staff are familiar with the *Guidelines on the Prevention of Challenging Behaviour*. Positive approaches to prevention form the major part of any programme which aims to control challenging behaviour.

(b) On rare occasions additional direct methods of controlling episodes of challenging behaviour may be necessary. Where episodes of challenging behaviour cannot be simply disregarded, behaviour techniques as described in 1(a) above may be appropriate to manage episodes when they occur and to facilitate change.

(c) **Programmes using these methods are a last resort and must only form a small part of the care plan.**

(d) Where the use of behavioural techniques as defined in paragraph 1(a) is being considered as a means of controlling episodes of challenging behaviour, the Head of Department/Care Area, in discussion with others, takes the decision to refer to the Behavioural Clinic.

(e) Before any programme using behavioural techniques to control behaviour, as described in 1(a), is implemented by Health Service staff, it must be agreed with and signed by the keyworker/primary nurse, a clinical psychologist, and the appropriate Nurse Manager/Head of Department and, in the case of in-patients, the responsible Medical Officer. Additional guidance is available in respect of community clients.

(f) Staff must observe the following when drafting such programmes:

   (i)   Resident's basic human rights must be protected. Programmes involving the denial or the threat of denial of food, water, shelter, clothing, warmth, personal dignity, access to friends or relations or to occupation or privacy (both physical and in relation to their personal thoughts and feelings) or confidentiality are not acceptable (Mental Health Act Code of Practice, Revised 1993).[32]

   (ii)   It is Trust policy that the use of physical punishment is not permitted in any circumstances.

   (iii) Programmes are so arranged as to enable residents to have access to additional positive reinforcement upon appropriate behaviour: such **additional positive reinforcement** being removed or restricted as a consequence of an episode of challenging behaviour.

   (iv) Where the use of aversive stimuli such as seclusion or restraint is necessary, the programme must adhere to the policies detailed in *Guidelines on the Management of Challenging Behaviour*.

   (v)   In all cases **before** any programme for controlling challenging behaviour is agreed, it is discussed fully with the client. Where possible the client's consent to the programme is obtained. Since the ultimate goal of services is to help clients to become responsible for their own behaviour and decisions, it is especially important that they become involved in devising management programmes.

   (vi) Where clients indicate disagreement either verbally or nonverbally with the proposed programme, the staff member who discussed the programme with the client is responsible for informing the Psychology Department of the disagreement within three working days. An appointment will be made at the next Psychology Clinic where the staff member and psychologist will meet with the client to discuss further courses of action.

   (vii) It is recognized at all times that staff have a duty to protect other clients themselves from physical injury.

   (viii) Programmes involving the removal of positive reinforcement are **only** related to the challenging behaviour.

(ix)   The consequences of any episode of challenging behaviour are dealt with in the environment in which they occurred.

(x)   In all cases the reason for restricting or removing positive reinforcement is explained to the client.

(xi)   Programmes are clearly written, easily accessible and readily understood by all members of staff, relatives, and where possible, clients themselves. Copies are sent to the relevant medical staff by the Psychology Department.

(xii) Detailed records are kept and are available to all relevant staff, Nurse Managers, Heads of Departments, Consultants and Psychologists. These records are dated and signed and include a full description of the challenging behaviour and the action taken in every instance when the agreed programme has been implemented.

(xiii) Programmes involving the use of behavioural techniques referred to in 1(a) above sometimes result in temporary increases in challenging behaviour. When the agreed programme results in a serious deterioration of behaviour which is not acceptable then the HOD/Care Area Manager may terminate the programme but is also responsible for ensuring that the Psychology Department and the Nurse Manager/Head of Department are informed that an appointment is being made to discuss alternative strategies at the next Psychology Clinic.

(xiv) Difficulty surrounding the development of any programme and its implementation should be communicated by relevant staff to the line manager and the Clinical Psychologist who are responsible for agreeing appropriate action.

(xv)   Data from monitoring systems will be reviewed at six-monthly intervals.

3. Procedure for Implementing the Policy on the Use of Behavioural Techniques to Control Challenging Behaviour

(a)   The attention of staff is drawn to paragraphs 2(c), 2(e), 2(f)(i), 2(f)(ii).

Where the policy specified in the above paragraphs is not followed, staff are advised that, after due consideration of all the facts and circumstances, action may be taken in line with the Leeds CMH Trust's disciplinary procedures.

(December 1994)

References

1. Potts M & Howard AF (1986) Psychology and community mental handicap. In Koch H (ed) *Community Clinical Psychology*. London: Croom Helm.
2. Ayllon T & Michael JL (1959) The psychiatric nurse as behavioural engineer. *Journal of the Experimental Analysis of Behaviour* **2**, 323–34.
3. Williams CD (1959) The elimination of tantrum behaviour by extinction procedures. *Journal of Abnormal and Social Psychology* **59**, 269–70.
4. Clarke ADB & Clarke AN (eds) *Mental Deficiency: the Changing Outlook*. London: Methuen.
5. Skinner BF (1938) *The Behaviour of Organisms*. New York: Appleton Century.
6. Skinner BF (1953) *Science and Human Behaviour*. New York: Macmillan.
7. Skinner BF (1957) *Verbal Behaviour*. New York: Appleton Century-Crofts.
8. Ayllon T (1963) Intensive treatment of psychotic behaviour by stimulus satiation and food reinforcement. *Behaviour Research and Therapy* **1**, 53–61.
9. Allyon T & Haughton E (1962) Control of the behaviour of schizophrenic patients by food. *Journal of the Experimental Analysis of Behaviour*, **5**, 343–52.
10. Ayllon T & Azrin NH (1968) *The Token Economy: A Motivational System for Therapy and Rehabilitation*. New York: Appleton Century-Crofts.
11. Bijou SW, Birnbrauer JS, Kidder JD & Tague CE (1966) Programmed instruction as an approach to the teaching of reading, writing and arithmetic to retarded children. *Psychological Record* **16**, 505–22.
12. Allen KE, Hart BM, Buell JS, Harris FR & Wolf MM (1964) Effects of social reinforcement on isolate behaviour of a nursery school child. *Child Development* **35**, 511–8.
13. Cliffe MJ, Gathercole C & Epling WF (1974) Some implications of the experimental analysis of behaviour for behaviour modification. *Bulletin of the British Psychological Society* **27**, 390–7.
14. McBrien J (1982) *Education of the Developmentally Young Mentally Handicapped Child: A Programme of Evaluated Dissemination and Research*. Final report to the Department of Education and Science, Hester Adrian Research Centre, University of Manchester. Manchester: University of Manchester.
15. Perkins EA, Taylor PD & Capie ACM (1976) *Helping the Retarded: a Systematic Behavioural Approach*. Kidderminster: BIMH Publications.
16. Shearer MS & Shearer DE (1972) The Portage Project: a model for early childhood education. *Exceptional Children* **36**, 210–7.
17. Honig WK (ed) (1966) *Operant Behaviour: Areas of Research and Application*. New York: Appleton Century-Crofts.
18. Honig WK & Staddon JR (eds) (1978) *Handbook of Operant Behaviour*. New York: Appleton Century-Crofts.
19. Kazdin AE (1980) *Behaviour Modification in Applied Settings* (revised edition). Homewood: Dorsey.
20. Presland JL (1989) *Overcoming Difficult Behaviour*. Kidderminster: BIMH Publications.
21. Tennant L, Cullen C & Hattersley J (1981) Applied behavioural analysis: intervention with retarded people. In Davey GCL (ed) *Applications of Conditioning Theory*. London: Methuen.
22. Meichenbaum D (1977) *Cognitive Behaviour Modification*. New York: Plenum.
23. Mackay TAWN (1981) Punishment viewed as a dignified alternative. *Apex* **9(1)**, 4–7.
24. Kohlenberg RB (1970) The punishment of persistent vomiting: a case study. *Journal of Applied Behaviour Analysis* **3**, 241–5.
25. Sajwaj T, Libet J & Agras S (1974) Lemon-juice therapy: the control of life-threatening ruminating in a six month old infant. *Journal of Applied Behaviour Analysis* **7**, 557–63.
26. Goldiamond IE (1974) Toward a constructional approach to social problems. *Behaviourism* **2**, 1–84.
27. McKeown D, Adams HE & Forehand R (1975) Generalisation to the classroom of principles of behaviour modification taught to teachers. *Behaviour Research and Therapy* **13**, 85–92.
28. Gardner JM (1972) Teaching behaviour modification to non-professionals. *Journal of Applied Behaviour Analysis* **5**, 517–21.
29. Milne D (1986) *Training Behaviour Therapists*. London: Croom Helm.
30. Keller FS (1968) Goodbye teacher … *Journal of Applied Behaviour Analysis* **1**, 79–89.
31. Mackrell K (1983) Teaching behaviour modification and behaviour analysis skills. *Behaviour Analysis* **4**, 2–17.
32. Department of Health and Welsh Office (1993) *Code of Practice, Mental Health Act*. London: HMSO.

14

Psychotherapy

Alexander Esterhuyzen and Sheila Hollins

Introduction

This chapter develops a rationale for the place of psychotherapy in promoting mental health for individuals with learning disabilities and their carers, by concentrating on issues related to attachment and its possible role in complicating their healthy development and individuation. It explores attachment theory and research in relation to learning disability in an effort to increase psychodynamic understanding of some of the common difficulties presented to community teams working with individuals who have a learning disability. Family responses to having a family member with a severe disability are discussed in a practical way, and some therapeutic approaches are outlined.

Children with disabilities are at greater risk for the development of emotional and behavioural disorders, particularly where the disability is associated with brain abnormalities.[1-4] There are many different mechanisms which may contribute to this increased risk of emotional and behavioural disorders. These include the direct effect of brain dysfunction, possible associated sensory deficits, a decrease in intellectual and physical ability and competence, all of which alter an individual's interaction with the environment and their capacity to use the environment for further development. Differences in appearance and ability will undoubtedly affect self-esteem and may engender social stigma. Family interactions may also be altered as a result of having to adapt to the disabled member of the family and their specific and often demanding needs. All of these may contribute to an increased risk of psychological as well as psychiatric disorders in this client group.[5]

Three 'anonymous' typical clinical vignettes of referrals to a community psychiatric team for people with learning disabilities are presented below. The discussion of attachment theory and research applied to individuals with learning disabilities that follows will be used to help understand some of the common problems which present to a community team from a psychodynamic perspective.

Clinical Vignettes

(1) 'Charles' is a 25-year-old man. He has a moderate learning disability and is a wheelchair user who has multiple physical disabilities, including congenital cardiac abnormalities and a

number of orthopaedic complications. He also has neurological disorders requiring specialist intervention. He is an engaging person with good speech and a number of interests outside his home. His referral was precipitated by the intense anxiety aroused in him and the surrounding system (paediatric team, parents and social workers) regarding transfer of his medical care to adult services. This transfer is taking place 9 years later than would normally be the case for people without learning disabilities. It is not unusual for any transition, such as the time of transfer from child to adult services, starting or changing schools or employment, leaving home, to generate anxiety in anyone, especially people with learning disability. However, the enormous anxiety generated in the system of carers around the person, such as in the case of Charles, warrants further exploration so as to increase our understanding of it, to contextualize it and deal with it more effectively.

(2) 'Michael' is a 45-year-old man with a severe learning disability. He has little speech and suffers from epilepsy. He was referred to the community team by his neurologist because of deterioration in the control of his epilepsy, which was not responding to medication and seemed to be aggravated by trips outside his home. On investigating there was no medical cause for this deterioration and there was some doubt as to whether Michael was always suffering genuine fits. After a home visit it was established that he had been kept at home from an early age after he had been labelled 'ineducable'. He never left home without one of his parents who devotedly cared for him. They were now becoming very elderly and father had recently developed a number of physical complaints which made him less mobile. The timing and circumstances of a referral such as this one is in no way unusual for a community team working in the field of learning disability. Examining it in the light of attachment theory helps to clarify the dynamics operating in this situation and enables use of this understanding in treatment.

(3) Moira is a 30-year-old woman. She has a moderate learning disability with fair speech and attends a day centre 3 days per week. The reason for her referral was her very difficult and conflicted relationship with her mother. Moira was often physically violent to her mother, who constantly contacted the community team insisting that her daughter must be mentally ill as she had been a 'sweet, obedient girl' until some years before. Her mother also logged a complaint against the team because she felt that her daughter's illness had not been properly investigated, despite many investigations including a computerized tomography (CT) scan which revealed no specific abnormalities that could account for her behaviour. While being investigated she was an inpatient, but was visited by mother and went home at weekends. Moira seemed unable to bear being with her mother yet

worried incessantly about her if away from home. Her aggressive behaviour was seldom expressed outside her relationship with her mother.

Attachment Theory and Research

Bowlby, linking his interest in psychoanalysis and ethology, first described how infant behaviours like sucking, crying, smiling, clinging and following become organized into attachment behaviour towards a specific care-giver.[6] This was elaborated and researched further by Ainsworth *et al.*,[7] among others; they categorized attachment behaviour into 'secure' and 'insecure', with the latter having a number of subcategories. The characteristics of attachment behaviour are listed in Table 14.1; attachment behaviour is activated particularly in the presence of external threat.

The relevance of attachment theory to individuals with learning disability is reinforced by the fact that attachment behaviour is evident in normal infants from the developmental level reached at 6 months of age. This implies that even those with severe learning disability may show attachment behaviour.

Bowlby not only described attachment behaviour, but also the consequences of separation from the attachment figure (i.e. when attachment behaviour is elicited but the attachment figure remains absent).[6] He divided the response to this separation into phases of protest, despair and reorganization.[8,9] During the protest phase the infant attempts to recover the lost object. There is weeping, searching, yearning for the lost object and anger. The aim of this behaviour is to reverse the loss. During the despair phase there is disorganization, a realization that the object is permanently absent and, with this, depression (see Table 14.2).

Table 14.1   The characteristics of attachment behaviour.

1. It involves a specific person as the attachment figure
2. Proximity seeking; actively seeking to be near the attachment figure
3. Secure base effect; the attachment figure is used as a secure base from which the environment is explored
4. Attachment behaviour is elicited by threat in the external or internal environment
5. Separation protest; occurs as a result of separation from the attachment figure
6. It is insensitive to experience with the attachment figure (i.e. persists even if the attachment figure is neglecting or abusing)
7. It persists and is not accessible to conscious control. (There is no habituation, even if there is an intellectual recognition that the attachment figure will not return and that an alternative attachment figure is available)

Table 14.2   Phases of separation.

1. Protest	(Related to separation anxiety)
2. Despair	(Related to mourning and grief)
3. Detachment/denial	(Related to defence)

During the reorganization phase, Bowlby[6] states that, if the phases of protest and despair are allowed to develop and the associated effects worked through, reorganization takes place and new patterns of attachment to new objects can take place. If not, yearning for the lost object persists unconsciously and is strongly defended. There follows a persistent striving to recover the lost object. This has important implications for individuals with learning disability where, because of the persisting level of dependence on attachment figures, separation responses may be particularly intense and opportunities for the expression and working through of effects associated with the separation are often minimal. Parkes elaborated the phases of the separation response to describe the phases of grief in normal adults.[10] He described four phases of grief in parallel to the separation reaction of infants separated from their attachment figure: (1) numbness, (2) yearning and protest, (3) disorganization and despair, and (4) reorganization.[10]

The milieu or pattern of the response between mother and infant contributes to the 'style' of attachment relationship (secure or insecure) between primary carer and infant. Bowlby suggests that the biological purpose of such early attachment relationships is to ensure survival of the helpless infant and to develop its emotional security and social autonomy. This fundamental style of relating forms the pattern for subsequent intimate relationships and is thought to extend beyond infancy. In effect, the attachment pattern becomes an internalized working model of relationships and is used unconsciously to predict expectations about care and intimacy with others.[11,12] However, little is known about how these internalized working models affect the behaviour of others.

Evidence exists that the attachment pattern predicts the future social competence of children, their approach to problem solving, and the affective quality of this interaction with others.[11,13,14] It also predicts the presence of psychological disorder in boys up to 5 years later.[15,16]

Children who are classified as having insecure attachment to their mothers at 18 months interact differently 2 or 3 years later with their peers from those with a secure attachment. The insecurely attached child interacts harmoniously with children who have secure attachments, but in a manner that victimizes, systematically exploits, demeans or otherwise mistreats their partner in play who has a history of insecure attachment.[13,17]

There is research into how maternal mental state, particularly depression might affect attachment patterns. Radke-Yarrow[18] found increased incidence of insecure attachment in the infants of depressed mothers. She found that those babies in her study group who showed a disorganized pattern of attachment behaviour had care-givers who had suffered a major loss. This issue was further investigated by Eichberg[19] and Ainsworth and Eichberg,[20] who found that care-givers who had a major loss but with resolved grief had infants with a normal range of attachment. Those care-givers with unresolved grief had infants with the disorganized pattern of attachment.

Intergenerational transmission of attachment patterns, although not necessarily indefinitely fixed, appears to be relatively consistent. Using the adult attachment schedule and the standardized strange situation infant observations, in 75% of cases the mother's own attachment pattern measured before birth is consistent with that of her child at 1 year and at 5 years of age.[12]

Application of Attachment Theory to Individuals with Learning Disability

Early Influences

It is possible that the lack of the usual pattern of turn-taking in communication in the neonate with delayed motor and neurological development could significantly affect the quality of attachment between mother and child. While the full repertoire of attachment behaviour as described by Bowlby[6] is present from 6 months of age, there are important precursors which depend on the degree of mutual mother–child responsiveness and the infant's expressiveness. These are clearly influenced by neurological and motor development which may be delayed or, in some instances, absent in the individual with a learning disability. This will be especially so if the expression and communication of important emotions such as fear or distress from the infant are modified because of the disability so that the parent has difficulty registering or interpreting them. This may be further complicated if the child is less able to interpret the parent's actions or regulate their own affective stage to the level that might be expected of their chronological age. The child may also be less able to orient or move towards the parent in response to internal security needs. All of these would require a capacity for the parent to be able to compensate for these deficits with increased sensitivity and responsiveness.[21–23] This is more likely to be possible if the parents themselves have a history of a secure attachment, have had experience of parenting, and are not subject to psychosocial deprivation. Parents of disabled children need a high level of skill to read emotional clues given by their child and to communicate with them in ways they can understand.[13,24] These important variables are likely to affect the quality of attachment between such infants and their mothers.

In addition to the parents' attachment pattern, their experience of child rearing (e.g. first child compared with subsequent children) and their temperament, there is also the question of the impact of a diagnosis of disability on the parent. Many authors describe a bereavement-like response – the loss of their idea of the expected normal child, and the subsequent grieving of this by the care-giver,[25] although there is evidence that mothers and fathers may differ significantly in their typical response.[26] A bereavement response may be expected to affect the attachment patterns developed between parent and child. In the case of the birth or later diagnosis of a child with severe disability the degree to which the mother's loss and unspoken grief and anxieties are acknowledged and worked through is variable in the extreme. Many articulate parents subsequently express their anger at the way in which this issue was dealt with at the time of diagnosis, only years later in the safety of self-support groups such as MENCAP. The loss and grieving of a mother who has given birth to a disabled child may affect the nature of attachment in the infant regardless of the mother's own attachment pattern. As noted earlier, the effects of loss and particularly unresolved loss or depression as studied in the general population can have lasting impact on a child's attachment pattern. Thus, it is proposed that learning disability in a new-born infant is likely to affect the quality of attachment between care-giver and infant, particularly if the mother has herself had an insecure attachment in her own infancy and especially if her own grief and loss due to this life event is unresolved. This is likely to be compounded further if the child needed neonatal intensive care.[27]

It is conceivable that in some cases this could contribute to an insecure or an over-anxious attachment pattern in the interaction between mother and infant. This is in accordance with research findings on the effect of unresolved loss on attachment described above. In individuals and their families who present with emotional, behavioural and/or psychological difficulties this important psychodynamic factor and its influence should be considered and included in the understanding of aetiology and treatment.

Life Transitions

The nature of the attachment pattern will affect the balance between the drives for independence or exploration, and the security needs of both the mother and infant. The factors which promote fading off of attachment to parents are listed in Table 14.3. It is self-evident that there are decreased opportunities for this natural fading to take place for adults with learning disability. Typically, more emphasis is laid on supporting the child's security needs than, for example, encouraging social and sexual maturation and independence, thus further complicating an already intense and possibly insecure attachment. Each life transition, for example, first attendance at school, changing school, leaving school, leaving home, facing loss or illness of a loved one, may re-evoke the feelings and anxieties associated with the particular attachment style that the individual has had with his primary carer. This is especially so where the individual with learning disability has not had the opportunity to develop a wide range of attachments in addition to that experienced with his or her primary carer. The perceived threat to the primary attachment at each life transition, on the

Table 14.3 Factors which promote fading of attachment to parents.

1. Sexual and social maturation of the individual
2. Increased capacity to recognize the limitation of parents
3. Displays of frailty of parents
4. Increased self-confidence and desire for independence
5. Distancing initiated by the parents

338   *Psychiatry in Learning Disability*

side of the carer and of the individual with learning disability, and the consequent protest and despair evoked will be dependent on the quality and nature of both of their attachment patterns. It should be noted that intense and complex emotions in individuals with learning disabilities are often acted out behaviourally owing to difficulties in articulating and acknowledging any powerful and possibly frightening emotions. If the importance and implications of these transitions are not recognized by carers and professionals an inordinate amount of anxiety can be generated in the client and the system involved with them.

Bereavement: An Important Example

Bereavement is a typical example of a life event which is likely to occur in the average life span of most people. Given the fundamental importance of attachment theory in describing and understanding the grief reaction, and particularly noting the fact that attachment behaviour is elicited from age 6 months, it seems entirely reasonable to expect that bereavement would have an impact on individuals who may have limited cognitive skills even though they do not have the intellectual capacity to comprehend some of the sophisticated concepts involved in understanding death and its implications (e.g. irreversibility, universality and nonfunctionality).[28] Lack of cognitive skills to understand what has happened will compound difficulties in coming to terms with the nonreturn of the attachment figure. If care-givers do not recognize the protest and despair for what it is and fail to facilitate working through of the associated affects, this may further impede reorganization and the capacity to form new and appropriate attachments. It may also lead to complicated grief which the client may express in ways which are not necessarily recognized as part of grieving (e.g. anger or other 'challenging behaviours').[29]

Evidence that insecure attachment affects future capacity to resolve losses and grief in the general population is given by Parkes *et al.* who cite an increase in psychiatric problems after bereavement if childhood attachment was insecure.[30] In the same text they also cite the work of Sable,[31] who found that in a sample of 81 widows, those with a secure childhood attachment pattern had a better outcome in ratings of anxiety and depression than the ones with insecure childhood attachment patterns. Marris[32] identified several factors that were more likely to be associated with depression in bereaved adults. These included: failure of early attachment; disruption of meaning in the individual's life; a sense of worthlessness; and, finally, paternalistic control by others of one's future. All of these factors are commonly observed in individuals with learning disabilities.

Thus, it is highly probable that many of them will be profoundly affected by bereavement, and specifically by the loss of a primary care-giver, despite their cognitive limitations. This discussion of attachment theory also highlights the fact that although the importance of research in this area has been recognized in the general population, none of this important dynamic work has been studied in individuals with learning disabilities.

The possible influence of insecure attachment and high levels of dependency in individuals with learning disability, many of whom have been – and continue to be – cared for at home for many years by carers who are now elderly has been alluded to above. It could also be argued that, because of a reduced social sphere and the limitations that are often placed on an individual with learning disability, the development of new relationships may be restricted. The breaking of their few, close bonds may have catastrophic consequences for both the internal and external life of that individual. It is vital for professionals to have a clear understanding of the nature of those important attachments, both to understand those relationships and to anticipate the likely consequences of their disruption. This understanding will shed light on the longer term use of these relationships as internal models that clients will use in subsequent intimate and important relationships (e.g. with key workers or residential cohabitees).

The situation for the individual with a learning disability following bereavement may be one of profound and multiple losses, including the person best able to understand their communications, disruption of their life patterns and environment. Preparation for separation, including death, is often minimal and there is a tendency to withhold information from the person with learning disability in a misguided attempt to 'protect' them. Part of the process of mourning involves the expression and working through of the protest and despair discussed above. Maeson *et al.*[33] have demonstrated the importance of exposure to cues relating to the deceased in facilitating resolution of grief. Yet, when death of a close family member occurs, it is common for a person with learning disability to be denied the opportunity to take part in the funeral. He or she may not be told about the death until weeks or months later, and sometimes not at all.[25,29,34]

Practice of Psychotherapy Using Attachment Theory

Clinical Vignettes

The implications of attachment theory for the clinical vignettes introduced earlier in the chapter will now be discussed.

(1) Charles

Charles was an only child who often had life-threatening illnesses from birth. His insecure anxious attachment to his mother and father was recreated in other important relationships. The professionals involved needed help to stand back and reflect on the anxiety that resulted in them treating this particular patient differently from other young people who were passed on to adult services at age 17. Work with Charles and his parents, but also including professionals such as his social worker, helped them to look at and understand some of their anxieties which were related to patterns established long ago and were no longer appropriate to a young man whose medical conditions were stable and well controlled. Much of his parents' loss – the loss of the perfectly healthy boy they had hoped for and the reminders to them and to himself at each milestone that he was disabled and different – had to be mourned and his gifts, including his warmth and humorous personality, appreciated so that they were able to go on to the next stage in his growing up. Careful planning of transfer of care, involving all the players in the system, with recognition and articulation of the underlying unconscious anxieties was necessary.

(2) Michael

Michael was found to be suffering from panic attacks rather than fits. These did not resolve until the whole system, in particular his parents, were included in regular treatment sessions with Michael. Work in these sessions included exploring their fears and anxieties for his future after his parents' death. After several months of family work using an understanding of attachment theory Michael began to attend the local day centre to learn basic self-care skills and cooking with the support of his parents. Gradually, he developed further independence and confidence and began to go on regular leisure excursions with a community volunteer.

(3) Moira

Moira's story demonstrates the tensions of separation/individuation in the context of an anxious attachment. Of interest is that her mother had had a difficult and disrupted childhood. She was also the last remaining member of her own family and her husband had died some years previously. No progress was made until Moira's mother was given individual psychotherapy sessions to deal with her own anxieties about separation which she was projecting onto her daughter. Gradually, Moira was able to use resources in the community and her mother was less anxious in her own involvement and contact with the community team. Ironically, Moira's mother then developed a life-threatening illness which involved Moira assisting in her physical care at home. This role reversal had to be managed carefully by the team in order to maintain Moira's independence and own individuation as well as addressing the possibility of her mother's death. Without a knowledge of the dynamics of attachment Moira may have been inappropriately labelled as having a psychiatric or behavioural problem, and/or the relationship between the team and her mother could have deteriorated seriously. It is of note that when Moira was a child her mother had commenced litigation in search of compensation for the imagined medical negligence which she assumed had caused Moira's disability. She did not pursue the claim after obtaining an expert legal opinion.

When to Refer for Psychotherapy and How to Support it

Pathways to specialist psychiatric and psychological care for people with learning disabilities are often impaired by failures of both relatives and professionals to recognize remediable problems in the community, and at the primary care and specialist health care filters.[35-37] The presenting problem is usually either disturbed behaviour or loss of skills in the child or adult with learning disability. These presenting features may be excused as being due to the condition such as fragile-X syndrome, which caused the learning disability, and such diagnostic overshadowing is probably the major barrier in accessing an adequate range of specialist mental health services for people with learning disabilities. Both individual and group analytic therapy work with the affect that the patient shows. Therapy is not an intellectual activity, and assessment of cognitive ability is irrelevant when considering someone's suitability. Psychotherapy should be a tertiary referral after a full biopsychosocial assessment has been completed because psychotherapeutic interventions will be unsuccessful if there are environmental or biological factors which are maintaining the symptoms for which a referral was made. The psychotherapist, whether offering individual, family or group therapy, will expect other factors and necessary support to be adequately addressed or provided by the community team, care manager or other supporter, so that the process of therapy will not be undermined. The psychotherapist will not intervene to sort out practical problems which develop in the individual's life during the timescale of the therapeutic contract. It is therefore essential that the referrer is in a position to deal with such practical matters. It is also important that they are committed to the referral themselves and will ensure adequate support to enable the person to attend their sessions regularly.

When Should Therapy End?

A common reason for therapy being discontinued is because an inexperienced carer is unable to tolerate any ambivalence which develops in the client about their therapy. Negotiations about the continuation or termination of therapy should take place in the session between the therapist and the 'patient'. Typically, termination is an issue from the first session. In some situations such as brief focal therapy, or, perhaps where the purchasers have restricted funding to a limited number of sessions, the contract will be agreed at the beginning, and the 'patient' may not even be involved in the negotiation.

Generally, it is impossible to anticipate the number of sessions which will be needed by any individual. Ending should, however, be anticipated and negotiated with the client well in advance so that the powerful affects associated with loss in this client group can be addressed during the process of ending therapy. Many individuals will show an increase in behavioural disturbance or depression as they develop insight about their inner world and their relationships. For an individual with an insecure attachment pattern, therapy provides an opportunity to act out their attachment pattern with the therapist and this may lead to erratic and ambivalent attendance patterns. The secure boundaries of the therapy session are designed to 'hold' the patient so that they can reorganize their inner world and develop more secure and healthy ways of relating to people from their past, present and future. The length of time that such reorganization can take varies enormously between individuals. Ideally, therapy continues until the individual has worked through their insecure attachments, and made new secure attachments in the real world.

Outcome measures of change following psychodynamic psychotherapy include continuing improvement in interpersonal functioning, and changes which are sustained for a longer period than are typically obtained for shorter behavioural interventions. Little research has been published about the efficacy of psychotherapy in people with learning disabilities other than detailed in case reports. Projective tests such as repertory grids have been used in a limited way but appear to confirm changes in an individual's inner world before and after group therapy.[38–42]

Therapeutic Approaches

Working with Families

Family therapy initially focused on work with families with children of different ages from toddlers to adolescence. Families were enabled to develop different coping strategies, and encouraged to involve individuals from their wider networks to help them. Concepts of 'scapegoating' and the 'identified patient' were developed, and the emphasis was shifted away from notions of pathology or blame. Work with families that had a disabled child was slow to develop. If the disability was permanent, it seemed that the focus would have to remain on the disabled child. The 'identified patient' remained the patient and there seemed no point in relocating any difficulties within the family system. If the child could not be cured, then it seemed that family therapy could have no role. Families referred for help were often irate that the professionals seemed to be blaming them for their child's disability, rather than offering the extra practical and understanding help they needed. Family therapists need an understanding of the context and system into which disability has arrived, and of the emotional tasks which families face at different stages.

Gradually, an awareness is growing about the importance of helping families at an early stage after diagnosis of disability to come to terms with the long-term implications of the particular diagnosis.[25,43]

This is preventative emotional work and is an effective early intervention which supports the development of healthy attachments. Separation or 'letting go' should begin in infancy with mothers allowing fathers to share in the child's care. Siblings can encourage contact with peers and even if the child attends a segregated special school, mainstream social and leisure opportunities will help to promote normal separation. Parents and siblings may need help to assert when their childs 'naughtiness' is due to the fact they are 3 years old, rather than to the fact they have Down's syndrome. Other enhancing experiences will include the support of family groups who have disabled children, the use of trusted baby sitters or, in the teenage and adult years, the 'Saturday night' pal. Few child development centres provide routine counselling to parents of children newly diagnosed with disabilities. Most medically led services still fail to offer a truly biopsychosocial approach, although the medical biological approaches and technologies are well advanced and the social and educational supports needed by disabled children have improved significantly. The essential psychological adaptations which are required are largely ignored, and parents do not usually take their own emotional needs to appointments with their child's paediatrician but instead recognize what is expected of them in different settings.

The strain caused by failure to deal with psychological issues associated with disability and difference are further compounded by the ordinary stresses and strains of family life. Families with a disabled member have to face life events similar to other families but with the hidden extras of either grief for their child's apparent loss of potential, or of guilt for their real or imagined role in causing the disability, or the challenge of seeking or refusing genetic counselling. They also have to face the additional burden of care which may include hard physical work with extra laundry, extended supervision and disturbed sleep.

The family may struggle with shame about the disabled child's difference, in terms of his/her appearance, behaviour or developmental age. Siblings may be embarrassed to bring their friends home, and parents may become increasingly isolated putting all their spare energy into 'child-centred' activities in the hope of enhancing his/her achievements. Bicknell[25] wrote eloquently in a classic inaugural lecture about the maladaptive responses of many families, and in particular she made the link with attachment theory in her description of overprotective parents and the failure of separation and individuation. Sadly, these can remain lifelong issues causing anxiety to widowed elderly carers coping on their own in their 80s and still confused about the future needs of their son or daughter. It follows that work with families with an adult family member will first need to look at early attachment to understand why they have become stuck in their current patterns of behaviour. Hollins and Grimer wrote about three 'secrets' in the lives of people with learning disability which appear to distort their emotional maturation and the fading of attachment to their parents.[44] These are the secrets of their disability and dependence, of their sexuality and of mortality, especially of their parents. More recently, the secret of sexuality has acquired increased significance as the high prevalence of abuse in disabled individuals is becoming apparent.

Family therapists will find it helpful to address each of these developmental issues with families before expecting any changes in family coping style to be sustainable.

Family Therapy – What to Expect

More experience of therapeutic work with families is now available and some specialist family therapy teams work with families who have a disabled family member of any age.[45,46]

In family therapy, the family members learn to 'dance a different dance'. The insights from a session (which may only be offered every 4–6 weeks) will inform and change the way the family lives and works together before the next session. Some therapists work on their own with the family and others as part of a team who watch and respond to the session from behind a one-way screen. In the latter case the therapist who is in the room will take a break to discuss the process of the session with the team. In some clinics the team will swap places with the family towards the end of the session and become a 'reflecting team', discussing their ideas about what is happening within the family system so that the family have the direct benefit of the discussion by listening to it together in private behind the screen. The therapist endeavours not to take sides but seeks to enlist the help of each family member. This may be achieved by giving the family a task, with some therapists choosing the controversial approach of paradoxical instruction. Sometimes simply revealing family secrets or clarifying misunderstandings can have a profound effect on family interactions and the presenting problem. The therapist may use circular questioning in which (s)he asks different members to find out what someone else thinks or feels. The therapist or family will sometimes invite someone from the extended family network or system to join one, or more sessions, or will decide to work with a subgroup of the family – perhaps the parents – on their own.

Two of the vignettes described earlier in this chapter benefited from a family therapy/systems approach.

The Secret of Mortality

In two of the cases described earlier anxiety about parental mortality was also a prominent feature. In another family the presenting patient was a 37-year-old man who was electively mute and anorectic. After many months of family therapy his father was able to make a will, and discuss the arrangements he had made for his son's future. Only then was the 'patient' able to communicate safely by talking, his previous communication being through painstakingly slow and primitive drawings.

The Secret of Sexuality

In a family that sought help for their adolescent daughter's disturbed behaviour at the time of menstruation, the need for a careful biopsychosocial approach was again presented. The possibility of premenstrual syndrome and a hormonal intervention had to be considered. However, at the assessment interview at home it was also apparent that the daughter's behaviour was challenging her mother's attempt to deny her sexuality and her adulthood. Her dependency on her mother for her sexual safety and her physical care, and her mother's inability to trust her daughter's leisure supervision to anyone else, was in contrast to the daughter's two wishes: to have a new tape (of romantic love), and to have a boyfriend. Her respite care and day-centre holidays were in women-only groups.

Working with Individuals

Parents have often found it difficult to tolerate the loss of their unique role as confidante for their child when (s)he enters therapy. The same is true for children and adults with learning disabilities. Suddenly, their son or daughter has secrets with another adult. Interestingly in terms of attachment theory, engagement in individual therapy can be seen as a therapeutic aid to the fading of attachment behaviour. Given the strength of the dependency experienced by many adolescents and adults with learning disability, it is understandable why their parents and carers may need extra support for themselves, so that they do not undermine the therapeutic process.

Psychoanalytic Psychotherapy – What to Expect

The therapist typically offers a 50-min session at the same time and in the same room at least once per week (or 90 min for a group). The familiarity of the time and the setting provides safe boundaries for the 'patient' to explore their inner world and the nature of their relationships, including the relationship with the therapist. The individual with a severe learning disability may not be able to manage a 50-min session, and the therapist may decide to set aside a shorter period of time, or to allow the individual to build up to using a full session later. Experimenting by the patient with the boundaries of the session may include coming early or late, leaving early or wanting to outstay the session, going out to the toilet frequently, and so on. This 'experimenting' must be understood by the therapist in the context of anxieties that are being raised by the therapeutic relationship and reflected back to the patient. If the individual is escorted to their sessions, it follows that the escort must remain in the waiting room throughout. One patient who did not need an escort regularly came late and left early until during a heavy snowfall he came to check whether the therapist had still turned up for the session. After this he seemed convinced of his therapist's reliability and began to arrive on time.

The therapist working with individuals with learning disabilities will talk to the patient even if they are nonverbal. They will also attend to their behaviour, posture, facial expression and other ways of communicating how they feel and what is important to them. The skilled therapist works with transference and counter-transference feelings in his/her relationship with the patient. In this way, the patient is enabled to differentiate their inner world from the outer reality of the actual relationship with the therapist. They may encourage the patient to use art or play materials in the manner of a child psychotherapist.

The therapist does not set an agenda for sessions but waits to see what is on the patient's mind. The exception to this would be if brief focal work has been proposed because of a particularly traumatic event such as the death of the main carer or a difficult relationship. In this case, the therapist would focus on material in the area of particular concern. Both individual and group therapy may have particular benefits in supporting the development of individuation, maturation and self-esteem.

The Secret of Disability

In individual therapy the therapist is confronted by the patient's disability without the mediating effect of family members or carers. Sometimes, the disability appears to be reduced as the therapeutic alliance develops, and the patient trusts the therapist enough to reveal his/her emotional intelligence. This seemed to be the case with a 27-year-old man with severe athetoid cerebral palsy who had no speech, and was assumed by his family not to know what was going on. His distress at his battered sister's state at the hands of his brother-in-law was therefore hard to explain until his own inadequacies as his sister's defender because of his disability had been explored in therapy.

Individual Therapy in a Residential Setting

Individuals with learning disability living in a residential setting staffed by professional carers face particular difficulties when they are referred for psychotherapy; there are issues about continuity of care and whose responsibility it is to know someone's life story and to support the referral. The support needs of the carer who is excluded from the therapeutic relationship must be attended to, especially as they may be the recipient of disturbed behaviour between sessions. They may become bored with the long-term responsibility of a process they do not understand, or undermine the time and space boundaries of the therapy, or try to break the confidentiality of the sessions by insisting on speaking to the therapist.

Changes of staff and of escorts during the life of the therapy are common. To avoid such challenges to the therapy, it is advisable to arrange for another team member to work with the staff (in a similar way as is traditional with parents of children in therapy directly to support, inform and receive relevant information about the 'patients' progress in their daily life. In some institutionalized settings the confidentiality of the treatment may provoke envy in staff who have been accustomed to knowing every intimate detail of an individual's life – again in a similar way to some parents of severely disabled people).

Group Therapy

Group therapy is not individual therapy of the group members conducted in a group session. The members of the group work on group ideas and themes and confront each other about inconsistencies in their stories. These meetings with peers enable them to reassess their relationships – real and imagined – and to re-evaluate their own abilities and disabilities. The therapists do not impose an agenda, as it is the process rather than the content of the sessions which is important. As with individual therapy, the boundaries of the session are important, with considerable attention paid to the holiday breaks or any unscheduled absences and the way in which the members are able to cope with these. For example, a group member who missed two sessions because her own escort was ill, was unable to look at the therapist in the next session until it was suggested that she was afraid they were angry with her for her absence and she was afraid they may have changed.

In group therapy the members support each other in broadening their potential for developing relationships in a way that seems particularly valuable. There is no scope for further development of the principles and practice of group therapy in this chapter and the interested reader is referred elsewhere.[41,47]

Conclusions

It must be emphasized that insecure attachment is no more nor less than a vulnerability factor and is not a diagnosis of pathology. There is no implication that the presence of learning disability will necessarily lead to an insecure attachment pattern, or difficulties with separation and bereavements and subsequent pathology. However, the importance of knowledge in this area when dealing with referrals of individuals who are presenting with difficulties, is emphasized.

There is a propensity to perceive behavioural problems in this client group purely in terms of learning theory and to attribute behavioural difficulties to organic or cognitive deficits. For the individual with learning disability, separation may present particular emotional problems which can present with increased aberrant behaviours which are not necessarily understood or recognized for what they are – responses to separation or the threat of separation from an attachment figure and/or part of the grieving process. While there is increasing recognition of behavioural phenotypes associated with some syndromes, it is equally important that psychodynamic understanding and research such as that on attachment and loss should be encouraged and developed in the field of learning disability so that it can take its rightful place within the biopsychosocial approach.

References

1. Seidel UP, Chadwick OFD & Rutter M (1975) Psychological disorders in crippled children. A comparative study of children with and without brain damage. *Developmental Medicine and Child Neurology* **17**, 563-73.
2. Breslau N (1985) Psychiatric disorder in children with physical disabilities. *Journal of the American Academy of Child Psychiatry* **24**, 87–94.
3. Shaffer D (1985) Brain damage. In Rutter M & Hersov L (eds) *Child and Adolescent Psychiatry: Modern Approaches*, pp. 129–51. Oxford: Blackwell.
4. Eiser C (1990) Psychological effects of chronic disease. *Journal of Child Psychology and Psychiatry* **31**, 85–98.

Psychiatry in Learning Disability

5. Bernal J & Hollins S (1995) Psychiatric illness and learning disability – a dual diagnosis. *Advances in Psychiatric Treatment* **1**, 138–45.
6. Bowlby J (1971) *Attachment and Loss*, Vols 1, 2 and 3. London: Hogarth Press.
7. Ainsworth MDS, Blehar MC, Waters E & Wall S (1978) *Patterns of Attachments: A Psychological Study of The Strange Situation.* Hillsdale: Erlbaum Association.
8. Robertson J & Bowlby J (1952) *Responses of Young Children to Separation from their Mothers.* Paris: Courier of the International Children's Centre.
9. Robertson J (1953) Some responses of young infants to loss of maternal care. *Nursing Care* **49**, 382–6.
10. Parkes CM (1972) *Bereavement: Studies of Grief in Adult Life.* London: Penguin.
11. Stroufe LA (1986) Bowlby's contribution to psychoanalytic theory and developmental psychology; attachment, separation, loss. *Journal of Child Psychology and Psychiatry and Allied Disciplines* **27(6)**, 841–9.
12. Fonagy I, Steele H & Steele M (1991) Maternal representations of attachment during pregnancy predict the organization of infant mother attachment at one year of age. *Child Development* **62**, 891–905.
13. Cox AD & Lambrenos K (1992) Childhood physical disability and attachment. *Developmental Medicine and Child Neurology* **34**, 1037–46.
14. Speltz M, Greenberg MT & Deklyen M (1990) Attachment in pre-schoolers with disruptive behaviour: a comparison of clinic referred and non problem children. *Developmental and Psychopathology* **2**, 31–46.
15. Emde MD (1988) The effect of relationships on relationships: a developmental approach to clinical intervention. In Hinde R & Stevenson-Hinde J (eds) *Relationships within Families: Mutual Influences*, pp. 354–64. Oxford: Oxford University Press.
16. Grossman KE, Fremmer-Bombik E, Rudolf J & Grossman J (1988) Maternal attachment representations as related to patterns of infant mother attachment and maternal care during the first year. In Hinde R & Stevenson-Hinde J (eds) *Relationships within Families: Mutual Influences*, pp. 241–60. Oxford: Oxford University Press.
17. Troy M & Stroufe LA (1987) Victimization among pre-schoolers: the role of attachment relationship history. *Journal of the American Academy of Child Psychiatry* **26**, 166–72.
18. Radke-Yarrow M (1991) Attachment patterns in children of depressed mothers. In Parkes CM, Stevenson-Hinde J & Marris P (eds) *Attachment Across the Life Cycle*, pp. 115–26. London: Routledge.
19. Eichberg CG (1987) Quality of infant–parent attachment: related to mother's representation of her own history and child care attitudes. In Parkes CM, Stevenson-Hinde J & Marris P (eds) *Attachment Across the Life Cycle*. London: Routledge.
20. Ainsworth MDS & Eichberg CG (1991) Effects on infant mother attachment of mother unresolved loss of an attachment figure, or other traumatic experience. In Parkes CM, Stevenson-Hinde J & Marris P (eds) *Attachment Across the Life Cycle*. London: Routledge.
21. Brooks-Gunn J & Lewis M (1982) Affective exchanges between normal and handicapped infants and their mothers. In Field T & Fogel A (eds) *Emotion and Interaction: Normal and High Risk Infants* Hillsdale: Erlbaum.
22. Brooks-Gunn J & Lewis M (1984) Maternal responsivity in interactions with handicapped infants. *Child Development* **55**, 782–93.
23. Goode D (1995) *A World Without Words: The Social Construction of Children Born Deaf and Blind.* Philadelphia: Temple University Press.
24. Chicchetti D & Schneider-Rosen K (1988) Theoretical and empirical considerations in the investigations of the relationship between affect and cognition in atypical populations of infants. In Izard C, Kagan J & Zajonc R (eds) *Emotion, Cognition and Behaviour.* New York: Cambridge University Press.
25. Bicknell J (1983) The psychopathology of handicap. *British Journal of Medical Psychology* **56**, 167–78.
26. Damrosch SP & Perry LA (1989) Self-reported adjustment, chronic sorrow and coping of parents of children with Down's syndrome. *Nursing Research* **38**, 25–9.
27. McFadyen AC (1994) *Special Care Babies and their Developing Relationships.* London: Routledge.
28. Bihm E & Elliot L (1982) Conception of death in mentally retarded persons. *Journal of Psychology* **56**, 167–78.
29. Esterhuyzen A & Hollins S (1997) Bereavement and grief in adults with learning disabilities. *British Journal of Psychology* (in press).

30. Parkes CM, Stevenson-Hinde J & Marris P (1991) *Attachment Across the Life Cycle*. London: Routledge.
31. Sable PO (1989) Attachment, anxiety and loss of a husband. *American Journal of Orthopsychiatry* **59(4)**, 550–6.
32. Marris P (1993) *Loss and Change*. London: Routledge.
33. Maeson D, Marks I, Ramm L & Stern RS (1981) Guided mourning for morbid grief: a controlled study. *British Journal of Psychiatry* **138**, 185–93.
34. Oswin M (1991) *Am I Allowed To Cry? A Study of Bereavement Amongst People who Have Learning Disability*. London: Souvenir Press.
35. Hollins S & Curran J (1996) *Understanding Depression in People with Learning Disabilities*. East Sussex: Pavilion Publishing.
36. Goldberg D & Huxley P (1980) *Mental Illness in the Community: The Pathway to Psychiatric Care*. London: Tavistock.
37. Goldberg D & Huxley P (1992) *Common Mental Disorders: A Bio-social Model*. London: Routledge.
38. Hollins S, Evans C & Evered C (1996) A repertory grid study of change in a psychotherapy group for young adults with learning disability. Unpublished data.
39. Sinason V (1992) *Mental Handicap and the Human Condition – New Approaches from the Tavistock*. London: Free Association.
40. Symington N (1981) The psychotherapy of a subnormal patient. *British Journal of Medical Psychology* **54**, 187–99.
41. Hollins S & Evered C (1990) Group process and content – the challenge of mental handicap. *Group Analysis* **23(1)**, 55–67.
42. Stokes J & Sinason V (1992) Secondary mental handicap as a defence. In Waitman A & Conboy-Hill S (eds) *Psychotherapy and Mental Handicap*, pp. 46–58. London: Sage.
43. Cunningham C & Davis H (1985) Early parent counselling. In *Mental Handicap – A Multidisciplinary Approach*. London: Baillière Tindall.
44. Hollins S & Grimer M (1988) *Going Somewhere: Pastoral Care for People with Learning Disabilities*. London: SPCK.
45. Goldberg D, Magrill L, Hale J, Damaskinidou K, Paul J & Tham S (1995) Protection and loss: working with learning disabled adults and their families. *Journal of Family Therapy* **17**, 263–80.
46. Cooklin A & Hollins S (1988) *Hugo Wasn't Invited*. An Institute of Family Therapy Teaching Tape. Available from the Institute of Family Therapy, 24–32 Stephenson Way, London NW1 2HX.
47. Pantlin AW (1985) Group analytic psychotherapy with mentally handicapped patients. *Group Analysis* **XVIII**, 44–53.

15

Physical Treatments

David Clarke

Introduction

This chapter reviews the use of medication and other physical treatments for psychiatric and behavioural disorders, and in the management of epilepsy. Other treatment and management strategies are addressed elsewhere in the text, and are not referred to here. The nature of learning disability is such that affected individuals often have many problems, with many factors contributing to their onset or maintenance. Combined treatments, involving the use of medication in combination with other strategies, are often indicated. The emphasis on physical treatments should not be taken as implying that such strategies are necessarily the most appropriate or the only approaches to the problems and disorders discussed. The use of medication in the treatment of severely self-injurious behaviour, for example, should be placed in the wider context of research integrating biological, social, and other factors.[1]

Drug Names

All drugs have at least two names: a nonproprietary or generic name indicating the compound (such as carbamazepine) and a proprietary name given to the preparation manufactured by a particular pharmaceutical company (such as Tegretol). Proprietary names may vary in different countries. The different proprietary formulations of a particular drug are listed in publications such as the *British National Formulary*.[2]

Concern about Medication-use, and Prescribing Surveys

The prescription of drugs, especially psychotropic drugs, to individuals with learning disability has long been a subject associated with much controversy and relatively few clear-cut answers. Many studies from different countries have shown that about one-third of individuals with learning disability resident in long-stay institutions receive psychotropic medication (predominantly antipsychotics). A similar proportion receive anticonvulsants. The latter observation probably reflects the high prevalence of epilepsy among people with severe learning disability. The high rate of prescribing antipsychotics has been variously interpreted (often as indicating that 'appropriate' psychological treatments are being neglected).

One study from the USA concluded that the decision to prescribe an antipsychotic was influenced as much by the nature of the facility in which clients resided as by their behaviour;[3] another US survey reached the opposite conclusion.[4] One series of studies in the UK found that 40.2% of people with learning disability in hospitals received drugs 'for behaviour', compared with 19.3% of people in Local Authority hostels or group homes and 10.1% of people living with their family.[5] However, antipsychotic prescribing did not alter following discharge from hospital to community, despite a mean follow-up of 25 months and evidence that general practitioners were actively reviewing and altering medication.[6]

Few would disagree with a philosophy of using drugs in the lowest dose and for the shortest time that is effective, of paying attention to the risk:benefit ratio and assessing the impact of prescribing, and of tailoring drugs to individuals as well as presenting problems. The complexity of learning disability (with regard to heterogeneity of aetiology and the presence of additional problems or disabilities in a sizeable proportion of people) is such that treatment may sometimes seem to be inappropriate to researchers who are unaware of the detailed needs of the individual prescribed for and the other options available.

The Appropriateness of Drug-based Treatments

It is sometimes thought that drug-based treatments are most appropriately used where problems are of 'organic' origin, and conversely that medication should not be used to help ameliorate problems with a large social component to their causation because this 'does not tackle the underlying cause'. In practice, the factors contributing to a maladaptive behaviour such as severely self-injurious behaviour may be difficult to identify with certainty, and of many different types. Self-injury may start immediately after a key-worker moves from the person's day centre, for example, but then come to assume a communicatory function or serve as a strategy for avoiding certain tasks. Secondary biological effects (such as changes in neuropeptide functioning causing altered pain sensation and leading to a state of 'dependence' on self-injury) may then come about.[7] The prescription of an opiate antagonist such as naltrexone may reduce self-injury by blocking the effects of endogenous opiates produced during self-injury, and help prevent tissue damage.[8] Such a prescription does not address the underlying cause of the behaviour, but impacts on one factor maintaining it. Provided that this does not expose the person with learning disability to risks that outweigh the benefits of a reduction in self-injury, most clinicians would be happy with this apparently 'inappropriate' use of medication.

Risks, Benefits, and Efficacy

Attention to the risk/benefit ratio is the key to optimizing the use of drugs employed in the psychiatry of learning disability. This chapter therefore separates the treatment of specific psychiatric disorders (such as depressive disorders) and of epilepsy, from the treatment of relatively non-specific 'challenging' behaviours (such as aggressive behaviours). The efficacy of drugs in the treatment of psychiatric disorders such as schizophrenia is well established,[9] whereas the efficacy of drugs in the treatment of maladaptive behaviours is much less well established, and often based on uncontrolled studies, case reports, or controlled studies with small samples. Even where several treatment studies have shown benefit and have been published in peer-reviewed journals, allowance has to be made for effects such as the greater probability of achieving publication for a report showing a positive effect of a treatment, rather than a negative outcome. This means that it is more difficult to be sure that a particular drug will work for most people with learning disability and a particular maladaptive behaviour (e.g. self-injury), rather than being of help for some people with a particular form of learning disability and the problem (e.g. men with fragile-X syndrome and hand-biting behaviour in the context of social anxiety or over-arousal). The use of drugs to treat behavioural abnormalities or problems occurring in association with learning disability is an under-researched area, partly because of ethical concerns about carrying out treatment trials and partly because of the heterogeneous nature of 'learning disability' and associated problems and disabilities. Clinicians are not infrequently asked to contribute to the management of behaviours (notably aggressive, self-injurious or inappropriate sexual behaviours) which have potentially very serious consequences for the person concerned. Other forms of management may not have worked, or not be available. Medication may have to be used for indications for which there is some evidence of efficacy (e.g. from published work) but for which the medication is not licensed. There is a pressing need for methodologically sound treatment trials in this area.

Responsibility for the Consequences of Behaviours

The issue of responsibility for 'problem' behaviours may prove difficult where a pharmacological approach is taken. Some individuals with learning disability and/or their carers regard drugs as removing responsibility from the individual. In practice, most 'challenging' behaviours fall in a spectrum somewhere between the individual retaining total control over the expression of the behaviour in all situations, to relatively rare conditions (such as unfocussed hitting out during a seizure) where the person has no control over their behaviour, which is effectively involuntary. The issue of responsibility may need to be addressed before prescribing.

Assessing the Impact of Medication

If a drug is used as part of the management of a behaviour for which there is some, but not overwhelming, evidence for its efficacy, a measure of change in the target behaviour may be valuable. This may be the carer's subjective opinion (rated from 1 to 10) on a daily basis, or some more concrete measure such as the area of tissue damage caused by persistent self-injury, or a score on a standardized instrument such as the Aberrant Behaviour Checklist or its community version.[10,11] The drug can then be withdrawn if there is no benefit.

Studies of drug monitoring and reduction programmes have shown that regular review, with feedback about behavioural change to prescribers, reduces psychotropic prescribing to people with learning disability. The involvement of a pharmacist in the review programme may be especially valuable.[12,13]

Adverse Effects

The adverse effects of the drugs reviewed in this chapter are not considered in detail. All treatments (including psychologically and socially based interventions) which are capable of producing beneficial change for some individuals may produce adverse effects for others, or in different situations. Most medications are known to be associated with a range of potential adverse effects, which are detailed in the manufacturers' data sheets.[14] Relatively few adverse effects will be referred to here, and readers are advised to consult data sheets for further information.

People with learning disability are particularly susceptible to adverse effects of medication, partly because of the coexistence of other disorders or problems (such as epilepsy, cerebral palsy or constipation) and partly because communication problems may limit their ability to describe bodily changes to their doctor or carer. Prescribers need to be alert to potential adverse effects, and should alert carers to the more common possibilities. Information can be given to carers who attend with the patient, but it may be valuable to provide written information about adverse effects in view of the limited amount of information people can absorb in the course of one consultation. Specially prepared material such as lithium information cards (available from NPA services, 38–42 St Peter's Street, St Albans, UK, AL1 3NP) may be helpful. Academic papers or educational videos may be helpful to some carers, and the involvement of a community nurse may be valuable. Some unwanted effects can be minimized by altering the dose or the time at which medication is given. It is important that individuals with learning problems are not denied potentially beneficial treatments because of undue concern about rare adverse effects.

Particular care is needed when prescribing for women of child-bearing age, because medication should not be taken during pregnancy. Some drugs (such as lithium and most anticonvulsants) are known to produce fetal abnormalities in a proportion of pregnancies. The danger of fetal abnormalities is usually greatest early in pregnancy, when a woman with learning disability or her carer may not be aware she is pregnant.

Investigations

It is sometimes necessary to ensure that certain body systems are performing adequately before prescribing a medication. Kidney function is routinely checked before starting treatment with lithium because it is excreted by the kidneys. Checks may be necessary to document pretreatment function, so that subsequent assessments can be made to ensure the medication is not having an adverse effect. Thyroid function tests are also performed before lithium treatment is started because lithium occasionally interferes with thyroid gland activity. Investigations during the course of treatment may also be necessary to detect rare but dangerous adverse effects at an early stage. This may be particularly relevant where someone with a severe communication problem is receiving several drugs for different indications, and the medications share adverse effects such as agranulocytosis (lack of production of white blood cells). Some relevant investigations are mentioned in connection with specific treatments, but it is not possible to list all advisable investigations.

Drug Treatments for Psychiatric Disorders

The classification and clinical features of psychiatric disorders are considered in other chapters, but it is relevant to note that classifications such as ICD-10[15] are based on clinical features that occur together (i.e. syndrome based), and empirical. Drugs are usually prescribed after diagnosis, but alter symptoms or specific features rather than syndromes. Antipsychotic drugs, for example, effectively reduce the impact of clinical features such as delusions and hallucinations in schizophrenic disorders, affective disorders, and acute and chronic organic psychotic disorders. Drugs may, therefore, be used effectively in some circumstances where the diagnosis is uncertain or is impossible to establish. The drugs used to treat psychiatric disorders are therefore surveyed by class of medication rather than by psychiatric diagnosis.

Antipsychotics

The antipsychotic drugs, also referred to as 'neuroleptics' and 'major tranquilizers', are relatively commonly prescribed for people with learning disability (see the introduction to this chapter). They are effective treatments for mental illnesses such as schizophrenia, delusional disorders, manic illnesses, and depressive states where hallucinations or delusions are prominent features. They are also used in the management of some maladaptive behaviours, and this use is reviewed later.

Antipsychotics are often divided into groups based on chemical structure, because drugs from similar groups have broadly similar therapeutic and adverse effects (with the exceptions of the 'miscellaneous' group). The aliphatic group includes chlorpromazine, the first antipsychotic widely

used in psychiatry; the piperidine group includes thioridazine; the piperazine phenothiazines include fluphenazine; the butyrophenones include
haloperidol; the thioxanthenes include flupenthixol; and the diphenylbutylpiperidines include pimozide. A miscellaneous group includes
'atypical' antipsychotics such as clozapine and risperidone, drugs with
novel structures and different adverse effect profiles from compounds in
the other groups.

The principal clinically relevant differences between antipsychotics are
in their potency (which correlates strongly with dopamine D_2 receptor
blocking activity) and their adverse effect profile. Older drugs such as
thioridazine affect neurotransmitter systems other than D_2 receptors and
are associated with anticholinergic effects such as dry mouth, blurred
vision, retention of urine and constipation. More specific and potent
dopamine antagonists such as haloperidol cause few anticholinergic-related
adverse effects, but are much more likely to result in extrapyramidal
adverse effects such as rigidity, tremor and acute dystonic reactions. The
use of haloperidol may therefore be preferable in an individual with
learning disability who has a psychotic illness and is prone to constipation,
whereas thioridazine would be preferable for an elderly man with learning
disability, Parkinson's disease and a psychosis.

Clozapine is an atypical antipsychotic and belongs to the dibenzazepine
group of compounds. It is highly effective in the management of treatment-
resistant schizophrenia. Between 30% and 60% of patients with symptoms
not controlled by conventional antipsychotics in adequate dose respond
to clozapine.[16] Clozapine has a beneficial effect on negative, as well as
positive, symptoms of schizophrenia, and often improves social functioning.[17] Common adverse effects include excessive salivation, weight gain, an
increase in pulse rate, and drowsiness. Convulsions are more likely to be
provoked by clozapine than by most other antipsychotics, especially where
doses above 600 mg per day are employed, and this will be of particular
concern where a patient with learning disability has epilepsy or a past
history of seizures. Extrapyramidal adverse effects are rare. Clozapine is
associated with a relatively high rate of agranulocytosis (about 10 times
higher than with other antipsychotics) and all patients receiving it must be
registered with the Clozaril Patient Monitoring Service, so that blood counts
are performed and recorded regularly. Clozapine must be stopped immediately if the total white cell count falls below $3 \times 10^9 \, l^{-1}$ or the neutrophil
count falls below $1.5 \times 10^9 \, l^{-1}$. Risperidone is a benzisoxazole compound
with both $5HT_2$ and D_2 antagonist properties. It may have a beneficial effect
on both negative and positive symptoms and have less prominent extrapyramidal adverse effects than standard antipsychotics.[18] The newer
antipsychotics and the issue of treatment resistance have been reviewed
recently.[19]

It is important that schizophrenia and related disorders are treated as
soon as possible after the diagnosis is established, because delay in initiating treatment is associated with a poorer long-term outcome.[20]

Antipsychotics are also used to calm patients with psychoses who
are extremely agitated or aggressive, when talking, distraction or other

measures have failed. If parenteral treatment is given, close monitoring of the individual's level of consciousness, respiration, pulse and blood pressure should be carried out. Antipsychotics should not be administered intravenously unless resuscitation equipment and appropriately skilled staff are available. Regimens include chlorpromazine 25–50 mg intramuscularly (i.m.), haloperidol 2–10 i.m. (repeated hourly if necessary to a maximum of 60 mg in 24 h) and droperidol (5–20 mg i.m.). Chlorpromazine is less likely to cause acute dystonic reactions, but may lead to hypotensions or arrrhythmias. Benzodiazepines may also be used, such as lorazepam 25–30 µg kg^{-1} body weight by intramuscular injection. Lorazepam be given in conjunction with an antipsychotic, and this may allow a lower dose of antipsychotic to be used.[21] Intramuscular administration of diazepam, however, is best avoided because such injections are poorly absorbed and may be painful.

The neuroleptic malignant syndrome (NMS) is a rare, idiosyncratic complication of treatment with antipsychotic drugs. NMS usually occurs early in treatment, or following large increases in dose or the addition of other medication. The cardinal features include muscular rigidity, raised temperature, a fluctuation in the level of consciousness, lability of blood pressure, and a rapid pulse. The syndrome may be fatal (through dehydration and muscle breakdown, leading to kidney failure). One review suggested that NMS had a fatal outcome in about 10% of cases.[22]

Route of Administration

Oral administration has the advantage that dose adjustments can be made quickly, and the sedative properties of some antipsychotics can be used to promote sleep while minimizing day-time drowsiness, where sleep problems are associated with psychotic phenomena. The oral route is preferred by some patients because they regard depot injections as undignified, fear intramuscular injections or choose to take day-to-day responsibility for their own treatment. Many individuals with mental retardation do not administer their own medication, and compliance is less often a problem than for people who have to remember to take their own oral medication.

Depot injections avoid the need to remember to take medication. They may also be more efficacious than oral medication in the prevention of relapses among patients who stop taking medication when psychotic symptoms result in loss of insight. Depot administration also results in a lower total drug dose being administered (because the metabolism which occurs in the gut and liver after oral administration is avoided). Toxicity, however, may be greater with depot preparations.[23,24] Antipsychotic drugs are stored in body fat, and after some weeks of oral administration the patient effectively has a depot store of antipsychotic, albeit with a more rapid loss of effect when treatment is stopped. The choice of route of administration should ideally be the patient's, informed by relevant advice from the psychiatrist.

The Parkinsonian-like effects of potent dopamine blockers can often be reversed by giving an anticholinergic drug (such as procyclidine). However, routine use of anticholinergics is not advisable because they may reduce the effectiveness of antipsychotics, cause sleep and other problems, be abused for euphoriant effects, and may cause acute confusional states in the elderly or if high doses are taken.[25,26] The resulting confusional state (atropine psychosis) may be misdiagnosed as a worsening of the psychotic disorder for which an antipsychotic was originally prescribed.

Antipsychotics lower the convulsive threshold. This effect is of concern when prescribing to people with learning disability and epilepsy, but the magnitude of the effect seems to be relatively small.[27] One author concluded that 'neuroleptic drug treatment of psychosis in persons with epilepsy can be undertaken with low probability of seizure exacerbation if therapeutic serum AED (antiepileptic drug) levels are maintained'.[28] Seizures are more likely if high doses of antipsychotic medication are employed, or where the dose is increased rapidly.[29] There is debate about the relative epileptogenicity of different antipsychotics. One study of 100 children and adults with epilepsy receiving anticonvulsants and thioridazine found that 64 had fewer seizures after thioridazine was introduced, and 36 had no change in seizure frequency.[30] Another study reported no change or an improvement in seizure frequency in 22 out of 23 children with epilepsy treated with thioridazine.[31]

Antidepressants

Tricyclic antidepressants (TCAs) were introduced shortly after the antipsychotic drugs, and proved effective in the treatment of moderate and severe depressive disorders. Double-blind, placebo-controlled trials have shown that between one-half and two-thirds of patients with depressive disorders experience remission of their illness after a TCA is prescribed (usually with a lag of about 2 weeks before any beneficial effect is seen).[32] TCAs are thought to exert their effect by blocking the reuptake of the neurotransmitters noradrenaline and serotonin at synapses in the central nervous system (CNS). The antidepressant effect is believed to mirror secondary changes in the number and/or sensitivity of functioning synaptic receptors (thus accounting for the delay in therapeutic effect). TCAs are very toxic if taken in overdose, with many deaths (often as a result of cardiotoxicity) among people with depression using them to commit suicide. It is particularly important to ensure that small numbers of tablets are prescribed initially (especially where the patient is responsible for their own medication), and that patients know that there will be a delay before the therapeutic effect becomes apparent. Many deaths by suicide occur when patients start to recover from depression because 'biological' features often respond more quickly than mood, and patients may regain energy and motivation (sometimes directed to ending their life) while still feeling low in mood. TCAs also cause relatively problematic adverse effects for a substantial proportion of patients receiving them, including postural hypotension, sedation, light-headedness, and anticholinergic effects (consti-pation, changes in visual accommodation, etc.). These adverse effects may lead patients to stop treatment.

Other types of antidepressant have been developed, including a group of medications called the specific serotonin reuptake inhibitors (SSRIs) which have become widely used over the past few years. The SSRIs, as the name implies, selectively prevent the reuptake of serotonin at synapses within the CNS. The SSRIs are as effective as the TCAs in the treatment of depression, but are much safer in overdose and are associated with fewer and less severe adverse effects for most people. An adverse effect common to many SSRIs when used to treat people with learning disability is agitation, although there are differences between compounds and the effect is sometimes transient. The SSRIs and other newer antidepressants are much more expen-sive than TCAs, prompting debates about cost-effectiveness and the factors that should be taken into account when assessing this. TCAs are poorly tolerated and as a result are less likely to be taken as prescribed; they sedate and increase road traffic and other accident rates, are more toxic and more effective as a means of committing suicide, and therefore their adverse effects will lead to the indirect costs of treating episodes of urinary retention, inappropriately reassessing visual accommodation, etc.

Some SSRIs have other effects, such as anti-obsessional effects and a posi-tive effect on the course of some eating disorders. In learning disability psy-chiatry, they have been used to treat severely self-injurious behaviour and some other repetitive, stereotyped behaviours. This use is reviewed below.

Many clinicians prefer to use SSRIs, rather than TCAs, for individuals with learning disability and depressive disorders, unless that individual has no other problems or disabilities relevant to the choice of an anti-depressant and has a carer to give medication and observe for potential adverse effects. Many people with learning disability also have congenital heart disease, epilepsy, a vulnerability to constipation, or other problems that TCAs may exacerbate.

One combined noradrenaline and serotonin reuptake inhibitor has been marketed, and other novel antidepressants are becoming available.

Both TCAs and SSRIs may induce seizures or worsen control of epilepsy, although the literature suggests that TCAs may be more epileptogenic. Estimates of the frequency with which TCAs induce seizures in people with no history of epilepsy range from 0.1% to 4%.[33]

All types of antidepressant medication may rarely cause a lowering of blood sodium concentration (hyponatraemia), leading to drowsiness, confusion or convulsions, especially in elderly patients.

Lithium

Lithium is a very different compound, widely used in psychiatry to treat bipolar (manic-depressive) illnesses. It is effective in the treatment of acute episodes of both mania and depression, and is of particular value in preventing relapse of unipolar and bipolar illnesses. Lithium is a naturally occurring element, and is used therapeutically in the form of its salts (lithium carbonate, lithium citrate, etc.). These salts are chemically similar to common salt, and have the advantage of being very cheap to produce.

The correct dose of lithium is ascertained by gradually increasing the dose and measuring the concentration of lithium achieved in blood, adjusting the dose until an optimal serum concentration (about 0.4–1.0 mmol l^{-1} 12 h after the last dose) is obtained. Lithium is usually safe and well tolerated when taken in therapeutic doses, and when the patient and carer are aware of situations in which lithium toxicity may develop. These include episodes of severe diarrhoea or vomiting, or other situations causing dehydration, fluid loss or electrolyte imbalance. Lithium serum concentrations may also rise to toxic levels (above 2 mmol l^{-1}) if the patient is prescribed, or buys at a pharmacy, a nonsteroidal anti-inflammatory drug (pain-killer such as ibuprofen) or diuretic (water tablet). Lithium information cards are available to give patients and/or their carers. One survey found individuals with mild learning disability and their carers to be about as knowledgeable regarding the lithium's action and dangers as people with long-term mental health problems.[34] Both groups included a small proportion of people with potentially dangerous gaps in their knowledge, and further educational measures such as the involvement of a community nurse may be helpful for this subgroup.

In therapeutic doses, lithium causes relatively few adverse effects; these include fine hand tremor, rashes or worsening of psoriasis, gastrointestinal disturbances, thirst, and an increase in urine volume. In toxic doses lithium causes neurotoxicity, with development of a coarse tremor, unsteadiness and lack of coordination, slurred speech, weakness, drowsiness, seizures, and eventually coma and death. Gastrointestinal signs of toxicity include anorexia, diarrhoea and vomiting.

Anxiolytics and Hypnotics

The benzodiazepines effectively reduce anxiety, and may be used to induce sleep. However, they are associated with tolerance (a larger dose being needed to maintain the wanted effect over time) and dependence, with unpleasant withdrawal symptoms. They do not appear to be used very much in learning disability psychiatry in the UK, other than as agents to terminate status epilepticus. They are relatively safe when taken orally, and effective if taken for short periods (a few days). They may produce paradoxical reactions, with disinhibition and aggression instead of sedation, in some people.

Benzodiazepines are also sometimes combined with antipsychotics in the management of serious episodes of aggressive behaviour where the person is obviously a danger to themselves or others, and has not responded to oral or injected antipsychotic agents alone. A combination of droperidol and lorazepam has been suggested for short-term use in such circumstances, and details of dose regimens are given in the section on antipsychotics.

Zolpidem hemitartrate is a relatively new hypnotic said to be free of the potential for dependence or abuse.

Anti-obsessional Agents and the
Treatment of Stereotyped Behaviours

Clomipramine is a tricyclic antidepressant with a potent serotonin reuptake blocking action. It has been used to treat obsessive–compulsive disorders, and has also been reported to be effective in the management of stereotyped, repetitive, maladaptive behaviours associated with learning disability, such as hair pulling[35] and nail biting.[36] It is a much more effective anti-obsessional agent than desipramine (a tricyclic with an effect predominantly on the reuptake of noradrenaline) or placebo. Gordon *et al.* carried out a double-blind comparison of clomipramine, desipramine, and placebo in the treatment of 24 autistic subjects (12 treated with clomipramine versus desipramine; 12 with clomipramine versus placebo).[37] The authors found a reduction in stereotyped behaviour, abnormal reciprocal social interaction, anger and compulsive behaviours when treatment was with clomipramine, but not when desipramine or placebo were used. Reductions in self-injury were also noted, but these were not systematically assessed. The authors concluded that there may be links between compulsive phenomena and stereotyped, repetitive behaviours associated with autistic disorders, and that controlled trials of other serotonin reuptake inhibitors, such as the SSRIs, in the treatment of autistic individuals with learning disability would be valuable. A double-blind placebo-controlled crossover trial of clomipramine in eight male and two female patients with learning disability (four of whom had autism) demonstrated a clinically significant improvement in one or more repetitive behaviours among the seven subjects who tolerated the drug. The subjects taking part had severe (four) or profound (six) learning disability, were aged between 18 and 42, and resided in a state facility for people with mental retardation in the USA. All had body rocking movements, six had object stereotypies (such as shaking toys), five had repetitive self-injury and three had compulsive behaviours such as checking, ordering or touching. The most prevalent adverse effect noted during clomipramine treatment was an increase in appetite (in four subjects). One person had a seizure, and two developed ataxia, flushing and a worsening of mood state with agitation and aggression.[38]

Mehlinger *et al.* described a 26-year-old white, autistic female with temper outbursts and aggressive behaviour at a sheltered workshop.[39] Her placement was in jeopardy because of a 2-month escalation in aggression. She had previously received imipramine, with an initial improvement followed by a reversion to her previous behaviour. When treated with fluoxetine (20 mg every other day) she became more interactive, socially appropriate and tolerant of human contact. Behaviours such as the ordering of subjects and other repetitive, stereotyped behaviours declined in frequency and severity, her temper outbursts became less frequent and her mood improved. When the dose was increased, her anxiety and stereotypies increased. The dose was subsequently reduced (to 20 mg per day) and improvement was maintained. The authors noted the use of fluoxetine to treat obsessive symptomatology, and speculated about similarities between the two disorders. Friedman suggested that the worsening of stereotypies noted after fluoxetine treatment may have been due to 'serotonergic-mediated inhibition of dopamine lateralized to the right hemisphere of the brain' and that it could be avoided by gradual dose titration.[40] Ghaziuddin *et al.*, however, reported four cases in which an autistic person had been treated with fluoxetine, and concluded that fluoxetine appeared to be most useful when a clear-cut superimposed depressive illness was present. They found little beneficial effect on compulsive rituals or stereotypies.[41]

Other Physical Treatments for Psychiatric Disorders

Electroconvulsive Therapy

Electroconvulsive therapy (ECT) consists of the induction of a seizure by the passage of electrical current through the brain. Electrical 'treatments' have a long history: Hippocrates and John Wesley were both advocates.[42] ECT is no exception, being one of the oldest psychiatric treatments still in regular use. In learning disability psychiatry, its use is confined mainly to the core group of patients for whom there is a reasonable consensus regarding its effectiveness; these being individuals with severe depressive disorders and an imminent and substantial risk of suicide, depressive stupor or danger to physical health. Most individuals with learning disability who receive ECT in the UK have stopped eating and/or drinking as a result of depression, or are in danger of self-harm. Most will have failed to respond to drug treatment, or cannot receive such treatment.[43]

ECT may be given bilaterally (electrodes being placed on both sides of the head) or unilaterally (both electrodes being placed over the nondominant hemisphere). An anaesthetic and muscle relaxant are always given before ECT in the UK. The Royal College of Psychiatrists has issued guidelines on the administration of ECT and the training of doctors who give it, emphasizing the need to reassure patients, minimize anxiety, and employ a standard and effective technique.

American[44] and UK[31] multicentre studies of ECT demonstrated that about 75% of patients (without learning disability) who had depressive disorders responded to ECT. This proportion is greater than the proportion of people responding to TCAs, and ECT usually has a much more rapid onset of antidepressant effect. Studies have usually shown that the convulsion is the effective component of ECT, although a small number of studies have reported few differences in outcome between patients given ECT and those given all components of the treatment except the convulsion. Relatively recent trials support the view that the main advantage of ECT is its rapid action. Johnstone and others randomly allocated 70 patients with depressive disorders to a course of eight bilateral ECT treatments or to eight simulated ECT sessions.[45] The initial improvement in the 'real ECT' group was greater, but there were no significant differences at 1 month and 6 months follow-up. West randomly assigned 22 people with major depression to real or simulated ECT.[46] Any patient who failed to respond after six sessions was switched to the other group. The improvement in the real ECT group after two or more treatments was greater (as rated by psychiatrists, nurses, and patients). Ten of the 11 people in the simulated group were switched to real ECT with subsequent relief of depressive symptoms. No patients needed to be switched from real to simulated ECT. Results were not given for follow-up. The benefits of ECT in the treatment of severe affective disorder therefore appear to be real, but may be relatively short-lived.

Studies of ECT are difficult to evaluate. Ethical considerations mean that the group most likely to receive ECT in learning disability practice (those who are severely depressed, at risk of harm, and where other treatments are not possible or associated with an unacceptable delay in effect) are least likely to be included in trials with randomization. A number of studies have suggested that ECT is of most benefit for individuals whose depression is so severe that it is associated with features such as delusions.[47] ECT is a relatively safe treatment for individuals without learning disability, with most complications arising from the use of an anaesthetic and muscle relaxant rather than the seizure. The death rate (estimated at about four deaths per 100 000 treatments)[48] is comparable to that associated with minor surgery. The mortality (death rate) associated with severe depression in the non-learning disabled population is about 10%,[49] mainly due to suicide or self-neglect. The main adverse effect of ECT is memory loss. Retrograde amnesia and deficits in retaining new information have been documented, although severe depression is also associated with cognitive abnormalities including memory deficits. Memory loss may be less troublesome after unilateral ECT.[50]

ECT is often portrayed as frightening or punitive (e.g. the infamous scene in the film *One Flew Over The Cuckoo's Nest*). One study of 166 patients receiving ECT in one year in a UK hospital found that 13% of patients would be reluctant to have ECT again, but only 18% regarded it as more upsetting than visiting the dentist; 50% regarding it as less upsetting.[51] Relatively few patients appeared to understand the nature and purpose of the treatment, possibly because ECT-associated memory impairments had negated the explanations given. The authors suggested that explanations regarding ECT may need to be repeated several times.

Light Therapy for Seasonal Affective Disorder

Kraepelin and Pilez described patients with seasonally related low mood in the early years of the twentieth century.[52] In 1984, Rosenthal and others described Seasonal Affective Disorder (SAD), characterized by recurrent depressive episodes in the winter months, and remission in spring (sometimes followed by hypomania).[53] It occurs most often in young adult women. The episodes of low mood are accompanied by anxiety and irritability, fatigue, loss of libido, and a profound reduction in socialization. Seasonally related affective disorder has been described in association with learning disability[54] and is probably under-diagnosed.

Patients with SAD respond to treatment with bright artificial light (phototherapy). A typical treatment regimen would consist of exposure to 2500 lux full spectrum light emitted from a fixture containing eight fluorescent tubes behind a plastic diffusing screen. The light source is placed at eye level, about 1 m from the patient, and administered for about 4 h per day in the evening or early morning. One study suggested that light applied to the eyes, rather than the skin, has a much greater antidepressant effect.[55]

Auditory Input or Masking in the Treatment of Auditory Hallucinations

Although antipsychotic drugs form the mainstay of treatment for schizophrenia and other disorders characterized by auditory hallucinations, they may not be effective for some patients, or may cause such severe adverse effects that their use is not appropriate. Other treatments have been developed for persistent auditory hallucinations, including the use of ear plugs,[56,57] auditory stimuli such as music played through headphones,[58,59] or vocalization tasks such as counting. Psychology services may be able to advise on the suitability and implementation of such nondrug physical treatments, which may also occasionally be useful adjuncts to pharmacological treatment.

Drug Treatments for Epilepsy

The pharmacology of epilepsy dates back to the introduction of bromides in 1857. For over 50 years, these were the only anticonvulsants in use. In 1912 the anticonvulsant properties of barbiturates were documented,[60] and a few years later the hydantoins were introduced.[61] From the 1950s onwards, anticonvulsant compounds have been developed with increasing frequency.

When treating epilepsy, the aim should always be to ensure the optimal balance between control of seizures and quality of life. The most satisfactory drug regimen is monotherapy (the use of one anticonvulsant). This minimizes adverse effects and potential for interactions with other drugs, and aids compliance. Some people with learning disability have seizures despite treatment with adequate doses of one or more anticonvulsants. Surveys of prescribing to individuals with learning disability in hospital and community settings indicate that most receive one or two anticonvulsants. A recent audit in a local service found a small proportion of in- and out-patients receiving three anticonvulsants, and evidence that clinicians had tried to simplify treatment regimens as much as possible. As with drugs prescribed for psychiatric disorder, there is a need to tailor the medication to the patient, rather than simply following accepted guidance about the first-line treatments for specific seizure types or syndromes, although such knowledge is important.

The diagnosis and classification of epilepsy are dealt with in Chapter 16. Correct diagnosis, both of epilepsy and of the seizure type(s) occurring, is an essential first step in deciding on drug treatment. In this context it should be remembered that 'one seizure does not mean epilepsy', and that some investigations (such as an electroencephalogram (EEG), computed tomography (CT) or magnetic resonance imaging (MRI) scan, and systemic tests) may be necessary to help decide on the most appropriate treatment, as well as to establish the diagnosis. Most patients seen by a specialist in the psychiatry of learning disability fall into the group of people with active epilepsy who are receiving drug treatment. The tasks to be performed when reviewing such patients include reviewing diagnosis, reviewing previous treatments and response, rationalizing drug treatment, assessing toxicity, providing information and counselling, and (if appropriate) considering neurosurgery.[62]

The most widely used first-line anticonvulsants are sodium valproate and carbamazepine. Both are associated with an increased risk of fetal abnormalities (notably neural tube defects) if taken during pregnancy. Sodium valproate is currently considered by many clinicians to be the first choice drug for the treatment of generalized seizures and syndromes, and carbamazepine the drug of first choice for partial (focal) seizures and syndromes. The older drugs phenytoin and phenobarbitone are very rarely used because phenobarbitone causes sedation, disinhibition and many other adverse effects, and phenytoin results in facial coarsening, gum hyperplasia, hirsutism (excessive hair growth) and has a very low therapeutic ratio (the ratio between the clinically effective dose and the dose causing toxic effects).

Carbamazepine

Carbamazepine is a tricyclic compound (with two benzene rings and one azepine ring), structurally related to tricyclic antidepressants, and licensed in the UK for the treatment of all forms of epilepsy except absence seizures. It is also licensed for the treatment of bipolar (manic-depressive) illness, and has been used to treat some forms of aggressive behaviour (the latter use is reviewed below). Clinical trials concerning the use of carbamazepine in epilepsy were reported in the 1960s, and it was introduced in Europe in 1973. Carbamazepine is usually well tolerated, but may cause dizziness, unsteadiness, gastrointestinal disturbances, rashes or problems with the formation of blood cells. Diplopia may occur and, like unsteadiness, may be related to high doses or peak plasma concentrations. Carbamazepine should not be given to patients with a history of certain types of heart abnormality (atrioventricular conduction abnormalities), porphyria or a history of bone marrow depression. The manufacturer recommends monitoring of blood count, kidney and liver function, although the *British National Formulary*[2] notes 'but evidence of practical value unsatisfactory . . . patients or their carers should be told how to recognize signs of blood, liver, or skin disorders, and advised to seek immediate medical attention if symptoms such as fever, sore throat, rash, mouth ulcers, bruising, or bleeding develop. Leucopenia which is severe, progressive or associated with clinical symptoms requires withdrawal (if necessary under cover of a suitable alternative)'. Carbamazepine serum concentrations can be assayed, and the serum level correlates with anticonvulsant activity. The usual adult dose is between 0.8 and 1.2 g daily, given in divided doses, although up to 2 g may be needed exceptionally when carbamazepine is used alone. A modified release preparation is available.

Sodium Valproate

Sodium valproate was first marketed in France in 1967, in the UK in 1974 and in the USA in 1978. It is an effective treatment for tonic clonic seizures, especially when these result from primary generalized epilepsy, for generalized absence seizures and for myoclonic seizures. It is also effective for many patients with partial (focal) seizures, and is usually well tolerated. It has widespread metabolic effects, and some adverse effects are dose related. The most dangerous adverse effects are rare, and include liver and pancreatic dysfunction or damage. For this reason, sodium valproate should not be prescribed to individuals with liver disease or a family history of serious liver disease. Liver damage appears to be more likely in children, people with learning disability and severe seizure disorders, and early in treatment. Liver function should be assessed before starting treatment and during the first 6 months of treatment, although elevated serum liver enzymes are not uncommon and are often transient. Patients should be monitored if such rises are observed, and treatment discontinued if there is evidence of an abnormal prolongation of prothrombin time. Common adverse effects include gastric irritation, nausea, weight gain, transient hair loss and inhibition of platelet aggregation. Treatment must be discontinued immediately if anorexia, vomiting, jaundice, drowsiness or loss of seizure control occur. The usual dose is between 1 and 2 g daily (maximum 2.5 g). A modified release preparation is available. Serum concentrations can be assayed, but are not a useful index of therapeutic effect. The serum concentration may be relevant if noncompliance is suspected, but routine monitoring has no value.

As with carbamazepine, patients or their carers should be told how to recognize signs of liver disease or blood dyscrasias, and told to seek medical advice immediately if they occur.

Lamotrigine

Lamotrigine is a phenyltriazine compound, found to have anticonvulsant properties during trials of potential antifolate compounds (in the 1960s, a hypothesis was advanced that antifolate activity was correlated with antiepileptic activity, a hypothesis that was subsequently disproved). After clinical trials, lamotrigine was introduced in the UK as an adjunctive treatment for partial seizures and secondarily generalized seizures not satisfactorily controlled by other anticonvulsants. It proved to be an effective antiepileptic, with the added advantages of not usually causing sedation or mental slowing, often being associated with an improvement in feelings of well-being and reducing the severity and impact of residual seizures. It is now licensed for the monotherapy of partial seizures, and primary and secondarily generalized tonic clonic seizures. Introduction has to be slow, and the dose regimen to be followed depends on whether the patient receives other anticonvulsant treatment. Guidance is given in the data sheet and the *British National Formulary*[2] regarding dose regimens suitable for introducing lamotrigine to patients receiving therapy with, and without, sodium valproate. Adverse effects are said to be less common than with other anticonvulsants. They include rashes, fever, malaise and influenza-like symptoms, and drowsiness. Other adverse effects occur more rarely, including liver dysfunction, Stevens–Johnson syndrome and other dermatological problems. It is necessary to monitor liver and kidney function and clotting parameters when initiating treatment, and to advise the patient or carer about potential adverse effects. Lamotrigine appears to be relatively well tolerated by many individuals with learning disability and epilepsy that is refractory to treatment with other drugs.

Gabapentin

Gabapentin is licensed for the adjunctive treatment of partial seizures (with or without secondary generalization) that are not satisfactorily controlled by other antiepileptics. Adverse effects include somnolence, dizziness, headache and tremor. An increase in seizure frequency has been reported rarely. Gabapentin has the advantage when used as adjunctive therapy that no interactions have been found with carbamazepine, sodium valproate or phenytoin.

Other anticonvulsants

Topiramate has recently been introduced for the adjunctive treatment of partial seizures with or without secondary generalization. Patients receiving topiramate should be advised to maintain an adequate fluid intake, to avoid kidney stones. Topiramate may be sedating, and dizziness, confusion, depression and emotional lability have been reported occasionally. Oral contraceptives taken by women using topiramate should contain at least 50 μg of oestrogen. Vigabatrin is used to treat epilepsy which is not satisfactorily controlled with other anticonvulsants, but its use for people with learning disability is limited by potentially adverse effects on behaviour (aggressive behaviour and psychotic symptoms appear to be not uncommon). Acetazolamide, a carbonic anhydrase inhibitor, is occasionally used as an anticonvulsant. Clobazam and clonazepam are benzodiazepine antiepileptics. They may be useful as adjuncts in the short-term management of epilepsy, but may be sedating or disinhibiting and tend to become less effective after many weeks of use. Ethosuximide is used to treat simple absence seizures. Its adverse effects include drowsiness, dizziness, mood changes and (rarely) psychotic symptoms.

Infantile spasms, which typically occur in the first 6–8 months of life, are usually treated with adrenocorticotrophic hormone (ACTH).

Lennox–Gastaux syndrome (LGS) is a severe epileptic syndrome of childhood, with intractable seizures of many types including tonic seizures; mental retardation and a characteristic EEG with diffuse bilateral slow spike and wave complexes during wakefulness and bilateral paroxysmal rapid rhythms during sleep. LGS is often treated with sodium valproate or benzodiazepine anticonvulsants.

Status epilepticus may be treated with rectal or intravenous diazepam, or intravenous lorazepam or clonazepam and, in hospitals where electrocardiogram (ECG) monitoring is possible, intravenous phenytoin and other drugs may be used to prevent recurrence. When benzodiazepines are given intravenously, trained staff and facilities for resuscitation must be on hand.

Surgery

Surgical treatments for epilepsy involve the removal or isolation of parts of the cortex forming foci for the onset of seizures. Surgery is thus most appropriate for people with partial (focal) epilepsy where the focus can be removed or isolated, or people with mixed or secondarily generalized epilepsy where hemispherectomy or corpus callosotomy may be feasible. Details of operative procedures are given in standard texts on epilepsy management.[63]

Drug Treatments for Maladaptive Behaviours

Aggressive Behaviour and Episodic Dyscontrol

Aggressive behaviour is one of the commoner reasons for individuals with learning disability being denied access to facilities or services, or being admitted to hospital under the provisions of the Mental Health Act. Aggression, although 'maladaptive', usually has a function. It is not always possible to determine this, or to change the underlying reasons for aggressive behaviour. Some individuals with brain injury or learning disability have episodes of loss of self-control, with sudden, explosive outbursts of temper (episodic dyscontrol). Episodic dyscontrol may be related (at least in part) to underlying brain dysfunction. A proportion of people with such problems have electroencephalographic abnormalities. Pharmacological strategies have been employed as part of the management of such behaviours, and some of the compounds used are reviewed.

Carbamazepine

Carbamazepine was developed as an anticonvulsant, but is also used to treat bipolar affective disorders (for which it is licensed) and episodic dyscontrol and some other behavioural abnormalities (for which it is not licensed). Its adverse effects are considered in the section on epilepsy.

Reports in the 1970s and 1980s that some individuals with episodic dyscontrol had EEG abnormalities[64] led to the use of carbamazepine both in patients with such abnormalities[65] and in those without them.[66] One review suggested that there was evidence for an effect of carbamazepine on aggressive behaviour regardless of the condition or abnormality with which the aggression was associated (abnormal EEG, a schizophrenic psychosis, etc.), but that further, placebo-controlled trials were necessary before the evidence could be considered conclusive.[67]

Some reports have suggested that carbamazepine is helpful for people with learning disability and aggressive behaviours, especially where these are 'explosive' in nature. Gupta and others described the treatment of episodic dyscontrol associated with Prader–Willi syndrome[68] and Buck and Havey the use of carbamazepine in combination with lithium.[69] Langee reported a retrospective study of 76 people with learning disability and maladaptive behaviours treated with carbamazepine.[70] The behaviours included aggression which 'did not appear to be under the patients' conscious control. That is, it was neither escape behaviour, manipulative, attention seeking, a product of physical distress, nor a response to environmental stimuli'. Of the 76 subjects, 30 experienced complete or almost complete loss of the target behaviour, 10 improved slightly, and 31 derived no benefit. Of the 30 responders, 29 had an abnormal EEG. Another author retabulated data from Langee's study, and suggested that carbamazepine was unlikely to benefit individuals without epilepsy and with normal EEGs, and that some of the observed effect may have been due to carbamazepine interacting with other drugs given concomitantly.[71]

Zuclopenthixol and Other Antipsychotics

Zuclopenthixol, an antipsychotic, has been found to reduce the frequency and severity of aggressive behaviours among people with learning disability in some studies.[72–75] Following reports that aggressive behaviour among people with schizophrenia improved when they were treated with zuclopenthixol, Yar-Khan reported a beneficial effect on the aggressive behaviour of 15 people with learning disability.[76] A further study by Mlele and Wiley found marked reductions in aggressive behaviour among 10 inpatients with learning disability, but the authors pointed out that other variables may also have influenced the subjects' behaviour (at the time of the study the wards in the unit were being refurbished).[72] One study compared the effects of zuclopenthixol or haloperidol (versus placebo) in a double-blind crossover trial involving 34 people with learning disability.[75] The authors reported reductions in scores of an instrument derived from the Schedule of Handicaps, Behaviours and Skills (HBS) but no change in scores obtained using the Clinical Global Improvement Scales. They also reported beneficial effects from relatively low doses of zuclopenthixol (the mean daily doses after 8 weeks of treatment were 5.5 mg and 5.13 mg for the two phases of the trial). Aggressive behaviour was a problem for 11 of the 34 subjects; other maladaptive behaviours included anxiety, psychomotor agitation, self-injury, and 'psychotic symptoms, halluci-nations or both'. In view of the established efficacy of antipsychotics in reducing psychotic phenomena, the results of this study pertaining to the treatment of nonpsychotic behaviour disorders such as aggression must be treated with caution. Further controlled studies with more tightly defined inclusion criteria are necessary before firm conclusions can be drawn about the benefits of zuclopenthixol in the treatment of aggressive behaviours. However, as antipsychotics are widely used to attempt to treat such dis-orders when other measures have proven ineffective or impractical, zuclopenthixol would appear to be one of the antipsychotics for which there is some evidence for efficacy. Other antipsychotics, notably thiori-dazine, haloperidol and chlorpromazine, are also widely used in the management of aggressive behaviours occurring in association with learning disability (see Chapter 6).

Lithium

From the 1970s onwards, reports have been published that suggest lithium may have a place in the management of aggressive and/or self-injurious behaviour among people with learning disability. An early case report described a woman with severe self-injury which responded well to treat-ment with lithium.[77] Her self-injury may, however, have been a manifes-tation of an underlying affective disorder, for which lithium is a well-recognized and effective treatment. Another report described (subjec-tively) an improvement in the behaviour of 10 people with severe learning disability and maladaptive behaviours.[78] In 1975, a report of the treatment of eight women with learning disability and aggressive behaviour was published.[79] This trial used double-blind methodology and placebo control, and the authors concluded that 'the group as a whole showed a reduction in aggression scores while on lithium ($P < 0.01$): three patients became less aggressive, one became worse and two were unchanged'. Eleven out of 15 individuals with learning disability and aggressive behaviour treated with lithium by Dale showed a reduction in aggressive behaviour,[80] although the study was not controlled, and ratings of aggressive behaviour were subjective, with an additional retrospective analysis of ward reports. A double-blind trial of the effect of lithium on 42 learning disabled individ-uals with aggressive behaviour found that 73% of those treated experi-enced a reduction in aggression during lithium treatment.[81] The trial was conducted at five centres, and care taken over methodological issues such as the standardization of behavioural assessments and the maintenance of blind status by the investigators. However, the patients treated had various combinations of aggressive and self-injurious behaviours, and the five-point scale used to assess behavioural change included relatively vague items such as 'mood uncertain'. A 10-year retrospective study of 74 institutionalized residents with severe or profound learning disability and 'behaviour disorders' that had not responded to other treatments found 'a sustained major reduction or elimination of behavioural symptoms' after lithium treatment; four of the 31 responders had aggressive behaviour, as had 11 of the 35 nonresponders.[82] The author concluded that older age and the presence of psychotic symptoms were associated with a better response to lithium. A review of the literature concerning the use of lithium to treat behavioural abnormalities associated with learning disability concluded that 'of the various indicators for lithium, the most solid are for aggression, although the type of aggression is not specified'.[83] The author noted that others had suggested the characteristic most likely to be associated with a good response of aggressive behaviour to lithium treatment was a 'short fuse', with sudden escalation. This resembles the conclusions of some of the studies relating to the use of carbamazepine reviewed above.

Self-injurious Behaviour

This description of the use of drugs in the management of severely self-injurious behaviour should be placed in the wider context outlined in the introduction to this chapter. Evidence suggests that drugs may be helpful for some individuals, and that biological factors may help to maintain self-injury. Psychological and social mediators may also be important, and psychological and biological factors maintaining self-injury would be expected to interact. The expression of the compulsive self-injury associated with Lesch–Nyhan disease, for example, is modified by environmental influences.

Opiate Antagonists

Naloxene and naltrexone reverse the effects of drugs such as morphine by competing for receptor sites. They also reverse the effects of naturally occurring opiate-like neuropeptides within the CNS and other body systems. Naloxone has to be given by intravenous, subcutaneous or intramuscular injection, whereas naltrexone can be given orally. Because they antagonize the effects of naturally occurring opioids, they cause hyperalgesia (increased sensitivity to pain). They occasionally cause other adverse effects such as vomiting, dizziness or drowsiness. The opiate-like neuropeptides consist of short chains of amino acids, derived from larger peptide precursors. β-Endorphin (BE) is one such neuropeptide with analgesic and euphoriant effects. It is a 31 amino acid fragment produced by cleavage of the precursor pro-opiomelanocortin (POMC). Studies have demonstrated that BE and other naturally occurring opioids induce dependence; the characteristic opiate withdrawal syndrome follows if they are administered for a period of time and then withdrawn.[84]

Similarities between behaviours seen in association with autism and those occurring during chronic opiate use have been pointed out by some authors.[85,86] Subsequent research has tended to support a connection between opioid dysfunction and the self-injury which is a problem for some people with autism, rather than a connection with autism *per se*.[87,88]

Two hypotheses have been advanced to account for the continuation of self-injurious behaviours despite significant tissue damage that would intuitively be associated with extreme pain and emotional distress. The analgesia hypothesis suggests that self-injury leads to the release of compounds such as BE inducing a state of analgesia and predisposing to further tissue damage. The addiction hypothesis suggests that the pleasurable euphoric effects of substances such as BE, released after tissue damage, result in a state of dependence on self-injury, with dysphoria experienced in their absence. The two hypotheses are not mutually exclusive: both are supported by recent research showing that plasma BE concentrations rise after self-injury, but there is no corresponding rise in substances such as ACTH that usually accompany BE.[7] β-Endorphin and ACTH are both derived from POMC and are usually co-released from the pituitary under the influence of a hypothalamic peptide (corticotrophic releasing hormone, CRH). A similar 'uncoupling' of BE and ACTH has been observed in individuals with opiate-dependence problems.[89]

Several studies of the effect of opiate antagonists such as naloxone and naltrexone on self-injury associated with learning disability have now been published. One study described a marked reduction in self-injury (and other stereotyped behaviours) in subjects.[90] Another reported a reduction in self-injury in one subject after naloxone treatment,[91] and a further study found that infusions of naloxone over 6 h for 2 days resulted in a 2-day cessation of self-injury.[92] Further reports of the effect of naloxone followed.[93,94] Naloxone's usefulness is limited by the need for parenteral administration and more recent studies have described the use of naltrexone. One group of authors treated seven autistic children aged between 3 and 7 years with naltrexone, and reported that five children benefited. Another group of researchers found a dose-linked reduction in self-injury among three children treated with naltrexone.[95] Double-blind studies have also been conducted;[96-98] some studies have failed to find a beneficial effect.[99] A review of the opiate hypotheses and relevant studies has recently been published.[8]

Specific Serotonin Reuptake Inhibitors

In addition to their efficacy in the treatment of depressive disorders, there is some evidence to suggest a beneficial effect of SSRIs for some individuals with learning disability and severe self-injurious behaviour.

The severely self-injurious behaviour associated with Lesch–Nyhan disease was found to improve following administration of 5-hydroxy tryptophan, a serotonin precursor, leading to suggestions that serotonin neural pathways may be implicated in the maintenance of such behaviours.[100] The similarities between stereotyped repetitive behaviours, obsessive–compulsive disorder and self-injury have been highlighted by some authors, and antidepressants have been found to reduce self-injury for some individuals.[101] Two trials have shown reductions in self-injury among individuals with learning disability following the use of fluoxetine, an SSRI.[102,103] Two case reports of a reduction in self-injury after treatment with fluvoxamine have been reported.[104] Fluoxetine has been reported to reduce the self-injury through skin picking associated with Prader–Willi syndrome when used alone or in combination with naltrexone.[105,106]

The reports published suggest that SSRIs may be helpful for some individuals with learning disability and severe self-injury. However, until more is known about the nature of self-injury and the factors which maintain it at a cellular level, the rational choice of treatment for individuals with such problems will be difficult. SSRIs, opiate blockers and dopamine antagonists may be helpful for some individuals, but there is no way of deciding which drug is most likely to succeed for a given individual. In such circumstances, clinicians' choices are influenced by the potential adverse effects of medication. SSRIs and opiate antagonists appear to compare favourably with antipsychotics, these being the drugs most commonly used in the adjunctive treatment of self-injury in the past. Biological factors influencing self-injury, and the implications for treatment, have been addressed by Winchel and Stanley.[100]

Inappropriate or Offending Sexual Behaviour

Drug treatments may play a role in the management of the inappropriate sexual behaviour of some people with learning disability. Most such behaviour results from a lack of understanding of the social framework surrounding the usual expression of sexuality, and is most appropriately addressed by education and other strategies outlined elsewhere. For some men with sexual behaviour which is not amenable to such interventions, especially where there is potential for conflict with the law, the prescription of a drug to lower libido may be of great help. Medication can lower sexual drive but will not change attitudes or sexual orientation.

There have been few studies of the effectiveness of antilibidinal medications for men with learning disabilities, but there is little reason to suppose that the outcome of treatment differs from that for men of normal intelligence. Motivation for change and commitment to the management programme are probably much more important influences on outcome than intellectual ability.

Of the drugs available in the United Kingdom at present, the evidence for efficacy is greatest for cyproterone acetate. Cyproterone acetate also effectively reduces female sexual drive, but it is not licensed for this indication and the drug should not be given to women who may become pregnant because of its feminizing effects on the fetus. Medroxyprogesterone acetate (MPA) is also an effective antilibidinal used in North America and occasionally in the UK. Benperidol appears to have a less certain antilibidinal effect. The adverse effect profile of benperidol resembles that of other butyrophenone antipsychotics.

Cyproterone Acetate

Cyproterone acetate (CPA) is a steroid analogue with progestogenic activity which is also a competitive antagonist of testosterone. Its progestogenic activity leads, through negative feedback, to decreased hypothalamic gonadotrophin release and hence decreased testosterone production. Its administration causes a fall in serum testosterone, luteinizing hormone and follicle-stimulating hormone and a rise in serum prolactin. Because hormonal influences do not entirely determine male human sexual behaviour, the effect of CPA varies from person to person and an antilibidinal effect cannot be guaranteed. However, there is good evidence from studies of men without learning disability that CPA is an effective antilibidinal,[107,108] and some evidence from studies including men with learning disability.[109]

CPA should not be given to young men whose bone or testicular development may not be complete. It is also contraindicated for men with malignant or wasting diseases, liver disease, or a history of thromboembolic disease. It inhibits spermatogenesis, and results in reversible infertility. Spermatogenesis usually returns to normal within months of treatment being discontinued. The commonest adverse effects are transient fatigue (for the first few weeks of treatment) and gynaecomastia (breast enlargement), which is a problem for about 20% of men receiving treatment. The manufacturers suggest investigations including a pretreatment sperm count, blood count, and biochemical profile.

Medroxyprogesterone Acetate

MPA is a progestogenic compound, and is an effective antilibidinal agent.[110,111] A double-blind trial of MPA and CPA in seven men with a diagnosis of paedophilia found the compounds to be equally effective, with reductions in sexual thoughts and fantasies, and also (variable) reductions in penile responsiveness.[112] The authors of the study noted, however, that 'only a minority of paedophiles are likely to accept libido-reducing drugs'. Gagne reported a positive effect of MPA in 40 out of 48 men with 'long-standing histories of deviant sexual behavior'.[113] The effect was usually rapid (within 3 weeks), with reductions in sexual fantasies and arousal, a decreased desire to engage in deviant sexual behaviour and improved psychosocial functioning. A study of 30 sex offenders (without learning disability) randomly allocated to treatment with MPA, imaginal desensitization or both found no significant differences in the responses to the three treatment options.[114] MPA has been used successfully in the treatment of unacceptable sexual behaviours among men with sex chromosome abnormalities,[115,116] dementing illnesses[117] and schizophrenia.[118]

Low oral doses (60 mg per day) may be as effective as higher ones (500–800 mg i.m. weekly),[111] but i.m. preparations have the advantage of aiding compliance and monitoring. The treatment of a 26-year-old man with an IQ of 76 and a 6-year history of paedophilia is described by Myers.[119]

Benperidol

Benperidol is closely related to the antipsychotic haloperidol. It was introduced as an antilibidinal after clinical trials showed a reduction in masturbatory activity among men with senile dementia when they received benperidol.[120] The mechanism by which it exerts an antilibidinal effect is uncertain; it may reduce sexual fantasies, rather than having an effect on potency.[121] The authors of a double-blind study concluded that the libido-reducing effects of benperidol were weak, and unlikely to be sufficient to control serious antisocial sexual behaviour.[122]

Benperidol has the adverse effects expected of an antipsychotic, notably sedation and movement disorders such as acute dystonias, Parkinsonian symptoms (cogwheel muscular rigidity and tremor), akathisia (restlessness) and tardive dyskinesia. The manufacturer suggests blood and biochemical monitoring.

Other Drugs

Goserelin acetate (GA) is a luteinizing hormone releasing-hormone analogue, administered by subcutaneous injection at 28-day intervals. GA has been used as an antilibidinal, although it is not licensed for this use in the UK.[109]

References

1. Oliver C & Head D (1990) Self-injurious behaviour in people with learning disabilities: determinants and interventions. *International Review of Psychiatry* 2, 99–114.
2. British Medical Association and the Royal Pharmaceutical Society of Great Britain (1995) *British National Formulary, Number 30* London: BMA & RPSGB.
3. Intagliata J & Rinck C (1985) Psychoactive drug use in public and community residential facilities for mentally retarded persons. *Psychopharmacology Bulletin* 21, 268–78.
4. Buck JA & Sprague RL (1989) Psychotropic medication of mentally retarded residents in community long-term care facilities. *American Journal of Mental Retardation* 93, 618–23.
5. Clarke DJ, Kelley S, Thinn K & Corbett JA (1990) Psychotropic drugs and mental retardation: 1. Disabilities and the prescription of drugs for behaviour and for epilepsy in three residential settings. *Journal of Mental Deficiency Research* 34, 385–95.
6. Thinn K, Clarke DJ & Corbett JA (1990) Psychotropic drugs and mental retardation: 2. A comparison of psychoactive drug use before and after discharge from hospital to community. *Journal of Mental Deficiency Research* 34, 397–407.
7. Thompson T, Symons F, Delaney D & England C (1995) Self-injurious behavior as endogenous neurochemical self-administration. *Mental Retardation and Developmental Disability Research Reviews* 1, 137–48.
8. Sandman CA & Hetrick WP (1995) Opiate mechanisms in self-injury. *Mental Retardation and Developmental Disability Research Reviews* 1, 130–6.

9. Davis JM & Casper RC (1978) General principles of the clinical use of neuroleptics. In Clark WG & Del Giudice J (eds) *Principles of Psychopharmacology*, pp. 511–36. New York: Academic Press.

10. Aman MG, Singh NN, Stewart AW & Field CJ (1985) The Aberrant Behavior Checklist: A behavior rating scale for the assessment of treatment effects. *American Journal of Mental Deficiency* **89**, 485–91.

11. Aman MG, Burrow WH & Wolford PL (1995) The Aberrant Behavior Checklist – community: factor validity and effect of subject variables for adults in group homes. *American Journal of Mental Retardation* **100**, 283–92.

12. Inoue F (1982) A clinical pharmacy service to reduce psychotropic medication use in an institution for mentally retarded persons. *Mental Retardation* **20**, 70–4.

13. Briggs R (1989) Monitoring and evaluating psychotropic drug use for persons with mental retardation: a follow-up report. *American Journal of Mental Retardation* **93**, 618–23.

14. Walker G (1995) *ABPI Data Sheet Compendium*. London: Datapharm Publications.

15. World Health Organization (1992) *The ICD-10 Classification of Mental and Behavioural Disorders: Clinical Descriptions and Diagnostic Guidelines*. Geneva: World Health Organization.

16. Drug and Therapeutics Bulletin (1991) Clozapine and loxapine for schizophrenia. *Drug and Therapeutics Bulletin* **29**, 41–2.

17. Kane J, Honigfield G, Singer J, Meltzer H & the Clozard Collaborative Study Group (1988) Clozapine for the treatment-resistant schizophrenic. A double-blind comparison with chlorpromazine. *Archives of General Psychiatry* **45**, 789–96.

18. Lieberman JA (1993) Understanding the mechanism of action of atypical antipsychotic drugs: a review of compounds in use and development. *British Journal of Psychiatry* **22** (Suppl.), 7–18.

19. Kane JM & Freeman HL (1994) Towards more effective antipsychotic treatment. *British Journal of Psychiatry* **25** (Suppl.), 22–31.

20. Crow TJ, MacMillan JF, Johnson AL & Johnstone EC (1986) The Northwick Park study of first episodes of schizophrenia. II. A randomised controlled trial of prophylactic neuroleptic treatment. *British Journal of Psychiatry* **148**, 120–7.

21. Drug and Therapeutics Bulletin (1995) The drug treatment of patients with schizophrenia. *Drug and Therapeutics Bulletin* **33**, 81–6.

22. Gratz SS & Simpson GM (1994) Neuroleptic malignant syndrome. Diagnosis, epidemiology and treatment. *CNS Drugs* **2**, 429–39.

23. Falloon I, Watt DC & Shepherd M (1978) A comparative controlled trial of pimozide and fluphenazine decanoate in schizophrenia. *Psychological Medicine* **8**, 59–70.

24. Rifkin A, Quitkin F, Rabiner C & Klein DF (1977) Fluphenazine decanoate, fluphenazine hydrochloride and placebo in remitted schizophrenics. *Archives of General Psychiatry* **34**, 43–7.

25. Johnstone EC, Crow TJ, Ferrier IN *et al.* (1983) Adverse effects of anticholinergic medication on positive schizophrenic symptoms. *Psychological Medicine* **13**, 513–27.

26. Arana GW, Goff DC, Baldessarini KJ & Keepers GA (1988) Efficacy of anticholinergic prophylaxis for neuroleptic-induced acute dystonia. *American Journal of Psychiatry* **145**, 993–6.

27. Cold JA, Wells BG & Froemming JH (1990) Seizure activity associated with antipsychotic therapy. *Drug Intelligence and Clinical Pharmacy* **24**, 601–6.

28. Scheur ML (1992) Medical aspects of managing seizures and epilepsy. In Pedley TA & Meldrum BS (eds) *Recent Advances in Epilepsy*, vol. 5, pp. 127–57. Edinburgh: Churchill Livingstone.

29. Logothetis J (1967) Spontaneous epileptic seizures and electroencephalographic changes in the course of phenothiazine therapy. *Neurology* **17**, 869–77.

30. Pauig PM, DeLuca MA & Osterheld RG (1961) Thioridazine hydrochloride in the treatment of behavior disorders in epileptics. *American Journal of Psychiatry* **117**, 832–3.

31. Baldwin RT & Kenny TJ (1966) Thioridazine in the management of organic behavior disturbances in children. *Current Therapeutic Research* **8**, 373–7.

32. Medical Research Council (1965) Clinical trial of the treatment of depressive illness. *British Medical Journal* **i**, 881–6.

33. Lowry MR & Dunner FJ (1980) Seizures during tricyclic therapy. *American Journal of Psychiatry* **137**, 1461–2.

34. Clarke DJ & Pickles J (1993) Lithium treatment for people with learning disability: patients' and carers' knowledge and attitudes to treatment. *Journal of Intellectual Disability Research* **38**, 187–94.

35. Swedo S, Leonard H, Rapoport JL *et al.* (1989) A double-blind comparison of clomipramine and desipramine in the treatment of trichotillomania (hair pulling). *New England Journal of Medicine* **321**, 497–501.
36. Leonard H, Lenane M, Swedo S *et al.* (1991) A double-blind comparison of clomipramine and desipramine in the treatment of onychophagia. *Archives of General Psychiatry* **48**, 821–7.
37. Gordon CT, State RC & Nelson JE *et al.* (1993) A double-blind comparison of clomipramine, desipramine, and placebo in the treatment of autistic disorder. *Archives of General Psychiatry* **50**, 441–7.
38. Lewis MH, Bodfish JW, Powell SB & Golden RN (1995) Clomipramine treatment for stereotypy and related repetitive movement disorders associated with mental retardation. *American Journal of Mental Retardation* **100**, 299–312.
39. Mehlinger R, Sceftner WA & Poznanski E (1990) Fluoxetine and autism. *Journal of the American Academy of Child and Adolescent Psychiatry* **29**, 985.
40. Friedman EH (1991) Adverse effects of fluoxetine. *Journal of the American Academy of Child and Adolescent Psychiatry* **30**, 508.
41. Ghaziuddin M, Tsai L & Ghaziuddin N (1991) Fluoxetine in autism with depression. *Journal of the American Academy of Child and Adolescent Psychiatry* **30**, 508.
42. Taylor PJ (1986) Electroconvulsive therapy. In Hill P, Murray R & Thorley A (eds) *Essentials of Postgraduate Psychiatry, 2nd edn*, pp. 667–81. London: Grune & Stratton.
43. Royal College of Psychiatrists (1989) *The Practical Administration of Electroconvulsive Therapy (ECT)*. London: Royal College of Psychiatrists.
44. Greenblatt M, Grosser GH & Wechsler H (1964) Differential response of hospitalised depressed patients to somatic therapy. *American Journal of Psychiatry* **120**, 935–43.
45. Johnstone EC, Deakin JFW & Lawler P *et al.* (1980) The Northwick Park electroconvulsive therapy trial. *Lancet* **ii**, 1317–20.
46. West ED (1981) Electric convulsion therapy in depression: a double-blind controlled trial. *British Medical Journal* **282**, 355–7.
47. Glassman A, Kantor SJ & Shostak M (1975) Depression, delusions and drug response. *American Journal of Psychiatry* **132**, 716–9.
48. Heshe J & Roeder E (1976) Electroconvulsive therapy in Denmark. *British Journal of Psychiatry* **128**, 241–5.
49. Winokur G & Tsuang M (1975) The Iowa 500: suicide in mania, depression and schizophrenia. *American Journal of Psychiatry* **132**, 650–1.
50. D'Elia G (1970) Unilateral electroconvulsive therapy. *Acta Psychiatrica Scandinavica* Supplement 215.
51. Freeman CPL & Kendell RE (1980) ECT: 1. Patients' experiences and attitudes. *British Journal of Psychiatry* **137**, 8–16.
52. Thompson C (1988) Seasonal affective disorders and phototherapy. In Granville-Grossman K (ed) *Recent Advances in Clinical Psychiatry*, vol. 6, pp. 209–26. Edinburgh: Churchill Livingstone.
53. Rosenthal NE, Sack DA & Gillin JC *et al.* (1984) Seasonal affective disorder: A description of the syndrome and preliminary findings with light therapy. *Archives of General Psychiatry* **41**, 72–80.
54. Arumainayagam M & Kumar A (1990) Manic-depressive psychosis in a mentally handicapped person. Seasonality: a clue to a diagnostic problem. *British Journal of Psychiatry* **156**, 886–9.
55. Wehr TA, Skwerer RG & Jacobsen FM *et al.* (1987) Eye versus skin phototherapy of seasonal affective disorder. *American Journal of Psychiatry* **144**, 753–7.
56. Birchwood M (1986) Control of auditory hallucinations through occlusion of monaural auditory input. *British Journal of Psychiatry* **149**, 104–7.
57. Done DJ, Frith CD & Owens DC (1986) Reducing persistent auditory hallucinations by wearing an ear plug. *British Journal of Clinical Psychology* **25**, 151–2.
58. Collins MN, Cull CA & Sireling L (1989) Pilot study of treatment of persistent auditory hallucinations by modified auditory input. *British Medical Journal* **229**, 431–2.
59. McInnis M & Marks I (1990) Audiotape therapy for persistent auditory hallucinations. *British Journal of Psychiatry* **157**, 913–4.
60. Hauptmann A (1912) Luminal bei Epilepsie. *München Medizinische Wochenschrift* **59**, 1907–9.
61. Werdnecke E (1916) Phenylathylhydantoin (Nirvanol), ein neues Schlaf- und Beruhigungsmittel. *Deutsche Medizinische Wochenschrift* **42**, 1193.

62. Oxley J, Espir M & Shorvon S *et al.* (1987) The framework of medical care for epilepsy. *Health Trends* **19**, 13–18.
63. Crandall PH, Risinger MW & Sutherling W *et al.* (1991) Surgical treatment of the partial epilepsies. In Dam M & Gram L (eds) *Comprehensive Epileptology*, pp. 683–714. New York: Raven Press.
64. Stone JL, McDaniel KD, Hughes JR & Hermann BP (1986) Episodic dyscontrol disorder and paroxysmal EEG abnormalities: successful treatment with carbamazepine. *Biological Psychiatry* **21**, 208–12.
65. Tunks ER & Dermer SW (1977) Carbamazepine in the dyscontrol syndrome associated with limbic system dysfuntion. *Journal of Nervous and Mental Disease* **164**, 56–63.
66. Mattes JA, Rosenberg J & Mayes D (1984) Carbamazepine vs. propranolol in patients with uncontrolled rage outbursts: a random assignment study. *Psychopharmacology Bulletin* **20**, 98–100.
67. Mattes JA (1986) Psychopharmacology of temper outbursts: a review. *Journal of Nervous and Mental Disease* **174**, 464–70.
68. Gupta BK, Fish DN & Yerevanian BI (1987) Carbamazepine for intermittent explosive disorder in a Prader–Willi syndrome patient. *Journal of Clinical Psychiatry* **48**, 423.
69. Buck OD & Havey P (1986) Combined carbamazepine and lithium therapy for violent behavior. *American Journal of Psychiatry* **143**, 1487.
70. Langee HR (1989) A retrospective study of mentally retarded patients with behavioral disorders who were treated with carbamazepine. *American Journal of Mental Retardation* **93**, 640–3.
71. Laminack L (1990) Carbamazepine for behavioral disorders. *American Journal of Mental Retardation* **94**, 563–4.
72. Mlele TJ & Wiley YV (1986) Clopenthixol decanoate in the management of aggressive mentally handicapped patients. *British Journal of Psychiatry* **149**, 373–6.
73. Izmeth MG, Khan SY & Kumarajeewa DI (1988) Neuroleptic treatment of oligophrenic patients. *Pharmatherapeutica* **5**, 217–27.
74. Singh I & Owino WJ (1992) A double-blind comparison of zuclopenthixol tablets with placebo in the treatment of mentally handicapped in-patients with associated behavioural problems. *Journal of Intellectual Disability Research* **36**, 541–9.
75. Malt UF, Nystad R & Bache T *et al.* (1995) Effectiveness of zuclopenthixol compared with haloperidol in the treatment of behavioral disturbances in learning disabled patients. *British Journal of Psychiatry* **166**, 374–7.
76. Yar Khan S (1981) The psychiatrically violent patient. *British Medical Journal* **282**, 1400–1.
77. Cooper AF & Fowlie HC (1973) Control of gross self-mutilation with lithium carbonate. *British Journal of Psychiatry* **122**, 370–1.
78. Miciev V & Lynch DM (1974) Effect of lithium on disturbed severely mentally retarded patients. *British Journal of Psychiatry* **125**, 110.
79. Worrall EP, Moody JP & Naylor GJ (1975) Lithium in non-manic-depressives: anti-aggressive effect and red cell values. *British Journal of Psychiatry* **126**, 464–8.
80. Dale PG (1980) Lithium therapy in aggressive mentally subnormal patients. *British Journal of Psychiatry* **137**, 469–74.
81. Craft M, Ismail IA & Krishnamurti D *et al.* (1987) Lithium in the treatment of aggression in mentally handicapped patients: a double-blind trial. *British Journal of Psychiatry* **150**, 685–9.
82. Langee HR (1990) Retrospective study of lithium use for institutionalized mentally retarded individuals with behavior disorders. *American Journal of Mental Retardation* **94**, 448–52.
83. Pary RJ (1991) Towards defining adequate lithium trials for individuals with mental retardation and mental illness. *American Journal of Mental Retardation* **95**, 681–91.
84. Wei E & Loh H (1976) Physical dependence on opiate-like peptides. *Science* **193**, 1262–3.
85. Kalat JW (1978) Speculations on similarities between autism and opiate addiction. *Journal of Autism and Child Schizophrenia* **8**, 477–9.
86. Deutsch SI (1986) Rationale for the administration of opiate antagonists in treating infantile autism. *American Journal of Mental Deficiency* **90**, 631–5.
87. Gillberg C, Terenius L & Lonnerholm G (1985) Endorphin activity in childhood psychosis. *Archives of General Psychiatry* **42**, 780–3.
88. Herman BH, Hammock MK, Egan J, Arthur-Smith A *et al.* (1989) Role for opioid peptides in self-injurious behaviour: dissociation from autonomic nervous system functioning. *Developmental Pharmacology and Therapeutics* **12**, 81–9.

89. Mutti A, Ferroni C & Vescovi PP *et al.* (1989) Endocrine effects of psychological stress associated with neurobehavioural performance. *Life Sciences* **44**, 1831–6.
90. Sandman CA, Datta P & Barron JL (1983) Naloxone attenuates self-abusive behavior in developmentally disabled clients. *Applied Research in Mental Retardation* **4**, 5–11.
91. Davidson PW, Kleene BM, Carroll M & Rockowitz RJ (1983) Effects of naloxone on self-injurious behavior: a case study. *Applied Research in Mental Retardation* **4**, 1–4.
92. Richardson JF & Zaleski WA (1983) Naloxone and self-mutilation. *Biological Psychiatry* **18**, 99–101.
93. Sandyk R (1985) Naloxone abolished self-injuring in a mentally retarded child. *Annals of Neurology* **17**, 520.
94. Bernstein GA, Hughes JR, Mitchell JE & Thompson T (1987) Effects of narcotic antagonists on self-injurious behavior: A single case study. *Journal of the American Academy of Child and Adolescent Psychiatry* **26**, 886–9.
95. Herman BH, Hammock MK & Arthur-Smith *et al.* (1987) Naltrexone decreases self-injurious behavior. *Annals of Neurology* **22**, 550–2.
96. Szymanski L, Kedesdy J, Sulkes S & Cutler A (1987) Naltrexone in treatment of self-injurious behavior: a clinical study. *Research in Developmental Disability* **8**, 179–90.
97. Barrett RP, Feinstein C & Hole WT (1989) Effects of naloxone and naltrexone on self-injury: a double-blind, placebo-controlled analysis. *American Journal of Mental Retardation* **93**, 644–51.
98. Sandman CA, Barron JL & Colman H (1990) An orally-administered opiate blocker, naltrexone, attenuates self-injurious behavior. *American Journal of Mental Retardation* **95**, 93–102.
99. Beckwith BE, Couk DI & Schumacher K (1986) Failure of naloxone to reduce self-injurious behavior in two developmentally disabled females. *Applied Research in Mental Retardation* **7**, 183–8.
100. Winchel RM & Stanley M (1991) Self injurious behavior. A review of the behavior and biology of self-mutilation. *American Journal of Psychiatry* **148**, 306–17.
101. Primeau F & Fontain R (1988) Obsessive disorder with self-mutilation: a sub-group responsive to pharmacotherapy. *Canadian Journal of Psychiatry* **33**, 331–2.
102. Markowitz PI (1990) Fluoxetine treatment of self injurious behaviour in mentally retarded patients. *Journal of Clinical Psychopharmacology* **10**, 299–300.
103. Markowitz PI (1992) Effects of fluoxetine on self injurious behaviour in the developmentally disabled: a preliminary study. *Journal of Clinical Psychopharmacology* **12**, 27–31.
104. Jawed SH, Krishnan VHR & Cassidy G (1994) Self-injurious behaviour and the serotonin link: two case illustrations and theoretical overview. *Irish Journal of Psychological Medicine* **11**, 165–8.
105. Benjamin E & Buot-Smith T (1993) Naltrexone and fluoxetine in Prader–Willi syndrome. *Journal of the American Academy of Child and Adolescent Psychiatry* **32**, 870–3.
106. Dech B & Budow L (1991) The use of fluoxetine in an adolescent with Prader–Willi syndrome. *Journal of the American Academy of Child and Adolescent Psychiatry* **30**, 298–302.
107. Bancroft J, Tennent G, Loucas K & Cass J (1974) The control of deviant sexual behaviour by drugs: 1. Behavioural changes following oestrogens and anti-androgens. *British Journal of Psychiatry* **125**, 310–5.
108. Cooper AJ (1981) A placebo-controlled trial of the antiandrogen cyproterone acetate in deviant hypersexuality. *Comprehensive Psychiatry* **22**, 458–65.
109. Clarke DJ (1989) Antilibidinal drugs and mental retardation: a review. *Medicine, Science and the Law* **29**, 136–46.
110. Cooper AJ (1986) Progestogens in the treatment of male sex offenders: a review. *Canadian Journal of Psychiatry* **31**, 73–9.
111. Gottesman HG & Schubert DSP (1993) Low-dose medroxyprogesterone acetate in the management of the paraphilias. *Journal of Clinical Psychiatry* **54**, 182–8.
112. Cooper AJ, Sandhu S & Loszytyn S *et al.* (1992) A double-blind placebo controlled trial of medroxyprogesterone acetate and cyproterone acetate with seven pedophiles. *Canadian Journal of Psychiatry* **37**, 687–93.
113. Gagne P (1981) Treatment of sex offenders with medroxyprogesterone acetate. *American Journal of Psychiatry* **138**, 644–6.
114. McConaghy N, Blaszczynski A & Kidson W (1988) Treatment of sex offenders with imaginal desensitization and/or medroxyprogesterone. *Acta Psychiatrica Scandinavica* **77**, 190–206.

115. Wiedeking C, Money J & Walker P (1979) Follow-up of 11 XYY males with impulsive and/or sex-offending behaviour. *Psychological Medicine* **9**, 287–92.
116. Blumer D & Mideon C (1975) Hormone and hormonal agents in the treatment of aggression. *Journal of Nervous and Mental Disease* **160**, 127–37.
117. Cooper AJ (1987) Medroxyprogesterone acetate (MPA) treatment of sexual acting out in men suffering from dementia. *Journal of Clinical Psychiatry* **48**, 368–70.
118. O'Connor M & Baker HWG (1983) Depo-medroxy progesterone acetate as an adjunctive treatment in three aggressive schizophrenic patients. *Acta Psychiatrica Scandinavica* **57**, 399–403.
119. Myers BA (1991) Treatment of sexual offences by persons with developmental disabilities. *American Journal of Mental Retardation* **95**, 563–9.
120. Sterkmans P & Geerts F (1966) Le benperidol (R4584) est-il le medicament specifique des comportements hypersexuels? *Acta Neurologica Belgica* **66**, 1030–40.
121. Haslam MT (1976) Psycho-sexual disorders and their treatment. Part III: Sexual deviation. *Current Medical Research and Opinion* **3**, 726–35.
122. Tennant G, Bancroft J & Cass J (1974) The control of deviant sexual behavior by drugs: a double blind controlled study of benperidol, chlorpromazine and placebo. *Archives of Sexual Behaviour* **3**, 261–71.

16

Epilepsy and Learning Disabilities

Pamela Crawford

Epilepsy is a common neurological disorder with a prevalence of 0.6 in 1000 individuals[1] and a lifetime prevalence of about 2%.[2,3] In individuals with learning disabilities, the prevalence of epilepsy is considerably greater. Overall about 25% of individuals with learning disabilities have epilepsy, but this figure is increased to about 50% of those with severe learning disabilities (Table 16.1).[4]

Epilepsy is defined as the tendency to recurrent seizures (two or more) unprovoked by any immediately identified cause.[5] Individuals with febrile convulsions or only neonatal seizures are excluded from the definition. One seizure does not equal epilepsy. An epileptic seizure is a clinical manifestation presumed to result from an abnormal and excessive discharge of a set of neurones in the brain.

Some specific epileptic syndromes are particularly associated with epilepsy and learning disabilities, such as infantile spasms (West syndrome) and Lennox–Gastaut syndrome. Many genetic, chromosomal and developmental disorders have a high prevalence of epilepsy in association with varying degrees of learning disabilities (Table 16.2).[6]

The association of epilepsy and learning disabilities means that all professionals dealing with people with learning disabilities need to be aware of the various forms of seizures and how to deal with them. Many absence and complex partial seizures go unnoticed by care staff as they are unaware of the protean manifestations of epilepsy. In particular, doctors dealing with people with learning disabilities need to be confident in the diagnosis and treatment of epilepsy, especially drug management. The recent introduction of four new anti-epileptic drugs has meant that there needs to be greater awareness of the use of these new agents in this particular group of people, who often have epilepsy that is difficult to treat.

Diagnosis

The diagnosis of epilepsy is the same for individuals with learning disability as those without these disabilities. It is a clinical diagnosis based on a personal or eyewitness description of the episodes. One of the major problems of diagnosis in individuals with learning disabilities is that they may be unable to give a description of what is actually happening to them

Table 16.1   Learning disabilities and epilepsy.[4]

	n	% with epilepsy
Children with mild/moderate learning disabilities	426	7%
Children with severe learning disabilities	126	26%
Children with mild/moderate learning disabilities and physical handicap	27	41%
Children with severe learning disabilities and physical handicap	64	67%

Table 16.2   Common conditions combining with learning disabilities and epilepsy.[6]

	Incidence of epilepsy
Chromosomal abnormalities	
Down's syndrome	5%
Fragile-X syndrome	25%
Angelman's syndrome	82%
Neurocutaneous syndromes	
Tuberous sclerosis	50–93%
Neurofibromatosis	5%
Sturge–Weber syndrome	75–90%
Neuronal migrational defects	
Lissencephaly/pachygyria	Most (infantile spasms)
Diffuse subcortical heterotopia	Some (Lennox–Gastaut syndrome)
Focal cortical dysplasia	Some

before or after an attack. Conversely, an eyewitness description of a classical tonic clonic seizure makes for easy diagnosis. There will be a description of falling to the ground, going stiff, shaking, often biting his/her tongue or being incontinent. Post-ictally there are often automatisms and the person frequently may sleep after the episode. Very few clinicians will have difficulty in making this diagnosis. Minor attacks such as absence or complex partial seizures are much more difficult to diagnose. Often, they may consist of staring episodes where the person is not responsive for a few seconds. These can be followed by automatisms or confusion, which are often quite short-lived.

An electroencephalogram (EEG) is useful for the classification of seizure type. Only rarely can it be used to make a diagnosis, i.e. if a seizure occurs while an EEG is being performed or specific EEG abnormalities occur such as generalized spike wave. One problem is that the more severe the learning difficulty, the more likely that the EEG will be abnormal due to the underlying brain disorder.

Differential Diagnosis

The main differential diagnosis with learning disabled people with suspected epilepsy is between epilepsy and behavioural episodes (Table 16.3). Occasionally syncope can be misdiagnosed. If a person feels faint

Table 16.3 Differential diagnosis of epilepsy.

Syncope
Panic attacks
Non-epileptic seizures
Behavioural problems
Migraine
Transient ischaemic attacks
Breath-holding attacks
Night terrors and nightmares
Movement disorders

and is kept upright a few myoclonic jerks can occur, or occasionally the episode can precipitate a tonic clonic seizure or incontinence. Stereotyped behavioural problems, especially in people with severe learning disabilities, can be mistaken for minor seizures. Repetitive head-banging or rhythmic rocking should not be mistaken for epilepsy but queries are occasionally raised. The individual is usually distractable, the episodes are long-lived and an EEG during the episode will not show any abnormal electrical activity (only movement artefact). Getting carers to video the episodes may sometimes be of value.

Nonorganic seizures often tend to occur in association with genuine epilepsy in people with learning disabilities. When witnessed, they do not usually look much like tonic clonic seizures. The seizures often include back arching or a lot of thrashing about. Around 10% of people with so-called 'drug resistant' epilepsy have nonorganic seizures.[7] If doubts exist, a video EEG recording is a worthwhile undertaking. It has to be remembered, however, that some frontal seizures may appear very bizarre with strange behaviour, such as cycling movements of the legs.

Nonconvulsive status epilepticus is not uncommon in people with learning disabilities and is frequently missed.[8] If a person with learning disabilities has sudden episodes of 'depression' lasting a few days or weeks, becomes unresponsive, incontinent and does not eat, it is worth obtaining an EEG during such an episode.

Seizure Classification

Epilepsy is classified in two ways. There is classification of the seizure itself (Table 16.4)[9] and there is syndromic classification (Table 16.5).[10] The syndromic diagnosis can be very useful for many individuals with learning disabilities as it gives an indication as to the choice of anti-epileptic drugs and prognosis.

Epilepsy is divided into two main groups. The generalized epilepsies occur when the abnormal electrical activity arises from both hemispheres together (generalized spike wave). Localization related epilepsy is when the abnormal electrical activity arises in one place in the brain and then spreads. Both forms of epilepsy can occur in people with learning disabilities, although both cannot exist in the same individual.

Table 16.4 Classification of seizures.[9]

I. Partial seizures	A.	Simple partial seizures
	B.	Complex partial seizures
		1. With impairment of consciousness at onset
		2. Simple partial onset followed by impairment of consciousness
	C.	Partial seizures evolving to generalized tonic clonic convulsions
		1. Simple evolving to generalized tonic clonic convulsion
		2. Complex evolving to generalized tonic clonic convulsion (including those with simple partial onset)
II. Generalized seizures	A.	1. Absence seizures
		2. Atypical absence
	B.	Myoclonic seizures
	C.	Clonic seizures
	D.	Tonic seizures
	E.	Tonic clonic seizures
	F.	Atonic seizures
III. Unclassified seizures		

Generalized Epilepsies

The generalized epilepsies are divided into two broad categories. Primary generalized epilepsy is a genetic disorder that manifests itself in various syndromes such as childhood absence epilepsy and juvenile myoclonic epilepsy. Various types of seizures can occur, such as absence seizures, myoclonic and tonic clonic seizures in association with generalized spike wave (3 per second) on the EEG. These syndromes tend to occur in individuals of normal intelligence. They respond best to treatment with sodium valproate, or lamotrigine as second line therapy. The outlook for total seizure control is excellent. The majority of children with childhood absence epilepsy will be seizure free and off treatment by adult life. Most patients with juvenile myoclonic epilepsy become seizure free but will relapse if treatment is stopped.

The second category is symptomatic generalized epilepsy, which is more commonly seen in people with learning disabilities. The classic 3 per second spike wave on the EEG does not occur. Instead the spike wave tends to be slower. This is often the most difficult form of epilepsy to treat and can be associated with quite severe learning disabilities. A typical person with symptomatic generalized epilepsy may begin with infantile spasms in infancy or the Lennox–Gastaut syndrome in childhood. A mixture of seizures occurs, including atypical absence seizures, myoclonic jerks, atonic and clonic seizures and tonic clonic seizures. The atonic attacks are particularly disabling as the person drops to the ground and often

384 Psychiatry in Learning Disability

Table 16.5 International classification of epilepsies, epileptic syndromes and related seizure disorders.[10]

1. Localization-related (focal, partial) epilepsies and syndromes	
1.1 Idiopathic (with age-related onset)	Benign childhood epilepsy with centrotemporal spikes
	Childhood epilepsy with occipital paroxysms
	Primary reading epilepsy
1.2 Symptomatic	Chronic progressive epilepsia partialis continua
	Syndromes characterized by seizures with various modes of precipitation
	Various syndromes based upon seizure types and anatomical localization
1.3 Cryptogenic	
2. Generalized epilepsies and syndromes	
2.1 Idiopathic (with age-related onset)	Benign neonatal familial convulsions
	Benign neonatal convulsions
	Benign myoclonic epilepsy in infancy
	Childhood absence epilepsy
	Juvenile myoclonic epilepsy
	Epilepsy with tonic clonic seizures on awakening
	Other generalized idiopathic epilepsies
	Epilepsies with seizures precipitated by specific modes of activation
2.2 Cryptogenic or symptomatic	West syndrome
	Lennox–Gastaut syndrome
	Epilepsy with myoclonic-astatic seizures
	Epilepsy with myoclonic absences
3. Epilepsies and syndromes undetermined whether focal or generalized	
3.1 With both generalized and focal seizures	Neonatal seizures
	Severe myoclonic epilepsy of infancy
	Epilepsy with continuous spike waves during slow-wave sleep

suffers frequent head injuries and fractures. Again, this seizure disorder responds best to sodium valproate and/or lamotrigine, although vigabatrin may prove useful in the treatment of infantile spasms.

Infantile Spasms (West Syndrome)

West syndrome consists of a characteristic triad of infantile spasms, arrest of psychomotor development, and hypsarrhythmia. Spasms may be flexor, extensor or nods. The peak onset is between 4 and 7 months and occurs before the age of 1 year. Boys are more commonly affected and the prognosis is poor. West syndrome is divided into two categories. The first is cryptogenic with no known aetiology while the other is symptomatic characterized by signs of brain damage or a known aetiology such as tuberous sclerosis.[11]

Lennox–Gastaut Syndrome

The Lennox–Gastaut syndrome manifests itself in children between the ages of 1 and 8 years, predominantly in preschool children. The most common seizure types are tonic, atonic and absence seizures but tonic clonic, myoclonic and partial seizures frequently occur. The seizure frequency is high and status epilepticus common. The EEG has abnormal background activity, slow spike waves and often multifocal abnormalities. During sleep, bursts of fast rhythms appear. In 60% of children, it is secondary to a previous encephalopathy. Seizures are difficult to control and cognitive impairment is common.[12]

Localization-related Epilepsy

In localization-related seizure disorders the abnormal electrical activity begins in one area of the brain and spreads. The seizure manifestations depend on the site of onset of the abnormal electrical activity and the rate of involvement and spread to other areas of the brain. For example, abnormal electrical activity arising in the temporal lobe may begin with a feeling of fear or déjà vu or an abnormal taste or smell. This is a simple partial seizure. As the abnormal electrical activity spreads, it involves more of the temporal lobe and consciousness is lost – a complex partial seizure. The individual may be seen to stare or gulp or swallow or perform repetitive movements or automatisms. If the abnormal electrical activity spreads to the other side of the brain, a tonic clonic seizure results. Therefore, tonic clonic seizures occur in both generalized and localization-related epilepsies. Localization-related epilepsies are divided into three categories: idiopathic, cryptogenic and symptomatic. Idiopathic epilepsies are those related to self (from the Greek 'idios' meaning self, own or personal) which have no underlying cause other than a possible heredi-tary predisposition. Idiopathic epilepsies are defined by age-related onset, clinical and EEG features and a presumed genetic aetiology. Cryptogenic refers to epilepsies where the cause is hidden or occult. They are presumed to be symptomatic but the aetiology is unknown. Symptomatic epilepsies are thought to be the consequence of a known disorder of the brain.

Investigations

An EEG is useful in trying to classify the type of seizure disorder and occasionally in diagnosis. Many patients without epilepsy will have minor abnormalities in their EEG. Between seizures, an individual with epilepsy can have a normal EEG, so an EEG should not be used for diagnosis.

Various other investigations are dependent on the likely aetiology of the seizures. In infancy or childhood, metabolic and storage disorders need to be excluded, as do chromosomal abnormalities.

A computed tomography (CT) scan or magnetic resonance imaging (MRI) scan can prove useful in determining the aetiology of both the seizure disorder and the learning disability. It has been discovered that many individuals with learning disabilities and epilepsy have migrational abnormalities that are detectable on MRI;[13] this is where islets of cortex remain in the white matter. Other abnormalities include the failure of the normal development of the cortex in certain areas and structural brain malformations. However, many people with learning disabilities will need a general anaesthetic or heavy sedation for an MRI scan to be undertaken, and the possible benefits have to be weighed against the risks. Knowing the correct aetiology of the cerebral disorder is unlikely to alter management because disorders such as tuberous sclerosis are usually diagnosable from additional systemic features or CT scan.

More detailed EEG investigations may be indicated either for diagnosis or if surgery is being considered (Table 16.6).[14] Sleep deprivation EEGs can give a higher yield of diagnostic abnormalities, helping to classify the seizure type. Obviously, this may be difficult to undertake in people with severe learning disabilities. If seizures are occurring at least weekly, ambulatory or, more profitably, video EEG recording can be undertaken. However, some individuals are obviously unsuitable if they are unable to tolerate EEG leads or likely to be destructive towards the monitoring equipment. Video EEG is very useful in the assessment of difficult to diagnose episodes as the attack can be watched on video and the electrical activity in the brain can be recorded at the same time.

Treatments

The principles of treatment for people with learning disabilities are identical to those for people with epilepsy without learning disabilities. The aim is monotherapy with an appropriate modern anti-epileptic drug such

Table 16.6 Types of EEG and their principal use in epilepsy.[14]

Type of EEG study	Principal indications
Routine EEG	Help confirm the diagnosis of epilepsy Classify the seizure disorder Look for photosensitivity Look for specific syndromes
Sleep/sleep-deprived	In patients with normal EEGs to help classify the seizure disorder
Ambulatory EEG	Detection/quantification of generalized spike wave discharges Diagnostic screening test in patients with paroxysmal attacks of unknown cause
Video-EEG telemetry	Diagnosis of paroxysmal attacks Seizure classification/quantification Presurgical evaluation

as sodium valproate or carbamazepine, in the lowest possible dose that will control seizures without side-effects.[15] However, individuals with learning disabilities and epilepsy present greater management problems in that their seizure disorders, on the whole, are more difficult to treat. They are also more prone to behavioral side-effects from the drugs.

Generalized Epilepsy

Sodium valproate is the drug of choice. Clobazam can be useful but tolerance tends to develop so it is best reserved for intermittent use. Vigabatrin has proved useful for babies with infantile spasms but in older people it can cause a deterioration, particularly in symptomatic generalized seizure disorders. Although there is no published data on topiramate, it is looking promising in primary generalized epilepsy; however, it is accompanied by a high incidence of side-effects.

Partial Epilepsy

All the main anti-epileptic drugs are equally effective (or ineffective) in the treatment of partial seizures, they just differ in their side-effects. First choice is between sodium valproate and carbamazepine. Carbamazepine is said to be the drug of choice for challenging behaviour although it can occasionally produce behavioural problems. Second line therapies include gabapentin, lamotrigine, vigabatrin and topiramate. Clobazam can be useful for predictable seizures such as perimenstrual seizures or when they occur in clusters.[15–17]

Anti-epileptic Drugs (Table 16.7)

Phenobarbitone

Phenobarbitone is an effective anti-epileptic drug but its use is accompanied by an unacceptably high incidence of behavioural problems and sedation. There are many new drugs that are just as effective but produce a much lower incidence of side-effects. Many specialist epilepsy units have the policy of trying to withdraw barbiturates in the majority of patients. The improvement in intellectual function and behaviour after withdrawal is often striking.[15]

Primidone

Primidone is a compound that is converted in the body to phenobarbitone. It has an even higher incidence of side-effects than phenobarbitone and should no longer be used.[17]

Table 16.7 Titration schedule for commonly used anti-epileptic drugs.

Drug	Dosage schedule (mg)			
	Start	Increments fortnightly	Maximum daily dosage	Frequency
Carbamazepine	100 B.D.[a]	100	800–1000	B.D.
Gabapentin	400 T.D.S.[c] over 1 week	400	2400	T.D.S.
Lamotrigine	50 I.D.	50	200–300	B.D.
with enzyme inducers	50 I.D.	50	400	B.D.
with sodium valproate	25 alternate nights	25	100–150	B.D.
Phenytoin	200 I.D.	50	400	I.D.[6]
Sodium valproate	200 B.D.	200	2500	B.D.
Topiramate	25	25	400–600	B.D.
Vigabatrin	500 I.D.	500	3000	B.D.

[a]B.D. = twice daily;
[b]I.D. = once during the day;
[c]T.D.S. = three times daily.

Phenytoin

Phenytoin is an effective anti-epileptic drug but appears to have a higher side-effect profile (Table 16.8) than some of the newer agents. It is a difficult drug to use because of its many interactions and saturable metabolism. Phenytoin has a narrow therapeutic range and nonlinear pharmacokinetics, so small increases in dosage can precipitate toxicity. It is a useful drug but some of the newer anti-epileptic drugs such as gabapentin and lamotrigine appear to be equally effective and have fewer side-effects, although there are no direct comparative studies.[15–19]

Carbamazepine

Carbamazepine is one of the first line drugs for the treatment of partial seizures. It can have a positive effect on behaviour. It is an hepatic micro-somal enzyme inducer and therefore speeds up the metabolism of other anti-epileptic drugs such as phenytoin, phenobarbitone and lamotrigine, as well as inducing its own metabolism. Its main side-effect is a rash which occurs in about 10% of people (Table 16.9). At high dosages there have been complaints of double vision and drowsiness. If this occurs after a dosage increase, it is worth waiting a week to see if symptoms resolve as induction occurs and blood levels fall. Maximum tolerated monotherapy dosages tend to be between 800 and 1200 mg daily. If dose-related side-effects are a problem then changing to carbamazepine retard can be helpful.

　Carbamazepine induces the metabolism of the combined oral contra-ceptive pill so a higher dose pill (50 μg or more of oestradiol) needs to be given. Women should be warned that even this dosage might not be 100%

Table 16.8   Side-effects of phenytoin.

CNS	Ataxia, cerebellar degeneration, confusion, dizziness, drowsiness, incoordination, involuntary movements, mental slowing, peripheral neuropathy, sedation
Skin	Acne, coarsening of facial features, gum hypertrophy, hirsutism
Haematological	Agranulocytosis, pseudolymphoma reaction, red blood cell aplasia, thrombocytopenia
Others	Decreased fertility, folate deficiency, hepatic failure hyposexuality, low Ig A levels, lupus-like reaction, myasthenia gravis, vitamin D deficiency

Table 16.9   Side-effects of carbamazepine.

Dose dependent	Ataxia, dizziness, double vision, drowsiness, nausea
Idiosyncratic	Behavioural changes, inappropriate ADH syndrome, leucopenia, rash, Stevens–Johnson syndrome

effective as contraception. Carbamazepine is at present the recommended anti-epileptic drug for partial seizures during pregnancy. However, many studies have suggested that all first line anti-epileptic drugs are equally teratogenic so preconception counselling should be given and pregnant women who receive carbamazepine should have ultrasound screening for spina bifida.

Sodium Valproate

Sodium valproate is the treatment of choice for the generalized epilepsies and the other first line drug for localization-related epilepsies. A recent American study suggested that sodium valproate was less effective than carbamazepine against complex partial seizures but other studies have failed to confirm these findings.

It is the drug of choice for women on the oral contraceptive pill as they can remain on a low dose preparation. Sodium valproate is teratogenic, particularly when combined with other anti-epileptic drugs, as it slows down the metabolism of drugs such as phenytoin and carbamazepine, leading to an increase in intermediary metabolites which are teratogenic. Sodium valproate should therefore only be used as monotherapy in women who wish to become pregnant and the fetus should be screened for spina bifida.

The main side-effects of sodium valproate are weight gain, tremor and hair loss at higher doses (Table 16.10). This weight gain can be a problem in young women and is due to stimulation of the appetite. About 60 cases of acute fatal hepatic failure have been reported with valproate therapy,

Table 16.10 Side-effects of sodium valproate.

Dose related	Alopecia/hair loss/curly hair, anorexia, dizziness, drowsiness, encephalopathy, nausea and vomiting, tremor, weight gain
Idiosyncratic	Acute hepatic failure, bone marrow aplasia, haemorrhagic pancreatitis, menstrual irregularities, thrombocytopenia

usually in children under the age of 2 years, with developmental delay. It tends to occur within 6 months of starting therapy. This idiosyncratic reaction may be the result of an underlying congenital metabolic disorder such as ornithine transcarbamalase deficiency. This problem should be differentiated from the benign elevation in liver enzymes that occurs in about 30% of patients treated with valproate.[15,16]

Gabapentin

Gabapentin is a new anti-epileptic drug that is structurally related to GABA. It is an effective anti-epileptic drug in partial seizures but does not appear to work in absence seizures and may exacerbate some symptomatic generalized seizure disorders. It has a low side-effect profile. The main side-effects reported are dizziness, drowsiness and light-headedness. Its benefits are its ease of use and lack of interaction with other anti-epileptic drugs and with other drugs generally, apart from a minor interaction with cimetidine. It is taken up by a specific amino acid transporter system in the gut so overdosage is not possible. Gabapentin is excreted unchanged in the urine. Doses therefore need to be modified in renal failure. Studies are under way looking at its use in people with learning disabilities. Behavioural side-effects have been reported but this does not appear to be a particular problem.[18]

Lamotrigine

Lamotrigine is a broad spectrum anti-epileptic drug like sodium valproate and is active against both generalized and partial epilepsies. It is well tolerated and has a low side-effect profile. Its main problems are those of rash and the interactions with other anti-epileptic drugs. This has meant that differing dosage schedules and maximum doses are used according to concomitant anti-epileptic drugs. Its half-life varies from 15 h, when used in combination with enzyme inducers such as phenytoin or carbamazepine, to 30 h when used as monotherapy and 72 h when combined with sodium valproate. Lamotrigine is now licensed in the UK as first line monotherapy medication. It appears to reduce inter-ictal seizure activity and many individuals with learning disabilities appear much brighter and more alert between seizures even though seizure frequency may not alter.[19]

An open study with 11 patients with Lennox–Gastaut syndrome reported excellent results using lamotrigine as add-on therapy. Ten of these patients experienced a greater than 50% reduction in seizures and no significant side-effects were reported.[20]

Vigabatrin

Vigabatrin is a GABA transaminase inhibitor and is active against partial seizures. It is also effective in infantile spasms. Its main problems are the psychiatric side-effects which include depression, anxiety and psychosis in particular and are detailed as follows:

- weight gain
- tolerance
- dizziness
- fatigue
- drowsiness
- mood changes
- depression
- confusion
- psychosis

Tolerance develops in about 40% of people treated with the drug. This limits vigabatrin use particularly in those with both learning disabilities and past history of psychosis. It requires judicial use but in selected patients it can be very effective.[15,16] In an open study in 22 patients with severe learning disabilities and epilepsy, 10 patients had a greater than 50% reduction in seizures over a 4-month period. However four patients had aggression and agitation problems and eight became more sedated.[21] Other studies have had similar findings.[22]

Topiramate

Topiramate is a new anti-epileptic drug that was licensed at the end of 1995 in the UK. However, there are few published studies and none specifically looking at its use in individuals with learning disabilities. It appears to be an effective anti-epileptic drug but does have a high side-effect profile, including mental slowing and difficulties in concentration. It would therefore be prudent to use it cautiously, if at all, in individuals with learning disabilities at present.

Clobazam

Clobazam is a 1,5-benzodiazepine specifically licensed for the treatment of epilepsy. It is used in a dose of 10–30 mg at night. Its main problem is that, if used daily, tolerance tends to develop in 30–70% of individuals. It is very useful for predictable seizures such as those around the time of menstruation or if seizures cluster. It can be used to terminate episodes of minor status epilepticus. It can be very useful in people with learning disabilities for special occasions as it may reduce or render a person seizure free for that period.[15]

Clonazepam

Clonazepam tends to be used for generalized epilepsies by paediatricians. It again has the problem of tolerance and appears to be more sedative and to have a greater incidence of behavioural side-effects than clobazam.[15]

Acetazolamide

Acetazolamide is of little value; tolerance tends to develop within 6 weeks of therapy.

Diazepam

Rectal diazepam can be of considerable value in terminating episodes of convulsive and nonconvulsive status epilepticus at home. It can be used in the community and the need for hospital admission may be avoided. A video is available from the manufacturers to instruct carers in the use of rectal diazepam.

Ethosuximide

Ethosuximide can be of value in absence and atypical absence seizures if sodium valproate and/or lamotrigine has failed. It is of no value in complex partial seizures.

Piracetam

Piracetam has recently been licensed for use in cortical myoclonus. The usual maintenance dose is 20 g daily in a twice or three times daily dose.

Drugs under Development

Tiagabine

Tiagabine is a GABA reuptake inhibitor that appears effective in partial seizures. It appears in clinical trials to have a low side-effect profile. It has not been evaluated in individuals with learning disabilities.

Remacemide

Remacemide is an NMDA receptor antagonist and decreases glutamate excitation. It is effective against drug-resistant partial seizures and appears to have a low side-effect profile. It has some interactions with carbamazepine and phenytoin, elevating concentrations. They in turn reduce remacemide concentrations. Formal studies in individuals with learning disabilities and epilepsy are needed to establish its role in this group of patients.

Oxcarbazapine

Oxcarbazapine is an analogue of carbamazepine. It has advantages over the parent compound in that it appears less sedative with a significant lower incidence of side-effects including rash. Its main drawback is that there is a higher incidence of hyponatraemia. Oxcarbazapine is effective against partial seizures. It has been licensed in the Netherlands for many years.

Anti-epileptic Drug Level Monitoring

In the majority of individuals this is a waste of time and money. People are their own *in vivo* drug assays. If someone is seizure free they are receiving the correct dosage of anti-epileptic drug and no alterations in dose are indicated. If seizures continue without side-effects then the dose can be increased. If dose-related side-effects occur, the dosage is too high. There is no bottom limit to the so-called therapeutic range and many people are able to tolerate plasma levels in excess of the top limit. Anti-epileptic drug levels are useful in checking compliance, a common reason for treatment failure. They can be of value for drugs such as phenytoin which have difficult pharmacokinetics and can be helpful in giving an idea of the scope for dose increments in someone with continuing seizures. However, in severely handicapped patients who are unable to communicate, anti-epileptic drug monitoring can be of value in detecting phenytoin and carbamazepine toxicity. Monitoring the blood levels of the other anti-epileptic drugs is not indicated.

Management of Drug-resistant Epilepsies

If seizures have failed to respond to a first line anti-epileptic drug, various questions need to be asked:

(1) Is this epilepsy?
(2) Is this the best anti-epileptic drug for the seizure type?
(3) Is it being prescribed at an adequate dosage?
(4) Is the individual actually taking the drug?

If someone has genuinely failed to respond, alternative therapies need to be considered. If seizures are predictable, intermittent clobazam is a useful adjunctive therapy. If not, another drug needs to be added, and the dosage increased until a response is obtained or side-effects develop. If the second drug is ineffective, then it should be stopped before another therapy is considered. If it is effective, then the first drug needs to be gradually withdrawn, as the aim of treatment is someone seizure free on monotherapy.[15]

Contraception

Many anti-epileptic drugs (barbiturates, phenytoin, carbamazepine and topiramate) interact with the combined oral contraceptive pill. They speed up the metabolism of the oestrogen and progesterone and therefore make the pill less effective. A higher dose combined oral contraceptive pill (i.e. one containing at least 50 μg of oestrogen) is therefore needed. If breakthrough bleeding occurs then higher doses of oestrogen than this may be indicated. There are no data looking at the effects of the enzyme inducing anticonvulsant drugs on the progestogen-only pill or medroxyprogesterone (Depo-Provera). Sodium valproate, gabapentin, lamotrigine and vigabatrin should not interfere with the metabolism of the combined oral contraceptive pill and one with a lower dose of oestrogen can be used.[23]

Pregnancy

Epilepsy itself is not a bar to having children, but it is one of the additional factors as to whether the mother would be able to cope with a child. All the first line anti-epileptic drugs (carbamazapine, sodium valproate, phenytoin and barbiturates) are teratogenic in animal models, as is topiramate. The risk of major malformation is increased at least twofold. If individuals with learning disabilities are contemplating pregnancy, they need to be on the lowest possible dose of a single drug. Drug combinations of sodium valproate with other anti-epileptic drugs in particular should be avoided. In addition to the risk of major malformations, there is a fetal anticonvulsant syndrome. This occurs in between 15% and 45% of babies exposed to anti-epileptic drugs *in utero*. It consists of mid-face abnormalities such as hypertelorism, a poorly formed nasal bridge, thin upper lip, etc. This may result from anti-epileptic drug exposure or be secondary to environmental factors. It is possible that gabapentin and lamotrigine will be the future drugs of choice for pregnancy as they do not appear teratogenic in animal studies but further clinical experience is needed.[24]

The genetics of the learning difficulty and the seizure disorder will also need to be taken into consideration. For example tuberous sclerosis is an autosomal dominant condition, so if one parent has this condition there is a 1:2 risk of the child inheriting the disease. The majority of inheritable syndromes, including epilepsy and learning disabilities, are autosomal recessive so there is a low risk of children developing the condition. The risk of a child developing epilepsy is related to the type of seizure disorder and the number of relatives affected. If the seizures are focal in onset the risk of subsequent children having epilepsy is low. A primary generalized seizure disorder carries a risk of about 1:10 of a child developing epilepsy, but this risk is increased if both parents have epilepsy or siblings develop epilepsy. If only the father has epilepsy there is a lower risk than if the mother has epilepsy that the child will develop seizures.[25]

Anticonvulsant Withdrawal

The MRC anti-epileptic drug withdrawal study[26] showed that neurological deficits and learning disabilities were not a bar to anticonvulsant withdrawal. In patients who were seizure free, at least 40% were able successfully to withdraw therapy. The longer the seizure-free period, the greater was the likelihood of successful withdrawal. Successful withdrawal was also related to the number of seizures before becoming seizure free and the number and dose of anti-epileptic drugs. The lower the number of seizures and the use of a single anti-epileptic agent were more likely to be associated with success.[26,27] An abnormal EEG is associated with an increased risk of relapse of the seizure disorder among those with learning disabilities.[28]

Surgery

Surgery for epilepsy is of two types. One is curative, such as resection of an epileptic focus, and the other is palliative, to try to improve seizure control. Temporal lobectomy is not of great value in people with learning disabilities as they have more diffuse brain damage, as indicated by the associated intellectual problems. Results are poor after temporal lobectomy compared with people with a normal intellect.[29]

Occasionally, resections of an epileptic focus such as in tuberous sclerosis may be of value in individual patients. Corpus callosotomy and hemispherectomy may be of value in severe intractable seizure disorders but the main treatment of epilepsy for people with learning disabilities continues to be drugs.

Sudden Epileptic Death

Sudden death in young people with epilepsy is a well-recognized phenomenon. Population-based studies suggest that the incidence is about 1:1000 per year. However, the incidence is much higher among individuals with severe uncontrolled seizure disorders. A study of pupils at a school for children with severe epilepsy and learning disabilities has suggested an incidence of 1:295 per year.[30]

Behavioural Problems and Epilepsy

There are specific areas of concern for individuals with learning disabilities when they are on anti-epileptic drugs. There is no increase in challenging behaviour among individuals with epilepsy and learning disabilities compared with those with only learning disabilities unless the epilepsy is severe. There is a high incidence of autistic behaviour among those who had infantile spasms particularly if secondary to tuberous sclerosis.[31-33]

All the anti-epileptic drugs can produce behavioural side-effects, but behavioural problems are particularly common with drugs such as phenobarbitone, primidone and clonazepam, especially in those with pre-existing behavioural problems.[6,15] Carbamazepine is said to have the least adverse effects on behaviour and is sometimes used to treat disturbed behaviour. However, it can occasionally precipitate a behavioural problem. Many behavioural side-effects begin within a few days of starting a new drug. It must also be remembered that drugs such as vigabatrin can occasionally precipitate psychosis many months after starting treatment.[16] The new anticonvulsant drugs have not been properly evaluated with regard to their effects on behaviour.

There is also a problem with what is called 'forced normalization'. This is when a person becomes seizure free as a result of adding a new anti-epileptic drug but the behaviour becomes intolerable. It appears that some people 'need' their seizures in order for them to have sociably acceptable behaviour.

If challenging behaviour is a problem, it is often worth trying to withdraw possible offending drugs as this may produce an improvement. Drugs rarely associated with behavioural side-effects are carbamazapine, sodium valproate and probably lamotrigine and gabapentin.

Management of Psychiatric Illness

The fact that a patient with epilepsy has developed a psychosis should not affect the specific management of the psychiatric disorder. Both the epilepsy and the psychosis should be treated conventionally. However, all the phenothiazines and butyrophenones decrease the seizure threshold and can increase seizure frequency. Anti-epileptic dosages may need to be adjusted and complete seizure control is often very difficult to achieve.[7]

Depression is best treated with 5HT reuptake inhibitors as these are felt to have the least effect on seizure threshold. If these fail then either a monoamine oxamine inhibitor or a tricyclic antidepressant should be used.[7]

It should be remembered that all drugs which lower seizure threshold can precipitate seizures in individuals who have never previously had seizures.

Social Issues

The combination of learning disabilities and epilepsy makes management more difficult. It often leads to overprotection and unnecessary restrictions.

Education of all those involved in caring for people with learning disabilities and epilepsy is needed, both about the disorder and about treatment. Anti-epileptic drug side-effects need to be explained and watched for as people with moderate and severe learning disabilities may not be able to complain about overdosage. This is one of the few situations where measuring anti-epileptic drug levels is indicated.

Carers are usually able to recognize tonic clonic seizures but the more subtle manifestations of absence and complex partial seizures are often missed, particularly episodes of nonconvulsive status.

In the UK, specialist education, treatment and assessments are available for children with epilepsy and learning disabilities and epilepsy at St Piers, Lingfield and the David Lewis Centre, Cheshire. Similar services exist for adults at the Chalfont Centre for Epilepsy and the David Lewis Centre. Providing joint clinics involving consultants in learning disabilities and neurologists seems to be a logical step forward and, where they have been established, they have been successful in improving seizure control in individuals with difficult to manage epilepsy. The Tuberous Sclerosis Society has funded assessment clinics for people with tuberous sclerosis and often specialist epilepsy advice is available.

References

1. Hall W & Chappell B (1997) Managing epilepsy in general practice: the dissemination and uptake of a free audit package and collated results from 12 practices in England and Wales. *Seizure* **6**, 9–12.
2. Hauser WA, Annegars JF & Kurland LT (1991) Prevalence of epilepsy in Rochester, Minnesota: 1940–1980. *Epilepsia* **32**, 429–45.
3. Hauser WA, Annegars JF & Kurland LT (1993) Incidence of epilepsy and unprovoked seizures in Rochester, Minnesota: 1935–1984. *Epilepsia* **34**, 453–68.
4. Shepherd C & Hosking G (1989) Epilepsy in school children with intellectual impairments in Sheffield: the size and nature of the problem and the implications for service provision. *Journal of Mental Deficiency Research* **33**, 511–4.
5. Hopkins A & Shorvon S (1995) Definitions and epidemiology of epilepsy. In Hopkins A, Shorvon S & Cascino G (eds) *Epilepsy*, 2nd edn, pp. 1–24. London: Chapman & Hall Medical.
6. Kirkham F (1995) Epilepsy and mental retardation. In Hopkins A, Shorvon S & Cascino G (eds) *Epilepsy*, 2nd edn, pp. 503–20. London: Chapman & Hall Medical.
7. Fenwick P (1995) Psychiatric disorder and epilepsy. In Hopkins A, Shorvon S & Cascino G (eds) *Epilepsy*, 2nd edn, pp. 453–502. London: Chapman & Hall Medical.
8. Besag FMC (1988) Cognitive detioration in children with epilepsy. In Trimble MR & Reynolds EH (eds) *Epilepsy, Behaviour and Cognitive Function*, pp. 113–28. Chichester: John Wiley.
9. Commission on Classification and Terminology of the International League against Epilepsy (1981) Proposal for revised clinical and electroencephalographic classification of epileptic seizures. *Epilepsia* **22**, 489–501.
10. Commission on Classification and Terminology of the International League against Epilepsy (1989) Proposal for revised classification of epilepsies and epileptic syndromes. *Epilepsia* **30**, 389–99.
11. Verity CM (1995) The epilepsy syndromes of infancy. In Hopkins A, Shorvon S & Cascino G (eds) *Epilepsy*, 2nd edn, pp. 355–94. London: Chapman & Hall Medical.
12. Tassinari CA, Rubboli & Michelucci R (1995) In Hopkins A, Shorvon S & Cascino G (eds) *Epilepsy*, 2nd edn, pp. 395–422. London: Chapman & Hall Medical.
13. Shorvon S & Cascino G (1995) (eds) *Epilepsy*, 2nd edn, pp. 25–34. London: Chapman & Hall Medical.

14. Fish D (1995) The role of electroencephalography. In Hopkins A, Shorvon S & Cascino G (eds) *Epilepsy*, 2nd edn, pp. 123–42. London: Chapman & Hall Medical.
15. Crawford PM (1994) Epilepsy. Managing therapy and possible problems. *Prescriber* 5, 31–6.
16. Shorvon S (1995) The drug treatment of epilepsy. In Hopkins A, Shorvon S & Cascino G (eds) *Epilepsy*, 2nd edn, pp. 171–214. London: Chapman & Hall Medical.
17. Mattson RH, Cramer JA & Collins JF *et al.* (1985) Comparison of carbamazepine, pheno-barbital, phenytoin and primidone in partial and secondary generalised tonic-clonic seizures. *New England Journal of Medicine* 313, 145–51.
18. Crawford PM (1996) The clinical efficacy of gabapentin. *Reviews in Contemporary Pharmacology*, 7, 215–26.
19. Johnson S & Johnson FN (eds) (1994) Lamotrigine. *Reviews in Contemporary Pharmacotherapy*. No. 2.
20. Timmings PL & Richens A (1992) Lamotrigine as an add-on drug in the management of Lennox–Gastaut syndrome. *European Neurology* 32, 305–7.
21. Armour DJ, Fidler C, Wright EC & Balarajan S (1992) Vigabatrin in adults with poorly-controlled epilepsy and learning disabilities. *Seizure* 1, 157–62.
22. Matilainen R, Pitkanen A & Ruutiainen T *et al.* (1988) Effect of vigabatrin on epilepsy in mentally retarded patients. *Neurology* 38, 743–7.
23. Orme M, Crawford P, Chadwick D & Back D (1991) Contraception, epilepsy and phar-macokinetics. In Trimble M (ed) *Women and Epilepsy*. Chichester: John Wiley.
24. Crawford PM (1992) Epilepsy and pregnancy. *Seizure* 2, 87–90.
25. Shorvon S (1995) The classical genetics of the epilepsies. In Hopkins A, Shorvon S & Cascino G (eds) *Epilepsy*, 2nd edn, pp. 87–92. London: Chapman & Hall Medical.
26. MRC Antiepileptic Drug Withdrawal Study (1991) Randomised study of antiepileptic drug withdrawal in patients in remission. *Lancet* 337, 1175–80.
27. Beghi E, Bollini P & Di Mascio R *et al.* (1987) Effects of rationalizing drug treatment of patients with epilepsy and mental retardation. *Developmental Medicine and Child Neurology* 29, 363–9.
28. Alvarez N (1989) Discontinuance of anti epileptic medications in patients with develop-mental disability and diagnosis of epilepsy. *American Journal of Retardation* 93, 593–9.
29. Cascino GD (1995) Surgical treatment of the epilepsies. In Hopkins A, Shorvon S & Cascino G (eds) *Epilepsy*, 2nd edn, pp. 221–42. London: Chapman & Hall Medical.
30. Nashef L, Fish DR, Garner S, Sander JWAS & Shorvon SD (1995) Sudden death in epilepsy: a study of incidence in a young cohort with epilepsy and learning difficulty. *Epilepsia* 36, 1187–94.
31. Espie CA, Pashley AS & Bonham KG *et al.* (1989) The mentally handicapped person with epilepsy: a comparative study investigating psychosocial functioning. *Journal of Mental Deficiency Research* 33, 123–35.
32. Riikonen R & Amnell G (1981) Psychiatric disorders in children with earlier infantile spasms. *Developmental Medicine and Child Neurology* 23, 747–60.
33. Hunt A & Dennis J (1987) Psychiatric disorder among children with tuberous sclerosis. *Developmental Medicine and Child Neurology* 29, 190–8.

Index

Bold page numbers refer to whole chapters in this book.